Prostate Cancer

Editors

MARC A. BJURLIN
SAMIR S. TANEJA

UROLOGIC CLINICS
OF NORTH AMERICA

www.urologic.theclinics.com

Consulting Editor
SAMIR S. TANEJA

November 2017 • Volume 44 • Number 4

ELSEVIER

1600 John F. Kennedy Boulevard • Suite 1800 • Philadelphia, Pennsylvania, 19103-2899

http://www.theclinics.com

UROLOGIC CLINICS OF NORTH AMERICA Volume 44, Number 4
November 2017 ISSN 0094-0143, ISBN-13: 978-0-323-54905-9

Editor: Kerry Holland
Developmental Editor: Alison Swety

Urologic Clinics of North America (ISSN 0094-0143) is published quarterly by Elsevier Inc., 360 Park Avenue South, New York, NY 10010-1710. Months of issue are February, May, August, and November. Business and Editorial Offices: 1600 John F. Kennedy Blvd., Suite 1800, Philadelphia, PA 19103-2899. Periodicals postage paid at New York, NY and additional mailing offices. Subscription prices are $360.00 per year (US individuals), $680.00 per year (US institutions), $100.00 per year (US students and residents), $415.00 per year (Canadian individuals), $850.00 per year (Canadian institutions), $515.00 per year (foreign individuals), $850.00 per year (foreign institutions), and $240.00 per year (Canadian and foreign students/residents). Foreign air speed delivery is included in all *Clinics* subscription prices. All prices are subject to change without notice. **POSTMASTER:** Send address changes to *Urologic Clinics of North America*, Elsevier Health Sciences Division, Subscription Customer Service, 3251 Riverport Lane, Maryland Heights, MO 63043. **Customer Service: 1-800-654-2452 (US). From outside the United States, call 1-314-447-8871. Fax: 1-314-447-8029. E-mail: JournalsCustomerServiceusa@elsevier.com (for print support)** and **JournalsOnlineSupport-usa@elsevier.com (for online support)**.

Reprints. For copies of 100 or more, of articles in this publication, please contact the Commercial Reprints Department, Elsevier Inc., 360 Park Avenue South, New York, New York 10010-1710. Tel.: 212-633-3874; Fax: 212-633-3820; E-mail: reprints@elsevier.com.

Urologic Clinics of North America is covered in MEDLINE/PubMed (*Index Medicus*), *Excerpta Medica, Current Contents/Clinical Medicine, Science Citation Index,* and *ISI/BIOMED.*

PROGRAM OBJECTIVE
The goal of *Urologic Clinics of North America* is to keep practicing urologists and urology residents up to date with current clinical practice in urology by providing timely articles reviewing the state of the art in patient care.

TARGET AUDIENCE
Practicing urologists, urology residents and other health care professionals practicing in the discipline of urology.

LEARNING OBJECTIVES
Upon completion of this activity, participants will be able to:
1. Review risk stratification and assessment for biopsies.
2. Discuss emerging methods for the management of prostate cancer.
3. Recognize approaches to high risk cancers and relapses.

ACCREDITATION
The Elsevier Office of Continuing Medical Education (EOCME) is accredited by the Accreditation Council for Continuing Medical Education (ACCME) to provide continuing medical education for physicians.

The EOCME designates this enduring material for a maximum of 15 *AMA PRA Category 1 Credit*(s)™. Physicians should claim only the credit commensurate with the extent of their participation in the activity.

All other health care professionals requesting continuing education credit for this enduring material will be issued a certificate of participation.

DISCLOSURE OF CONFLICTS OF INTEREST
The EOCME assesses conflict of interest with its instructors, faculty, planners, and other individuals who are in a position to control the content of CME activities. All relevant conflicts of interest that are identified are thoroughly vetted by EOCME for fair balance, scientific objectivity, and patient care recommendations. EOCME is committed to providing its learners with CME activities that promote improvements or quality in healthcare and not a specific proprietary business or a commercial interest.

The planning committee, staff, authors and editors listed below have identified no financial relationships or relationships to products or devices they or their spouse/life partner have with commercial interest related to the content of this CME activity:
Omar Alghazo, MBBS; Marc Bjurlin, DO, MSc; Michael Chaloupka, MD; Matthew R. Cooperberg, MD, MPH; Clemens C. Cyran, MD; Melvin D'Anastasi, MD; Shivashankar Damodaran, MBBS, MCh; Hasan Dani, MD; Renu S. Eapen, MD; Eric Edison, MA(Cantab), MBBS, MRCS; Scott E. Eggener, MD; Anjali Fortna; Nicholas Geurts, MD, FEBU; Christian Gratzke, MD; Jeremy Grummet, MBBS, MS, FRACS; Annika Herlemann, MD; Kerry Holland; Elias Hyams, MD; Harun Ilhan, MD; David F. Jarrard, MD; Adam Kibel, MD; Lauren Klotz, MD, FRCSC; Ross E. Krasnow, MD; Christos E. Kyriakopoulos, MD; Wayne Lam, FRCS (Urol), MSc; Benjamin Lamb, FRCS (Urol), PhD; Nathan Lawrentschuk, MBBS, PhD; Stanley L. Liauw, MD; Leah Logan; Matthew Mossanen, MD; Declan G. Murphy, MB BCh, FRACS, FRCS (Urol); Rajesh Nair, FRCS (Urol), FEBU, MSc; Paul L. Nguyen, MD; Mark Preston, MD, MPH; Joseph F. Rodriguez, MD; Christian G. Stief, MD; Kelly Stratton, MD; Samir S. Teneja, MD; Quoc D. Trinh, MD; Vignesh Viswanathan; Annah Vollstedt, MD; Samuel L. Washington III, MD.

The planning committee, staff, authors and editors listed below have identified financial relationships or relationships to products or devices they or their spouse/life partner have with commercial interest related to the content of this CME activity:
Hashim U. Ahmed, BM, BCh, MA, PhD, FRCS(Urol) is a consultant/advisor for Sophiris Bio, Corp., and has research support from SonaCare Medical, LLC; Sophiris Bio, Corp.; Trod Medical; Wellcome Trust; and Medical Research Council.
Michael Cookson, MD, MMHC is a consultant/advisor for Astellas Pharma US, Inc; Myovent Sciences; TesoRx LLC; MDxHealth; Janssen Global Services, LLC; and Pacific Edge.
Stacy Loeb, MD, MSc is a consultant/advisor for Genomic Health, Inc and Eli Lilly and Company.
Taimur Tariq Shah, MBBS, BSc, MRCS has research support from St Peters Trust Company Limited; Astellas Pharma US, Inc; Ferring Pharmaceuticals; and Galil Medical Inc.

UNAPPROVED/OFF-LABEL USE DISCLOSURE
The EOCME requires CME faculty to disclose to the participants:
1. When products or procedures being discussed are off-label, unlabelled, experimental, and/or investigational (not US Food and Drug Administration [FDA] approved); and
2. Any limitations on the information presented, such as data that are preliminary or that represent ongoing research, interim analyses, and/or unsupported opinions. Faculty may discuss information about pharmaceutical agents that is outside of FDA-approved labelling. This information is intended solely for CME and is not intended to promote off-label use of these medications. If you have any questions, contact the medical affairs department of the manufacturer for the most recent prescribing information.

TO ENROLL

To enroll in the *Urologic Clinics of North America* Continuing Medical Education program, call customer service at 1-800-654-2452 or sign up online at http://www.theclinics.com/home/cme. The CME program is available to subscribers for an additional annual fee of USD $270.

METHOD OF PARTICIPATION

In order to claim credit, participants must complete the following:
1. Complete enrolment as indicated above.
2. Read the activity.
3. Complete the CME Test and Evaluation. Participants must achieve a score of 70% on the test. All CME Tests and Evaluations must be completed online.

CME INQUIRIES/SPECIAL NEEDS

For all CME inquiries or special needs, please contact elsevierCME@elsevier.com.

Contributors

CONSULTING EDITOR

SAMIR S. TANEJA, MD
The James M. Neissa and Janet Riha
Neissa Professor of Urologic Oncology,
Professor of Urology and Radiology
Director, Division of Urologic Oncology,
Co-Director, Department of Urology,
Smilow Comprehensive Prostate Cancer
Center, NYU Langone Orthopedic Center,
New York, New York, USA

EDITORS

MARC A. BJURLIN, DO, MSc, FACOS
Director of Urologic Oncology, Clinical
Assistant Professor, Department of Urology,
NYU Langone Hospital, Brooklyn, New York,
USA

SAMIR S. TANEJA, MD
The James M. Neissa and Janet Riha Neissa
Professor of Urologic Oncology, Professor of
Urology and Radiology Director, Division of
Urologic Oncology, Co-Director, Department
of Urology, Smilow Comprehensive Prostate
Cancer Center, NYU Langone Orthopedic
Center, New York, New York, USA

AUTHORS

**HASHIM U. AHMED, BM, BCh, MA, PhD,
FRCS(Urol)**
Professor of Urology, Division of Surgery,
Department of Surgery and Cancer, Imperial
College London, Chair of Urology and
Consultant Urological Surgeon, Imperial
Urology, Imperial College Healthcare NHS
Trust, London, United Kingdom

OMAR ALGHAZO, MBBS
Fellow in Robotics and Uro-Oncology, Division
of Cancer Surgery, Peter MacCallum Cancer
Centre, Melbourne, Victoria, Australia

MARC A. BJURLIN, DO, MSc, FACOS
Director of Urologic Oncology, Clinical Assistant
Professor, Department of Urology, NYU
Langone Hospital, Brooklyn, New York, USA

MICHAEL CHALOUPKA, MD
Department of Urology,
Ludwig-Maximilians-University Munich,
Munich, Germany

MICHAEL COOKSON, MD, MMHC
Professor and Chair, Department of Urology,
Stephenson Cancer Center, University of
Oklahoma Health Sciences Center, Oklahoma
City, Oklahoma, USA

MATTHEW R. COOPERBERG, MD, MPH
Departments of Urology, and Epidemiology
and Biostatistics, University of California San
Francisco, Helen Diller Family Comprehensive
Cancer Center, San Francisco, California,
USA

CLEMENS C. CYRAN, MD
Institute for Clinical Radiology,
Ludwig-Maximilians-University Munich,
Munich, Germany

MELVIN D'ANASTASI, MD
Institute for Clinical Radiology,
Ludwig-Maximilians-University Munich,
Munich, Germany

SHIVASHANKAR DAMODARAN, MBBS, MCh
Fellow, Urologic Oncology, Department of
Urology, University of Wisconsin–Madison
School of Medicine and Public Health,
Madison, Wisconsin, USA

HASAN DANI, MD
The James Buchanan Brady Urological
Institute and Department of Urology, The
Johns Hopkins University School of Medicine,
Baltimore, Maryland, USA

RENU S. EAPEN, MD
Department of Urology, University of California
San Francisco, Helen Diller Family
Comprehensive Cancer Center, San
Francisco, California, USA

ERIC EDISON, MA(Cantab), MBBS, MRCS
Department of Urology, Kingston Hospital,
London, United Kingdom

SCOTT E. EGGENER, MD
Professor of Surgery and Radiology, Section of
Urology, The University of Chicago, The
University of Chicago Medicine, Chicago,
Illinois, USA

NICOLAS GEURTS, MD, FEBU
Fellow in Robotics and Uro-Oncology, Division
of Cancer Surgery, Peter MacCallum Cancer
Centre, Melbourne, Victoria, Australia

CHRISTIAN GRATZKE, MD
Department of Urology, Comprehensive
Cancer Center, Ludwig-Maximilians-University
Munich, Munich, Germany

JEREMY GRUMMET, MBBS, MS, FRACS
Urologist, Adjunct Clinical Associate Professor,
Department of Surgery, Central Clinical
School, Monash University, Caulfield North,
Victoria, Australia

ANNIKA HERLEMANN, MD
Department of Urology, University of
California San Francisco, Helen Diller Family
Comprehensive Cancer Center, San
Francisco, California, USA; Department of
Urology, Ludwig-Maximilians-University of
Munich, Munich, Germany

ELIAS HYAMS, MD
Assistant Professor of Surgery, Section of
Urology, Dartmouth Geisel School of Medicine,
Dartmouth College, Dartmouth-Hitchcock
Medical Center, Lebanon, New Hampshire,
USA

HARUN ILHAN, MD
Department of Nuclear Medicine,
Ludwig-Maximilian-University Munich,
Munich, Germany

DAVID F. JARRARD, MD
Professor Urologic Surgery, Vice Chair,
John P. Livesey Chair in Urologic Oncology,
Associate Director for Translational Research,
Carbone Cancer Center, University of
Wisconsin–Madison School of Medicine and
Public Health, Madison, Wisconsin, USA

ADAM S. KIBEL, MD
Division of Urology, Brigham and Women's
Hospital and Dana-Farber Cancer Institute,
Harvard Medical School, Boston,
Massachusetts, USA

LAURENCE KLOTZ, MD, FRCSC
Professor of Surgery, Sunnybrook Health
Sciences Centre, University of Toronto,
Toronto, Ontario, Canada

ROSS E. KRASNOW, MD
Fellow, Division of Urology, Brigham and
Women's Hospital, Harvard Medical School,
Boston, Massachusetts, USA

CHRISTOS E. KYRIAKOPOULOS, MD
Assistant Professor, Department of Medicine,
University of Wisconsin–Madison School of
Medicine and Public Health, Madison,
Wisconsin, USA

WAYNE LAM, FRCS (Urol), MSc
Assistant Professor, Department of Urology,
The University of Hong Kong, Hong Kong SAR,
China

BENJAMIN W. LAMB, FRCS (Urol), PhD
Fellow in Robotics and Uro-Oncology,
Division of Cancer Surgery, Peter
MacCallum Cancer Centre, Melbourne,
Victoria, Australia

NATHAN LAWRENTSCHUK, MBBS, PhD
Associate Professor of Urology, Division of
Cancer Surgery, Peter MacCallum Cancer
Centre, Melbourne, Victoria, Australia;
Department of Surgery, Austin Health, The
University of Melbourne, Parkville, Victoria,
Australia

STANLEY L. LIAUW, MD
Associate Professor, Department of Radiation
and Cellular Oncology, The University of
Chicago, The University of Chicago Medicine,
Chicago, Illinois, USA

STACY LOEB, MD, MSc
Departments of Urology and Population
Health, New York University, Department of
Urology, Manhattan Veterans Affairs Medical
Center, New York, New York, USA

MATTHEW MOSSANEN, MD
Fellow, Division of Urology, Brigham and
Women's Hospital, Harvard Medical School,
Boston, Massachusetts, USA

**DECLAN G. MURPHY, MB BCh, FRACS,
FRCS (Urol)**
Associate Professor of Urology, Division of
Cancer Surgery, Peter MacCallum Cancer
Centre, Melbourne, Victoria, Australia; Sir Peter
MacCallum Department of Oncology,
University of Melbourne, Parkville, Victoria,
Australia

RAJESH NAIR, FRCS (Urol), FEBU, MSc
Fellow in Robotics and Uro-Oncology,
Division of Cancer Surgery, Peter
MacCallum Cancer Centre, Melbourne,
Victoria, Australia

PAUL L. NGUYEN, MD
Department of Radiation Oncology, Brigham
and Women's Hospital and Dana-Farber
Cancer Institute, Harvard Medical School,
Boston, Massachusetts, USA

MARK PRESTON, MD, MPH
Division of Urology, Brigham and Women's
Hospital and Dana-Farber Cancer Institute,
Harvard Medical School, Boston,
Massachusetts, USA

JOSEPH F. RODRIGUEZ, MD
Resident Physician, Section of Urology, The
University of Chicago, The University of
Chicago Medicine, Chicago, Illinois, USA

CHRISTIAN G. STIEF, MD
Department of Urology, Comprehensive
Cancer Center, Ludwig-Maximilians-University
Munich, Munich, Germany

KELLY STRATTON, MD
Assistant Professor, Department of Urology,
Stephenson Cancer Center, University of
Oklahoma Health Sciences Center, Oklahoma
City, Oklahoma, USA

SAMIR S. TANEJA, MD
The James M. Neissa and Janet Riha Neissa
Professor of Urologic Oncology, Professor of
Urology and Radiology Director, Division of
Urologic Oncology, Co-Director, Department
of Urology, Smilow Comprehensive Prostate
Cancer Center, NYU Langone Orthopedic
Center, New York, New York, USA

TAIMUR TARIQ SHAH, MBBS, BSc, MRCS
Division of Surgery and Interventional Science,
University College London, Department of
Urology, Whittington Health NHS Trust,
London, United Kingdom

QUOC D. TRINH, MD
Division of Urology, Brigham and Women's
Hospital and Dana-Farber Cancer Institute,
Harvard Medical School, Boston,
Massachusetts, USA

ANNAH VOLLSTEDT, MD
Section of Urology, Dartmouth-Hitchcock
Medical Center, Lebanon, New Hampshire,
USA

SAMUEL L. WASHINGTON III, MD
Department of Urology, University of California
San Francisco, Helen Diller Family
Comprehensive Cancer Center, San
Francisco, California, USA

Contents

This article describes markers used for prostate biopsy decisions, including prostrate-specific antigen (PSA), free PSA, the prostate health index, 4Kscore, PCA3, and ConfirmMDx. It also summarizes the use of nomograms combining multiple variables for prostate cancer detection.

Until recently, prostate biopsy for the detection of prostate cancer has been performed transrectally and in an untargeted sampling fashion. Consequently, the procedure has suffered a small but significant risk of severe morbidity through infection, and low diagnostic accuracy, with undergrading and missed diagnosis being common. MRI is revolutionizing prostate cancer diagnosis by improving detection accuracy via targeted biopsy. Transperineal biopsy is eradicating sepsis as a risk of prostate biopsy, while avoiding the need for broad-spectrum or combination prophylactic antibiotics. This article analyzes the data on the various current methods of performing prostate biopsy and recommends an optimal technique.

Prostate MRI is commonly used in the detection of prostate cancer to reduce the detection of clinically insignificant disease; maximize the detection of clinically significant cancer; and better assess disease size, grade, and location. The clinical utility of MRI seems to apply to men with no prior biopsy, men who have had a previous negative biopsy, and men who are candidate for active surveillance. In conjunction with traditional clinical parameters and secondary biomarkers, MRI may allow a more accurate risk stratification and assessment of need for prostate biopsy.

Management of prostate cancer presents unique challenges because of the disease's variable natural history. Accurate risk stratification at the time of diagnosis in clinically localized disease is crucial in providing optimal counseling about management options. To accurately distinguish pathologically indolent tumors from aggressive disease, risk groups are no longer sufficient. Rather, multivariable prognostic models reflecting the complete information known at the time of diagnosis offer improved accuracy and interpretability. After diagnosis, further testing with genomic assays or other biomarkers improves risk classification. These postdiagnostic risk assessment tools should not supplant shared decision making but rather facilitate risk classification and enable more individualized care.

Prostate-specific membrane antigen (PSMA) PET has been recently introduced for the diagnosis of patients with metastatic prostate cancer (PCa). Until today, staging of patients with PCa relied mostly on morphologic features, such as size or shape, resulting in low detection rates in disease recurrence. PSMA PET imaging provides molecular information and, in combination with conventional imaging, offers improved sensitivity and specificity. This article discusses the benefits and limitations of PSMA imaging in the setting of primary staging and detection of recurrent disease in comparison with standard-of-care imaging techniques.

This article is a summary of the rationale for conservative management, the molecular biology of low-grade cancer, the principles of management, the expected outcome of surveillance, unanswered questions, and research opportunities.

Prostate cancer lesions smaller than 0.5 m^3, or Gleason pattern 3, are likely clinically insignificant. Clinically significant disease is often limited to a single index lesion. Focal ablation targets this index lesion, maintains oncologic control, and minimizes complications by preserving healthy prostate tissue. Template mapping biopsy or multiparametric MRI-targeted biopsies are used to identify appropriate index lesions. Multiple energy modalities have been tested, including high-intensity frequency ultrasound, cryoablation, laser ablation, photodynamic therapy, focal brachytherapy, radiofrequency ablation, and irreversible electroporation. Outcome is assessed by biopsy of the target area, triggered by prostate-specific antigen measurements or MRI imaging, or performed per protocol at 12 months.

Pelvic lymph node dissection (PLND) at the time of radical prostatectomy is the most accurate method of lymph node staging in prostate cancer. Although there are varied practices in the anatomic extent of PLND, evidence favors an extended PLND (ePLND) including external iliac, obdurator, and internal iliac nodes. Removing presacral or common iliac nodes to the ureteric crossing can improve staging. The oncologic benefits of extended dissection are unclear based on methodologic limitations and bias in the available evidence. Diverse nomograms may clarify which patients warrant ePLND. Higher level evidence is needed to clarify the therapeutic effects of ePLND and who benefits most.

Men classified as having high-risk prostate cancer warrant treatment because durable outcomes can be achieved. Judicious use of imaging and considerations of risk factors are essential when caring for men with high-risk disease. Radical prostatectomy, radiation therapy, and androgen deprivation therapy all play pivotal roles in the management of men with high-risk disease, and potentially in men with metastatic disease. The optimal combinations of therapeutic regimens are an evolving area of study, and future work looking into therapies for men with high-risk disease will remain critical.

Since 2010, 5 new agents have been approved for advanced prostate cancer treatment. The American Urologic Association (AUA) published guidelines for the management of castration-resistant prostate cancer in 2013. These guidelines identify 6 index patients to consider when selecting the most appropriate treatment. No comparative trials have provided an approach to optimize the sequencing of these drugs. For the urologist, incorporating the guidelines into clinical practice typically requires a multidisciplinary team. This article provides an algorithmic approach based on indication and mechanism of action that complements the AUA guidelines to ensure patients receive the most optimal care.

UROLOGIC CLINICS OF NORTH AMERICA

Preface
Prostate Cancer

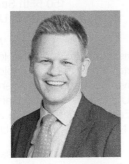
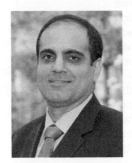

Marc A. Bjurlin, DO, MSc, FACOS   Samir S. Taneja, MD
Editors

Prostate cancer remains the most common malignancy diagnosed in men and is the third leading cause of cancer death among men in the United States. In the aftermath of the US Preventative Services Task Force grade D recommendation against prostate cancer screening, there has been an early observation of increasing detection of advanced disease in the face of decreased utilization of prostate-specific antigen (PSA) testing. On this basis, it is anticipated by many that the rates of prostate cancer mortality may rise in years to come, removing many of the advances made against the disease in recent decades. As such, a number of new challenges have emerged in prostate cancer, forcing urologists to consider new paradigms in disease management: both to improve methods of detection and to be more effective in managing the likely increasing numbers of men with advanced disease.

Screening and detection of prostate cancer have historically been performed through the use of PSA and systematic transrectal ultrasound–guided biopsy among all men with perceived elevation of PSA level. This diagnostic model has likely fueled much of the ongoing criticism of prostate cancer screening by contributing to overdiagnosis through random detection of indolent cancer, repetitive biopsy due to concerns of missed high-grade tumors, and overtreatment due to a lack of confidence in the accuracy of risk assessment. To address these concerns, the field of prostate cancer detection and diagnosis has now focused on improved baseline risk stratification through use of imaging, serum and urine biomarkers, and genomic testing. Disease management has been radically altered through better understanding of the disease biology and its natural history.

As editors of this issue of *Urologic Clinics*, it is our goal to provide readers a timely summary of some of the key advancements in prostate cancer early detection and risk stratification, active surveillance strategies, focal treatment, and management of metastatic and recurrent disease. The field of prostate cancer management has dramatically evolved over the past decade, largely owing to an increasing knowledge of disease biology and new tools for disease interrogation and treatment.

Articles in this issue explore new biomarkers, risk calculators, and evidence supporting their ability to assist in the decision of whom to biopsy, as well as emerging biopsy techniques, including controversies in attendant infection risks of the transrectal and transperineal approaches. Prostate MRI offers increasingly reliable visualization of potentially significant prostate cancers, thereby guiding biopsy to allow better sensitivity and negative predictive value, ultimately leading to better selection of patients for biopsy and to identify lesions for biopsy. These topics, taken together, have now begun to shift the paradigm to selective identification of only those cancers that may cause harm rather than diagnosing all cancers of the prostate.

As we learn more about the biology of prostate cancer, the criteria for active surveillance as a management strategy have expanded, resulting in its adoption in updated guidelines as the preferred approach to low-risk disease. Advancing imaging techniques have facilitated the implementation of focal therapy as an approach

Urol Clin N Am 44 (2017) xv–xvi
http://dx.doi.org/10.1016/j.ucl.2017.08.001
0094-0143/17/© 2017 Published by Elsevier Inc.

urologic.theclinics.com

allowing for cancer control while limiting side effects, aggressive treatment of oligometastases through improved detection of low-volume metastatic disease, and therapeutic targeting through functional imaging techniques. This issue reviews the evolution of treatment paradigms, including surgical approach, multimodal therapy, approach to the high-risk patient, and emerging approaches to castration-resistant disease, based upon increasing knowledge of disease biology.

The authors of these articles include some of the most knowledgeable thought leaders in the field. We are indebted to these experts for their contributions to this issue and are extremely appreciative of the insight that they have provided on these critically important topics. We expect these articles will be of great interest to a diverse readership.

Marc A. Bjurlin, DO, MSc, FACOS
Director of Urologic Oncology
Department of Urology
NYU Langone Hospital-Brooklyn
150 55th Street
Brooklyn, NY 11220, USA

Samir S. Taneja, MD
Division of Urologic Oncology
Co-Director, Department of Urology
Smilow Comprehensive Prostate Cancer Center
NYU Langone Medical Center
150 East 32nd Street, Suite 200
New York, NY 10016, USA

E-mail addresses:
marc.bjurlin@nyumc.org (M.A. Bjurlin)
samir.taneja@nyumc.org (S.S. Taneja)

Whom to Biopsy
Prediagnostic Risk Stratification with Biomarkers, Nomograms, and Risk Calculators

Stacy Loeb, MD, MSc[a,b,c,*], Hasan Dani, MD[d]

KEYWORDS

- Prostate cancer • Prostate-specific antigen • Biomarkers • Prostate biopsy • Nomograms

KEY POINTS

- Free prostate-specific antigen (PSA), phi, and the 4Kscore are blood tests that are more specific than PSA and can be used as reflex tests prior to initial or repeat biopsy decisions.
- Prostate cancer antigen 3 (PCA3) is a US Food and Drug Administration-approved and widely available urinary marker to aid in repeat biopsy decisions, but it is inferior to several new markers for predicting clinically significant prostate cancer.
- ConfirmMDx is a tissue marker using epigenetic changes to predict the risk of occult cancer that was not sampled on previous biopsy.
- A multivariable approach to prostate cancer detection is recommended that combines multiple clinical variables to provide patients with more individualized risk estimates.

INTRODUCTION

Historically, prostate biopsy was performed because of a prostate-specific antigen (PSA) level exceeding a specific threshold or suspicious findings on digital rectal examination. However, this approach lacks specificity, and more recently there has been an expansion in the availability of new blood, urine, and tissue tests that can be used to help with prostate biopsy decisions. In addition, the movement toward personalized medicine has led to an effort to develop prediction tools that can incorporate multiple variables together to provide more individualized risks of detecting prostate cancer on biopsy.

The purpose of this article is to describe currently available marker tests and multivariable nomograms that can be used in prostate biopsy decisions. This is a critical issue in patient management, because prostate biopsy is an invasive procedure with potential associated risks, such as infection, hematuria, hematospermia, pain, and lower urinary tract symptoms.[1] Further downstream, a critical issue is the overdiagnosis of clinically indolent prostate cancer resulting in unnecessary decrement in quality of life for a tumor that would not have caused harm. These considerations highlight the importance of using the best possible information to help patients and physicians make decisions about prostate biopsy.

Disclosure Statement: S. Loeb reports the following disclosures: Boehringer Ingelheim (honorarium for lecture, reimbursed travel to conference), Minomic (reimbursed travel to conference), MDxHealth (honorarium for lecture), Astellas (honorarium, reimbursed travel), and Lilly (consulting fees).

[a] Department of Urology, New York University, New York, NY, USA; [b] Department of Population Health, New York University, New York, NY, USA; [c] Department of Urology, Manhattan Veterans Affairs Medical Center, New York, NY, USA; [d] Department of Urology, SUNY Downstate College of Medicine, Brooklyn, NY, USA
* Corresponding author. 550 1st Avenue (VZ 30, #612), New York, NY 10016.
E-mail address: stacyloeb@gmail.com

Urol Clin N Am 44 (2017) 517–524
http://dx.doi.org/10.1016/j.ucl.2017.07.001
0094-0143/17/© 2017 Elsevier Inc. All rights reserved.

BLOOD BIOMARKERS
Total Prostate-Specific Antigen

Most prostate cancer is currently diagnosed through screening with PSA. The PSA test was initially used in forensics and was subsequently found to be elevated in the blood from men with prostatic disease. It is approved by the US Food and Drug Administration (FDA) for monitoring of prostate cancer after diagnosis and as an aid to early prostate cancer detection.

There have been several randomized trials of PSA-based screening. The largest studies of these trials, the European Randomized Study of Screening for Prostate Cancer (ERSPC), showed that screened men have a lower risk of metastatic disease and prostate cancer death, but this comes at a cost of unnecessary biopsies and overdetection of indolent tumors.[2] In the core age group of 55 to 69 years, PSA screening reduced PCA-specific mortality by 21% after 13 years of follow-up. This study primarily used a PSA level of 3 ng/mL as the threshold for performing prostate biopsy.

By contrast, the US Prostate, Lung, Colorectal and Ovarian (PLCO) screening trial found no significant difference in prostate cancer death between the screening and usual care arms.[3] However, more than 90% of men in the usual care arm received PSA tests before or during the trial, due to the widespread use of PSA screening in the United States already during the time of the study.[4] This study used a PSA of 4 ng/mL as the threshold for biopsy, although there were issues with biopsy compliance.

Although the initial FDA approval of PSA used a threshold of 4 ng/mL, there are a substantial proportion of cancers found at lower PSA levels. In practice, PSA is a continuous variable, and the selection of any particular cutoff involves a trade-off between sensitivity and specificity. Data from the Prostate Cancer Prevention Trial (PCPT) indicated that the risk of clinically significant cancer (ie, Gleason ≥ 7) with a PSA between 2.1 and 3.0 ng/mL and 3.1 and 4.0 ng/mL was 4.6% and 6.7%, respectively.[5] The PCPT also demonstrated that a PSA level greater than 10 ng/mL has a specificity of 99.5% for Gleason greater than or equal to 7 PCA.[6] These findings suggest that PSA is an excellent tool for biopsy decisions in men with significantly elevated PSA (ie, >10 ng/mL), but further risk stratification may be necessary prior to biopsy in men with moderately elevated PSA (ie, 2–10 ng/mL).

PSA values may also be confounded by numerous benign conditions and instrumentation of the urinary tract. Previous studies have shown that even assay standardization can have a substantial impact on the results, presenting a pseudoacceleration or pseudodeceleration that could potentially falsely influence clinical decisions.[7] Important recommendations to reduce confounding are to avoid checking PSA in the setting of recent urinary tract infections or procedures, to use the same laboratory for serial measurements, and to repeat abnormal values after a short period of observation, which itself can reduce unnecessary biopsies. Despite these efforts, however, there remain drawbacks to basing prostate biopsy decisions exclusively on total PSA values, and there has been intensive investigation into alternative markers that can be used in prostate cancer detection.

Free Prostate-Specific Antigen

PSA circulates in 2 forms, either complexed to proteins, or free (unbound) PSA. The percent of free PSA (%fPSA) is a way to distinguish benign from malignant conditions, wherein a higher % fPSA indicates a lower risk of significant prostate cancer.[8] A prospective, multicenter study of men with PSA levels of 4 to 10 ng/mL found that using a 25% fPSA cutoff would detect 95% of prostate cancers and avoid 20% of unnecessary biopsies.[9] Other studies have shown that %fPSA can also help distinguish benign versus malignant disease in men with PSA levels less than 4 ng/mL.[10,11]

Free PSA is approved by FDA, and it is widely available in clinical practice. In the 2016 National Comprehensive Cancer Network Guidelines, % fPSA is listed among the reflex testing options for men with a PSA greater than 3 ng/mL considering initial prostate biopsy, and for men with previous negative biopsy considering repeat biopsy.[12] Free PSA is also a component of 2 other new markers used as reflex tests, the prostate health index (phi) and 4Kscore.

Prostate Health Index

Phi is a newer prostate cancer marker test that measures 3 different forms of PSA: total PSA, free PSA, and [-2]proPSA, which is an isoform that is more specific for prostate cancer. It is calculated using the following formula: $([-2]proPSA/fPSA) \times \sqrt{PSA}$. Phi improves the specificity of prostate cancer detection, and it was approved by the FDA in 2012 for men with PSA levels between 4 and 10 ng/mL. The current National Comprehensive Cancer Network (NCCN) guidelines offer phi as an optional reflex test to help decide on initial or repeat prostate biopsy.[12] Phi has been validated in high-risk populations including men who are obese, African

American men, or men with a positive family history.[13-16]

Multiple prospective studies have shown that phi outperforms total and free PSA for prostate cancer detection on biopsy.[17-21] It is also associated with prostate cancer aggressiveness. In 658 men with PSA levels between 4 and 10 ng/mL, phi was compared with its individual variables for the prediction of clinically significant cancer.[18] Phi was the most accurate predictor, with an area under the curve (AUC) of 0.707 for Gleason greater than or equal to 7 cancer (vs AUC 0.661, 0.558, and 0.551 for %fPSA, [-2]proPSA, and PSA, respectively) and AUC of 0.698 for Epstein significant cancer (vs AUC 0.654, 0.550, and 0.549 for %fPSA, [-2]proPSA, and PSA, respectively). By reducing the number of unnecessary biopsies, phi as a reflex test prior to prostate biopsy can improve cost-effectiveness of PCA screening.[22]

Higher phi levels also predict a greater risk of adverse pathology at radical prostatectomy, including high-grade disease, larger tumor volume, extracapsular extension, and seminal vesicle invasion.[23] Phi has also been shown to predict biopsy reclassification during active surveillance.[24,25]

Recent studies have explored different methods of employing phi. Like PSA, phi can be considered in the context of other variables such as prostate volume (ie, to calculate a phi density). One study evaluated phi density in 118 men with PSA greater than 2 ng/mL who were undergoing prostate biopsy.[26] For the detection of clinically significant PCA, phi density demonstrated a higher AUC than PSA, PSA density, %fPSA, the product of %fPSA and prostate volume, and phi. Other studies have evaluated phi in conjunction with multiparametric MRI (mpMRI), with 1 study finding a negative predictive value of 97% for clinically significant PCA in men undergoing repeat biopsy.[21,27] This suggests that phi remains useful in an MRI-based detection paradigm.

4Kscore

The 4Kscore is a new marker test that combines 4 kallikrein markers (tPSA, fPSA, intact PSA, and human kallikrein 2) along with age, digital rectal examination (DRE), and prior biopsy results into a proprietary algorithm to predict the risk of high-grade PCA on biopsy. The 4Kscore is a Clinical Laboratory Improvement Amendments (CLIA)-certified test that is commercially available in multiple countries. In the NCCN guidelines, it is also an optional second-line test to help with initial or repeat prostate biopsy decisions.[12]

The 4Kscore has been shown consistently to improve the specificity of screening for both initial biopsy and repeat biopsy.[28-32] The 4-kallikrein panel was measured in 6129 men with elevated PSA undergoing biopsy in the ProtecT trial.[29] Performance of the base model including age and PSA was compared with that of the base model with %fPSA and the base model with the 4-kallikrein panel. The model incorporating the 4-kallikrein panel had an AUC of 0.820 for high-grade PCA (vs 0.799 and 0.738 for %fPSA and PSA models, respectively; P<.001). One head-to-head study by Nordström and colleagues[33] demonstrated that the 4-kallikrein panel and phi had similar performance for identifying high-grade prostate cancer on biopsy.

The 4Kscore has also been shown to predict aggressive pathology at prostatectomy[34] and future risk of metastatic disease.[35] The baseline 4Kscore also predicted reclassification on the first biopsy during active surveillance, although it did not add incremental value for prediction of subsequent surveillance biopsy outcomes.[36]

URINE BIOMARKERS
Prostate Cancer Antigen 3

PCA3 is a prostate-specific, noncoding mRNA that is overexpressed in PCA tissue relative to benign tissue.[37] In clinical practice, PCA3 is measured in the urine following a vigorous DRE in men suspected of harboring PCA.

A well-supported indication for PCA3 is in the setting of repeat biopsy. Several studies have demonstrated that PCA3 is a stronger predictor of PCA on repeat biopsy than either PSA or %fPSA.[38-41] Such evidence has led to approval by the FDA in 2012 and its inclusion in the NCCN guidelines as a testing option for men with a prior negative biopsy and continued suspicion of PCA.[12]

Some studies suggest that PCA3 in conjunction with PSA prior to initial biopsy improves overall PCA detection,[41-43] but its value is less evident for the detection of high-grade cancer.[43,44] A large multicenter study measured PCA3 levels in men scheduled for either initial or repeat biopsy.[44] Using PCA3 to determine need for repeat biopsy would avoid a substantial number of unnecessary biopsies while rarely missing the diagnosis of a high-grade PCA. In contrast, applying that same PCA3 cutoff for initial biopsy would significantly underdiagnose high-grade cancer.

The relationship between PCA3 score and clinically significant cancer detected on needle biopsy has not been clearly established.[38,40,43,45] However, several studies suggest that higher PCA3 does not predict disease progression on active surveillance, and there are conflicting data on its relationship to aggressive pathology at radical prostatectomy.[46–49] In fact, a recent study of 10,382 radical prostatectomy specimens and 1694 samples from initial biopsy suggested that more aggressive tumors have lower tissue PCA3 expression.[50] In this large sample of prostate tumors, Alshalalfa and colleagues found a bimodal expression of PCA3. Analysis of PCA3 expression in specific Gleason score subgroups revealed that Gleason 9 and 10 tumors had predominantly low PCA3 expression, whereas Gleason 3 + 3 and 3 + 4 tumors had predominantly high PCA3 expression. Low PCA3 expression was associated with high Gleason scores on initial biopsy and radical prostatectomy specimens. Furthermore, low PCA3 expression predicted increased likelihood of adverse pathologic features at radical prostatectomy, biochemical recurrence, metastatic disease at 5 years, and PCA-specific mortality at 10 years. Although this study examined PCA3 expression in tissue, other studies have similarly provided conflicting data on the performance of the urinary PCA3 assay to predict clinically significant prostate cancer.

Head-to-head comparisons of phi and PCA3 indicate that phi more accurately identifies clinically significant PCA on biopsy and radical prostatectomy pathology.[51,52] Another study demonstrated that preoperative MRI and phi predicted clinically significant PCA in patients undergoing radical prostatectomy, but PCA3 held no predictive value.[53] These findings suggest that PCA3 alone may be insufficient to select patients at risk for high-grade disease.

PCA3 appears most valuable when used alongside other available tools. Its use with either MRI or real-time elastography has demonstrated increased accuracy in detecting clinically significant PCA.[54,55] Multivariable nomograms that incorporate PCA3 have been internally and externally validated and are discussed in further detail in the nomogram section.[44,56–59]

Prostate Cancer Antigen 3 and TMPRSS2:ERG (T2:ERG)

T2:ERG is a gene fusion that is commonly found in PCA.[60] Like PCA3, its mRNA can be detected in urine after DRE.[61] Urinary T2:ERG levels predict clinically significant PCA on both core needle biopsy and radical prostatectomy pathology.[62] Although T2:ERG has a high specificity for PCA, it is present in only 50% of localized PCA. Thus, it has been combined with PCA3 to improve its sensitivity.[63]

Mi-Prostate Score (MiPS) is a commercially available tool that combines serum PSA and urinary PCA3 and T2:ERG. A prospective study by Tomlins and colleagues[64] evaluated MiPS in 1244 men undergoing initial or repeat prostate biopsy. Specifically, they compared the prediction of high-grade PCA by MiPS, PCA3 with PSA, T2:ERG with PSA, and PSA alone. MiPS was the most accurate predictor with an AUC of 0.772 versus 0.747, 0.729, and 0.651 for PSA + PCA3, PSA + T2:ERG, and PSA, respectively.

SelectMDx

Another recently developed tool is SelectMDx, which measures mRNA of PCA-associated genes (HOXC6 and DLX1) in urine collected after a DRE. It incorporates age, family history, DRE findings, history of prostate biopsy, PSA, and PSA density with urinary mRNA levels to predict a patient's risk of low-grade and high-grade PCA.

In a multicenter, prospective study of men undergoing initial or repeat biopsy, this model was developed and validated in consecutive cohorts of 519 and 386 men, respectively.[65] The model demonstrated an AUC of 0.90 (95% CI 0.85–0.95) in the validation cohort; it outperformed the base model of only clinical parameters, the Prostate Cancer Prevention Trial (PCPT) risk calculator, and the PCPT risk calculator with PCA3. Subgroup analysis in men with PSA less than 10 ng/mL revealed that SelectMDx remained a strong predictor for high-grade PCA. If SelectMDx were used to select which patients to biopsy in the validation cohort, 42% of biopsies would be avoided while missing the diagnosis of 2% of high-grade PCA.

ExoDx Prostate IntelliScore

Present in blood and urine, exosomes are vesicles that contain RNA, proteins, and other molecules derived from their cell of origin. ExoDx Prostate (IntelliScore) is a urine-based test that analyzes exosomal RNA of 3 genes associated with PCA (ERG, PCA3, and SPDEF). Using these measurements in combination with clinical variables such as PSA, age, race, and family history, this assay predicts risk of high-grade PCA in men undergoing their first biopsy. In a validation study of 519 men undergoing initial or repeat biopsy, the urine exosome gene expression assay outperformed the base model of clinical variables (AUC 0.73 vs 0.63, $P<.001$).[66] An advantage of this test is that it does not require a DRE prior to collecting urine. Future studies are needed to evaluate the comparative performance of the multiple new urine-based markers.

TISSUE BIOMARKERS
ConfirmMDx

Prostate biopsy samples a small fraction of the total prostate tissue. For men with a previous negative biopsy, the tissue from that biopsy can be examined for epigenetic changes suggestive of a nearby occult prostate cancer that was not sampled. This is the basis behind the ConfirmMDx test which specifically examines hypermethylation of GSPT1, APC, and RASSF1. ConfirmMDx is commercially available and suggested as an optional test by the NCCN guidelines for men under consideration for repeat biopsy.[12]

In the MATLOC study, 498 subjects from the United Kingdom and Belgium underwent repeat prostate biopsy, and the epigentic assay was a significant independent predictor of biopsy outcome.[67] The assay demonstrated a negative predictive value of 90%. A multicenter validation study (DOCUMENT) tested the epigenetic assay in 350 patients with prior negative biopsy from 5 US institutions.[68] Similarly, they found that the epigenetic assay was a significant independent predictor of biopsy outcome, with a negative predictive value of 88%.

NOMOGRAMS AND RISK CALCULATORS

There is increasing recognition that prostate biopsy decisions are not one-size-fits all and that a multivariable approach is important. Multiple guidelines now recommend using this type of approach to prostate biopsy decisions. The Melbourne Consensus Statement recommends that PSA testing should not be considered on its own, but rather as part of a multivariable approach to early prostate cancer detection.[69] The statement mentions 3 different risk calculators that may be used for this purpose: the ERSPC, PCPT and Canadian risk calculators.

The ERSPC risk calculator was first developed in 2006 based on data from Dutch men participating in the European Randomized Study of Screening for Prostate Cancer. Currently, multiple versions are available online for men at different stages of the screening process and with different types of information available. Risk calculator 1 is for men who do not have a PSA result available, and provides an estimate of general prostate cancer risk based on age, family history, and urinary symptoms. Risk calculator 2 uses PSA levels to estimate prostate cancer risk. Whereas these are meant to be used by laypeople, risk calculators 3 and 4 were designed for health care professionals to help with decision-making by estimating the risk of biopsy-detectable and significant prostate

cancer. The risk calculator has also been updated to include new markers such as phi, which improved its detection of clinically significant PCA. This calculator is available in a smartphone application format for ease of use.[70]

The PCPT risk calculator was initially developed in 2006 based on data from American men from the placebo group of the Prostate Cancer Prevention Trial. The first version included PSA, family history, DRE, and history of a prior negative biopsy, which together were used to estimate the risk of prostate cancer detection on biopsy. The PCPT risk calculator was subsequently updated to also include an estimate of the risk of high-grade cancer on biopsy. Recently, urinary biomarkers have been incorporated into the PCPT risk calculator in an effort to increase its predictive accuracy for high-grade PCA. Wei and colleagues[44] demonstrated that addition of PCA3 to the PCPT risk calculator improved its detection of high-grade PCA on both initial and repeat biopsies. Similarly, MiPS was added to the PCPT risk calculator and compared with PCPT + PCA3, PCPT + T2:ERG, and PCPT alone.[64] For the detection of high-grade cancer, both PCPT + PCA3 and PCPT + T2:ERG outperformed the PCPT risk calculator, and MiPS + PCPT was superior to the other 3 models. Similarly, the addition of phi to the PCPT improves its prediction of aggressive PCA.[71]

Finally, the Sunnybrook prostate cancer risk calculator was based on data from Canadian men undergoing prostate biopsy. It uses age, urinary symptoms, PSA, free PSA, ethnic background, family history, and DRE findings to provide an estimate of prostate cancer risk. Performance of nomograms across different populations may vary, making external validation of these tools essential.

It is noteworthy that several of the new marker tests discussed already incorporate a multivariable approach by combining the marker results with clinical variables directly in their algorithms. Examples of such tests include the 4Kscore, MiPS, SelectMDx, and ExoDx Prostate (IntelliScore). By contrast, other tests like phi and PCA3 do not include clinical variables into their formula, but the results of these tests can be incorporated into external nomograms. In addition to the risk calculators described previously, several other groups have created different nomograms using phi to predict overall or clinically significant prostate cancer on biopsy.[72,73] For example, a new nomogram combining continuous values of phi with age, prior biopsy, prostate volume, and PSA was shown to outperform the PCPT and ERSPC risk calculators for predicting aggressive disease on biopsy.[71]

SUMMARY

For both initial and repeat biopsy decisions, there are now multiple second-line tests available that outperform PSA for the prediction of detecting any prostate cancer and/or high-grade disease. A multivariable approach is also recommended that combines each patient's risk factors together to help inform more personalized biopsy decision making.

REFERENCES

1. Loeb S, Vellekoop A, Ahmed HU, et al. Systematic review of complications of prostate biopsy. Eur Urol 2013;64(6):876–92.

2. Schroder FH, Hugosson J, Roobol MJ, et al. Screening and prostate cancer mortality: results of the European Randomised Study of Screening for Prostate Cancer (ERSPC) at 13 years of follow-up. Lancet 2014;384(9959):2027–35.

3. Andriole GL, Crawford ED, Grubb RL 3rd, et al. Prostate cancer screening in the randomized prostate, lung, colorectal, and ovarian cancer screening trial: mortality results after 13 years of follow-up. J Natl Cancer Inst 2012;104(2):125–32.

4. Shoag JE, Mittal S, Hu JC. Reevaluating PSA testing rates in the PLCO trial. N Engl J Med 2016;374(18):1795–6.

5. Thompson IM, Pauler DK, Goodman PJ, et al. Prevalence of prostate cancer among men with a prostate-specific antigen level < or =4.0 ng per milliliter. N Engl J Med 2004;350(22):2239–46.

6. Thompson IM, Ankerst DP, Chi C, et al. Operating characteristics of prostate-specific antigen in men with an initial PSA level of 3.0 ng/ml or lower. JAMA 2005;294(1):66–70.

7. Loeb S, Chan DW, Sokoll LJ, et al. Differences in PSA measurements due to assay standardization bias. J Urol 2008;179(4):721.

8. Christensson A, Bjork T, Nilsson O, et al. Serum prostate specific antigen complexed to alpha 1-antichymotrypsin as an indicator of prostate cancer. J Urol 1993;150(1):100–5.

9. Catalona WJ, Partin AW, Slawin KM, et al. Use of the percentage of free prostate-specific antigen to enhance differentiation of prostate cancer from benign prostatic disease: a prospective multicenter clinical trial. JAMA 1998;279(19):1542–7.

10. Catalona WJ, Smith DS, Ornstein DK. Prostate cancer detection in men with serum PSA concentrations of 2.6 to 4.0 ng/mL and benign prostate examination. Enhancement of specificity with free PSA measurements. JAMA 1997;277(18):1452–5.

11. Haese A, Dworschack RT, Partin AW. Percent free prostate specific antigen in the total prostate specific antigen 2 to 4 ng/mL range does not substantially increase the number of biopsies needed to detect clinically significant prostate cancer compared to the 4 to 10 ng./ml. range. J Urol 2002;168(2):504–8.

12. National Comprehensive Cancer Network Guidelines: prostate cancer early detection 2016. Available at: http://www.nccn.org/professionals/physician_gls/pdf/prostate_detection.pdf. Accessed March 14, 2016.

13. Lazzeri M, Haese A, Abrate A, et al. Clinical performance of serum prostate-specific antigen isoform [-2]proPSA (p2PSA) and its derivatives, %p2PSA and the prostate health index (PHI), in men with a family history of prostate cancer: results from a multicentre European study, the PROMEtheuS project. BJU Int 2013;112(3):313–21.

14. Schwen ZR, Tosoian JJ, Sokoll LJ, et al. Prostate health index (PHI) predicts high-stage pathology in African American men. Urology 2016;90:136–40.

15. Fossati N, Lazzeri M, Haese A, et al. Clinical performance of serum isoform [-2]proPSA (p2PSA), and its derivatives %p2PSA and the Prostate Health Index, in men aged <60 years: results from a multicentric European study. BJU Int 2015;115(6):913–20.

16. Abrate A, Lazzeri M, Lughezzani G, et al. Clinical performance of the Prostate Health Index (PHI) for the prediction of prostate cancer in obese men: data from the PROMEtheuS project, a multicentre European prospective study. BJU Int 2015;115(4):537–45.

17. Catalona WJ, Partin AW, Sanda MG, et al. A multicenter study of [-2]pro-prostate specific antigen combined with prostate specific antigen and free prostate specific antigen for prostate cancer detection in the 2.0 to 10.0 ng/mL prostate specific antigen range. J Urol 2011;185(5):1650–5.

18. Loeb S, Sanda MG, Broyles DL, et al. The prostate health index selectively identifies clinically significant prostate cancer. J Urol 2015;193(4):1163–9.

19. de la Calle C, Patil D, Wei JT, et al. Multicenter evaluation of the prostate health index to detect aggressive prostate cancer in biopsy naive men. J Urol 2015;194(1):65–72.

20. Guazzoni G, Nava L, Lazzeri M, et al. Prostate-specific antigen (PSA) isoform p2PSA significantly improves the prediction of prostate cancer at initial extended prostate biopsies in patients with total PSA between 2.0 and 10 ng/mL: results of a prospective study in a clinical setting. Eur Urol 2011;60(2):214–22.

21. Tosoian JJ, Druskin SC, Andreas D, et al. Use of the prostate health index for detection of prostate cancer: results from a large academic practice. Prostate Cancer Prostatic Dis 2017;20(2):228–33.

22. Heijnsdijk EA, Denham D, de Koning HJ. The cost-effectiveness of prostate cancer detection with the

use of prostate health index. Value Health 2016; 19(2):153–7.

23. Cantiello F, Russo GI, Ferro M, et al. Prognostic accuracy of prostate health index and urinary prostate cancer antigen 3 in predicting pathologic features after radical prostatectomy. Urol Oncol 2015;33(4): 163.e15-23.

24. Tosoian JJ, Loeb S, Feng Z, et al. Association of [-2] proPSA with biopsy reclassification during active surveillance for prostate cancer. J Urol 2012; 188(4):1131–6.

25. Hirama H, Sugimoto M, Ito K, et al. The impact of baseline [-2]proPSA-related indices on the prediction of pathological reclassification at 1 year during active surveillance for low-risk prostate cancer: the Japanese multicenter study cohort. J Cancer Res Clin Oncol 2014;140(2):257–63.

26. Tosoian JJ, Druskin SC, Andreas D, et al. Prostate health index density improves detection of clinically significant prostate cancer. BJU Int 2017 Jun;20(2): 228–33.

27. Gnanapragasam VJ, Burling K, George A, et al. The Prostate Health Index adds predictive value to multiparametric MRI in detecting significant prostate cancers in a repeat biopsy population. Sci Rep 2016;6: 35364.

28. Vickers AJ, Cronin AM, Aus G, et al. A panel of kallikrein markers can reduce unnecessary biopsy for prostate cancer: data from the European Randomized Study of Prostate Cancer Screening in Goteborg, Sweden. BMC Med 2008;6:19.

29. Bryant RJ, Sjoberg DD, Vickers AJ, et al. Predicting high-grade cancer at ten-core prostate biopsy using four kallikrein markers measured in blood in the ProtecT study. J Natl Cancer Inst 2015;107(7) [pii: djv095].

30. Parekh DJ, Punnen S, Sjoberg DD, et al. A multi-institutional prospective trial in the USA confirms that the 4Kscore accurately identifies men with high-grade prostate cancer. Eur Urol 2015;68(3): 464–70.

31. Vickers A, Cronin A, Roobol M, et al. Reducing unnecessary biopsy during prostate cancer screening using a four-kallikrein panel: an independent replication. J Clin Oncol 2010;28(15):2493–8.

32. Gupta A, Roobol MJ, Savage CJ, et al. A four-kallikrein panel for the prediction of repeat prostate biopsy: data from the European Randomized Study of Prostate Cancer screening in Rotterdam, Netherlands. Br J Cancer 2010;103(5):708–14.

33. Nordström T, Vickers A, Assel M, et al. Comparison between the four-kallikrein panel and prostate health index for predicting prostate cancer. Eur Urol 2015; 68(1):139–46.

34. Carlsson S, Maschino A, Schroder F, et al. Predictive value of four kallikrein markers for pathologically insignificant compared with aggressive prostate cancer in radical prostatectomy specimens: results from the European Randomized Study of Screening for Prostate Cancer section Rotterdam. Eur Urol 2013;64(5):693–9.

35. Stattin P, Vickers AJ, Sjoberg DD, et al. Improving the specificity of screening for lethal prostate cancer using prostate-specific antigen and a panel of Kallikrein Markers: a nested case-control study. Eur Urol 2015;68(2):207–13.

36. Lin DW, Newcomb LF, Brown MD, et al. Evaluating the four Kallikrein panel of the 4Kscore for prediction of high-grade prostate cancer in men in the canary prostate active surveillance study. Eur Urol 2016 [pii:S0302–2838(16)30850-8].

37. Bussemakers MJ, van Bokhoven A, Verhaegh GW, et al. DD3: a new prostate-specific gene, highly overexpressed in prostate cancer. Cancer Res 1999;59(23):5975–9.

38. Marks LS, Fradet Y, Deras IL, et al. PCA3 molecular urine assay for prostate cancer in men undergoing repeat biopsy. Urology 2007;69(3):532–5.

39. Gittelman MC, Hertzman B, Bailen J, et al. PCA3 molecular urine test as a predictor of repeat prostate biopsy outcome in men with previous negative biopsies: a prospective multicenter clinical study. J Urol 2013;190(1):64–9.

40. Haese A, de la Taille A, van Poppel H, et al. Clinical utility of the PCA3 urine assay in European men scheduled for repeat biopsy. Eur Urol 2008;54(5): 1081–8.

41. Bradley LA, Palomaki GE, Gutman S, et al. Comparative effectiveness review: prostate cancer antigen 3 testing for the diagnosis and management of prostate cancer. J Urol 2013;190(2):389–98.

42. Deras IL, Aubin SM, Blase A, et al. PCA3: a molecular urine assay for predicting prostate biopsy outcome. J Urol 2008;179(4):1587–92.

43. Chevli KK, Duff M, Walter P, et al. Urinary PCA3 as a predictor of prostate cancer in a cohort of 3,073 men undergoing initial prostate biopsy. J Urol 2014; 191(6):1743–8.

44. Wei JT, Feng Z, Partin AW, et al. Can urinary PCA3 supplement PSA in the early detection of prostate cancer? J Clin Oncol 2014;32(36):4066–72.

45. Aubin SM, Reid J, Sarno MJ, et al. PCA3 molecular urine test for predicting repeat prostate biopsy outcome in populations at risk: validation in the placebo arm of the dutasteride REDUCE trial. J Urol 2010;184(5):1947–52.

46. Tosoian JJ, Loeb S, Kettermann A, et al. Accuracy of PCA3 measurement in predicting short-term biopsy progression in an active surveillance program. J Urol 2010;183(2):534–8.

47. Hessels D, van Gils MP, van Hooij O, et al. Predictive value of PCA3 in urinary sediments in determining clinico-pathological characteristics of prostate cancer. Prostate 2010;70(1):10–6.

48. Liss MA, Santos R, Osann K, et al. PCA3 molecular urine assay for prostate cancer: association with pathologic features and impact of collection protocols. World J Urol 2011;29(5):683–8.

49. van Gils MP, Hessels D, Hulsbergen-van de Kaa CA, et al. Detailed analysis of histopathological parameters in radical prostatectomy specimens and PCA3 urine test results. Prostate 2008; 68(11):1215–22.

50. Alshalalfa M, Verhaegh GW, Gibb EA, et al. Low PCA3 expression is a marker of poor differentiation in localized prostate tumors: exploratory analysis from 12,076 patients. Oncotarget 2017. [Epub ahead of print].

51. Seisen T, Roupret M, Brault D, et al. Accuracy of the prostate health index versus the urinary prostate cancer antigen 3 score to predict overall and significant prostate cancer at initial biopsy. Prostate 2015; 75(1):103–11.

52. Ferro M, Lucarelli G, Bruzzese D, et al. Improving the prediction of pathologic outcomes in patients undergoing radical prostatectomy: the value of prostate cancer antigen 3 (PCA3), prostate health index (phi) and sarcosine. Anticancer Res 2015; 35(2):1017–23.

53. Porpiglia F, Cantiello F, De Luca S, et al. In-parallel comparative evaluation between multiparametric magnetic resonance imaging, prostate cancer antigen 3 and the prostate health index in predicting pathologically confirmed significant prostate cancer in men eligible for active surveillance. BJU Int 2016; 118(4):527–34.

54. Fenstermaker M, Mendhiratta N, Bjurlin MA, et al. Risk stratification by urinary prostate cancer gene 3 testing before magnetic resonance imaging-ultrasound fusion-targeted prostate biopsy among men with no history of biopsy. Urology 2017;99:174–9.

55. Nygard Y, Haukaas SA, Halvorsen OJ, et al. A positive real-time elastography (RTE) combined with a Prostate Cancer Gene 3 (PCA3) score above 35 convey a high probability of intermediate- or high-risk prostate cancer in patient admitted for primary prostate biopsy. BMC Urol 2016;16(1):39.

56. Hansen J, Auprich M, Ahyai SA, et al. Initial prostate biopsy: development and internal validation of a biopsy-specific nomogram based on the prostate cancer antigen 3 assay. Eur Urol 2013;63(2):201–9.

57. Elshafei A, Chevli KK, Moussa AS, et al. PCA3-based nomogram for predicting prostate cancer and high grade cancer on initial transrectal guided biopsy. Prostate 2015;75(16):1951–7.

58. Rubio-Briones J, Borque A, Esteban LM, et al. Optimizing the clinical utility of PCA3 to diagnose prostate cancer in initial prostate biopsy. BMC Cancer 2015;15:633.

59. Greene DJ, Elshafei A, Nyame YA, et al. External validation of a PCA-3-based nomogram for predicting prostate cancer and high-grade cancer on initial prostate biopsy. Prostate 2016;76(11):1019–23.

60. Tomlins SA, Rhodes DR, Perner S, et al. Recurrent fusion of TMPRSS2 and ETS transcription factor genes in prostate cancer. Science 2005;310(5748): 644–8.

61. Tomlins SA, Bjartell A, Chinnaiyan AM, et al. ETS gene fusions in prostate cancer: from discovery to daily clinical practice. Eur Urol 2009;56(2):275–86.

62. Tomlins SA, Aubin SM, Siddiqui J, et al. Urine TMPRSS2:ERG fusion transcript stratifies prostate cancer risk in men with elevated serum PSA. Sci Transl Med 2011;3(94):94ra72.

63. Hessels D, Smit FP, Verhaegh GW, et al. Detection of TMPRSS2-ERG fusion transcripts and prostate cancer antigen 3 in urinary sediments may improve diagnosis of prostate cancer. Clin Cancer Res 2007;13(17):5103–8.

64. Tomlins SA, Day JR, Lonigro RJ, et al. Urine TMPRSS2:ERG plus PCA3 for individualized prostate cancer risk assessment. Eur Urol 2016;70(1):45–53.

65. Van Neste L, Hendriks RJ, Dijkstra S, et al. Detection of high-grade prostate cancer using a urinary molecular biomarker-based risk score. Eur Urol 2016; 70(5):740–8.

66. McKiernan J, Donovan MJ, O'Neill V, et al. A novel urine exosome gene expression assay to predict high-grade prostate cancer at initial biopsy. JAMA Oncol 2016;2(7):882–9.

67. Stewart GD, Van Neste L, Delvenne P, et al. Clinical utility of an epigenetic assay to detect occult prostate cancer in histopathologically negative biopsies: results of the MATLOC study. J Urol 2013;189(3):1110–6.

68. Partin AW, Van Neste L, Klein EA, et al. Clinical validation of an epigenetic assay to predict negative histopathological results in repeat prostate biopsies. J Urol 2014;192(4):1081–7.

69. Murphy DG, Ahlering T, Catalona WJ, et al. The Melbourne consensus statement on the early detection of prostate cancer. BJU Int 2014;113(2):186–8.

70. Foley RW, Maweni RM, Gorman L, et al. European Randomised Study of Screening for Prostate Cancer (ERSPC) risk calculators significantly outperform the prostate cancer prevention trial (PCPT) 2.0 in the prediction of prostate cancer: a multi-institutional study. BJU Int 2016;118(5):706–13.

71. Loeb S, Shin SS, Broyles DL, et al. Prostate health index improves multivariable risk prediction of aggressive prostate cancer. BJU Int 2017;120(1):61–8.

72. Lughezzani G, Lazzeri M, Larcher A, et al. Development and internal validation of a prostate health index based nomogram for predicting prostate cancer at extended biopsy. J Urol 2012;188(4):1144–50.

73. Lughezzani G, Lazzeri M, Haese A, et al. Multicenter European external validation of a prostate health index-based nomogram for predicting prostate cancer at extended biopsy. Eur Urol 2014;66(5):906–12.

How to Biopsy
Transperineal Versus Transrectal, Saturation Versus Targeted, What's the Evidence?

Jeremy Grummet, MBBS, MS, FRACS

KEYWORDS

- Transperineal prostate biopsy • Transrectal prostate biopsy • Targeted prostate biopsy
- Saturation prostate biopsy • Template prostate biopsy • MRI • Prostate cancer

KEY POINTS

- Transrectal biopsy has an increasing rate of infection because of increasing multiresistant rectal flora. Targeted prophylaxis with prior rectal swab and/or other methods must be used because standard quinolone prophylaxis is no longer adequate.
- Transperineal biopsy has a near-zero risk of sepsis. A single dose of first-generation cephalosporin only is recommended as prophylaxis, obviating concerns over increasing antibiotic resistance.
- MRI-targeted biopsy increases detection of significant prostate cancer over standard 12-core biopsy.
- It remains unknown if one method of MRI-targeted biopsy is superior to another for detection of significant prostate cancer.
- Combined targeted and template biopsy provides maximal detection of significant prostate cancer, at the cost of increasing detection of indolent disease.

INTRODUCTION

Prostate biopsy remains the gold standard for the diagnosis of prostate cancer (PC).[1] In the workup to determine if a man has PC, the biopsy is the first test along the diagnostic pathway that is truly invasive. In the present era of patient-centered care, it is of utmost importance that this invasive test is performed with optimal comfort, safety, and diagnostic accuracy.

Depending on how it is performed, however, prostate biopsy can cause pain, can miss or undergrade clinically significant cancer, and pose a risk of serious complications. The currently accepted minimum standard for prostate biopsy is to take 10 to 12 random cores transrectally with ultrasound guidance.[2] Although periprostatic infiltration of local anesthesia is the minimum standard in transrectal (TR) biopsy analgesia, it often fails to provide adequate cover, causing unnecessary pain, anxiety, and embarrassment to patients,[3] which has stimulated recent and current studies to improve the patient's biopsy experience.[4,5] This untargeted sampling method has also been shown to miss significant prostate cancer (SPC) up to nearly 30% of the time.[6] As a result, men are often subjected to multiple sets of biopsies until the

Disclosure Statement: Biobot Surgical (iSR'obot Mona Lisa): Travel and accommodation provided to attend UAA ASM in Singapore 2016. Scanmedics (BK Ultrasound): Honorarium for delivering Transperineal Biopsy Workshop in Melbourne 2014.
Department of Surgery, Central Clinical School, Monash University, 125 Balaclava Road, Caulfield North, Victoria 3161, Australia
E-mail address: jpgrummet@hotmail.com

Urol Clin N Am 44 (2017) 525–534
http://dx.doi.org/10.1016/j.ucl.2017.07.002

clinician is either satisfied there is no cancer, or that SPC is eventually found. Each of these invasive procedures puts patients at risk of complications, the most morbid of which is sepsis.[7] It is these shortcomings of traditional biopsy methods that have been cited as part of the reason for both the US and Canadian Preventive Services Task-forces'[8,9] recommendations against prostate-specific antigen (PSA) screening, because of harms outweighing benefits.

Multiparametric MRI, with its now standardized acquisition and reporting system (PIRADS),[10] has garnered much interest as a way of relatively reliably *seeing* SPC for the first time, and therefore, significantly increasing diagnostic accuracy.[11] When positive, MRI allows for targeted biopsies, which can be performed in a variety of ways (see later discussion) instead of, or in addition to, random biopsies. The burgeoning evidence of MRI's utility, as discussed elsewhere in this issue, has caused it to gradually work its way into official guidelines in specific clinical contexts.[1,2,12]

However, assessing MRI's accuracy is hampered by the constantly shifting definition of SPC, which is becoming increasingly restricted over time.[11] The confusion is evidenced by at least one study that has examined MRI accuracy using 4 different definitions of SPC,[13] and the recent PROMIS study even used Gleason score $\geq 4 + 3 = 7$ and cancer core length ≥ 6 mm.[14] This changeable definition is due to the combination of a growing recognition that Gleason pattern 3 is practically never metastatic,[15] and to current targeted biopsy methods now allowing regular detection of the longest cores of highest-grade tumor present in the gland.[14,16,17] This should be taken into account in the comparisons of diagnostic accuracy of the current array of biopsy methods discussed later.

Transperineal (TP) biopsy is also finally receiving increasing attention as a method of avoiding the risk of sepsis associated with TR biopsy.[18] This risk has been well documented as increasing in recent years because of the increase in multidrug resistance in rectal flora.[7] To date, TP biopsy has typically been performed under general anesthesia and is therefore a painless procedure; however, this has major implications for health resource use. Alternative methods for reducing the sepsis risk in TR biopsy have therefore also been advanced and are discussed later. A comparison of TP biopsy to the TR route in relation to diagnostic accuracy is also discussed later.

Multiparametric MRI and TP biopsy have added a vast array of options for prostate biopsy. The spectrum spans from the traditional hand-held random TR biopsy to now robotic MRI-targeted TP biopsy via just 2 skin punctures.[19] MRI and TP biopsy have the potential to minimize inaccuracy and risk to patients in the diagnostic workup of PC. These are critical advances in clinical practice that help to reverse the risk:benefit ratio, because harms must be outweighed when testing for PC.

PATIENT SAFETY AND COMFORT

Prostate biopsy, when performed optimally, provides clinicians with arguably the most important information for making management decisions in PC: tissue. However, it is an invasive procedure. It can cause pain, anxiety, and embarrassment,[3] as well as hematuria, hematochezia, hematospermia, erectile dysfunction, lower urinary tract symptoms (LUTS), and urinary retention.[7] Apart from hematochezia, both TR and TP biopsy can cause all of the above side effects to varying degrees. However, there is another complication risk where the choice of biopsy approach may have by far the most profound impact: infection. Infection can manifest from a simple urinary tract infection, epididymoorchitis, or bacterial prostatitis, through to life-threatening sepsis.

Potential side effects of prostate biopsy include the following:

- Pain
- Anxiety
- Embarrassment
- Hematuria
- Hematochezia
- Hematospermia
- Erectile dysfunction
- LUTS
- Urinary retention
- Infection/sepsis

TR biopsy has always been subject to the risk of sepsis. By passing the biopsy needle from the fecally contaminated rectum to the sterile prostate, the procedure contravenes the basic surgical principle of sterile technique. However, it is quick and convenient because it is usually performed under local anesthesia. In the past, sepsis risk has been kept low by covering the contamination by prophylactic broad-spectrum antibiotics. The drug family of choice remains quinolones.[3]

However, it is now clear that TR biopsy sepsis rates are increasing, in line with the increase in multi-drug-resistant and particularly quinolone-resistant rectal flora.[18] In a Canadian population-based study of more than 75,000 patients, Nam and colleagues[20] reported an increase from 0.6% to 3.6% of postprostate biopsy hospital admissions for infection over 10 years to 2005. In another study of nearly 200,000 patients on the English National Cancer Registry, Anastasiadis and colleagues[21] reported an increase of infective hospital admissions of 70% following prostate biopsy in 8 years to 2008. Most recently, Gershman and colleagues[22] reported on more than 100,000 men undergoing prostate biopsy in the United States from 2005 to 2014. Despite the absolute rate of biopsy decreasing as much as 33%, thought to be due mainly to recommendations against PSA testing, there was a significant increase from 14% to 18% in postbiopsy complications of those biopsied, which was driven by infection. Prior quinolone use was a predictor, suggesting quinolone resistance as an underlying factor.

It is therefore no longer adequate to simply administer a prophylactic quinolone antibiotic to all men presenting for TR biopsy.[7,18,23] In addition, in July 2016, the US Food and Drug Administration upgraded their warning on the use of quinolones because of the risk of permanent disabling side effects, advising that quinolones only be prescribed when there is no alternative available.[24]

Alternative methods to minimize or avoid altogether the risk of sepsis from TR biopsy are as follows:

- Rectal swab and targeted antibiotic prophylaxis
- Multidrug prophylaxis
- Carbapenem prophylaxis
- Rectal/needle disinfection
- TP biopsy
- MRI-targeted only biopsy
- No biopsy (if prior was MRI negative and other risk factors low)

Targeted and Multidrug Prophylaxis

Roberts and colleagues[25] performed a meta-analysis in 2014 of 9 studies comprising more than 2500 patients undergoing TR biopsy. They found a rate of 0.3% infection when using targeted prophylaxis based on prior rectal swab compared with 3.3% with empirical prophylaxis. Similarly, in 2016, Cussans and colleagues[26] reported their systematic review of 9 studies comprising more than 4500 patients. Postbiopsy infection was significantly lower in the targeted prophylaxis group (0.72% vs 4.55%). Concerned about the increasing rate of antibiotic resistance, the Michigan Urological Surgery Improvement Collaborative conducted a statewide intervention in prostate biopsy antibiotic prophylaxis for 2 years to 2014.[27] In using either multi-drug or targeted prophylaxis, they observed a significant 53% decrease in postbiopsy infective hospital admission from 1.19% to 0.56%.

The results of these reports support targeted or multidrug antibiotic prophylaxis for TR biopsy. Targeted prophylaxis is also consistent with antibiotic stewardship, which aims to optimize tradeoff between efficacy and preventing stimulation of further resistance.[28] However, these methods fail to achieve a zero infection rate. Furthermore, multidrug prophylaxis goes against antibiotic stewardship, because it is well established that unnecessary antibiotic use is the most important factor that leads to increasing resistance.[29]

Carbapenem Prophylaxis

Further evidence for concern about infection risk in TR biopsy is evidenced by the increasing use of carbapenem antibiotics for prophylaxis. In an Australian study, Leahy and colleagues[30] found an increase from 0% to 13% in the use of carbapenems for TR biopsy prophylaxis in nearly 2000 patients in 4 years to 2012. The rate of sepsis in the overall cohort was 1.2%, but none of those receiving carbapenem suffered infection. In New Zealand, Losco and colleagues[31] also found no patients with sepsis when using carbapenem prophylaxis. The "high-risk" sample group of 80 receiving carbapenem was small, but the 90 "low-risk" patients receiving standard prophylaxis with ciprofloxacin plus amoxicillin-clavulanate had a sepsis rate as high as 6.7%. The investigators comment that risk stratification based on known risk factors was clearly unhelpful in determining who should receive carbapenem prophylaxis and therefore recommend carbapenems for all.

The concern if carbapenems were to be used on a grand scale (>2 million prostate biopsies are performed every year[7]) is that it may lead to carbapenem resistance. With this in mind, in an elegant study, the same New Zealand group recently reported 326 patients receiving carbapenem prophylaxis for TR biopsy. None were found to have developed carbapenem-resistant bacteria on repeat postbiopsy rectal swabs. However, in this cohort, sepsis was not eliminated, occurring in 0.9%. Notwithstanding the lack of carbapenem resistance found in this relatively small cohort, it is recognized that unnecessary carbapenem use may lead to the further development of carbapenem-resistant Enterobacteriaceae, 1 of only 3 bacteria listed by the US Centers for Disease Control and Prevention (CDC) as an Urgent Threat, with a mortality of 50% when cultured in blood.[29] The CDC therefore strongly recommends against any use of carbapenems where alternative options are available.

Rectal/Needle Disinfection

Standard rectal enemas may improve the ultrasound images obtained but have not been shown to reduce TR biopsy sepsis.[32] However, another method investigated is by attempting to disinfect the rectal wall or the biopsy needle. It is an ambitious aim to counteract the natural environment of the rectum, being a storage facility for feces; however, there is some evidence to suggest efficacy.

In 2013, Abughosh and colleagues[33] reported a randomized controlled trial comparing 865 men with or without rectal cleansing with povidone-iodine. They found an encouraging 42% reduction in infection from 4.5% in the rectal cleansing group to 2.6% in the group without, but it was not statistically significant. Pu and colleagues[34] performed a systematic review and meta-analysis of rectal cleansing using a povidone-iodine enema for TR biopsy in 2014. In 7 studies comprising more than 2000 patients, they found significant reductions in fever, bacteremia, and bacteriuria in those using povidone-iodine enemas. However, it is not stated how these metrics translated to clinical diagnoses of infection. The investigators also comment on the need for large prospective studies because of the poor quality of the evidence.

Disinfection of the biopsy needle using formalin has also been investigated. In more than 1600 patients in whom the biopsy needle was dipped in formalin between each core taken, Issa and colleagues[35] found a sepsis rate of just 0.1%, and formalin exposure was reported to be safe and negligible. The overall 0.3% rate of infection was about one-third that of a historical cohort of nearly 1000 patients who did not have formalin needle disinfection (0.8%); however, it was not statistically significant. Further support for formalin needle disinfection was published recently by Singla and colleagues.[36] Of 756 patients undergoing TR biopsy, 253 received formalin needle disinfection. None of the 8 patients requiring hospital admission had formalin, and the 2.3% infection rate in the formalin group was less than half of the nonformalin group (5.2%), but this again failed to reach statistical significance.

Transperineal Biopsy

Notably, all of the above methods still require the use of broad-spectrum antibiotics, which in large scale use may lead to further development of antibiotic resistance. The World Health Organization has cautioned that if this kind of practice is continued, we risk entering a postantibiotic era.[37] However, TP biopsy, where the rectum and its flora are avoided altogether, is distinct in that it can be performed using only a single dose of a first-generation cephalosporin as prophylaxis and still achieve a zero rate of sepsis.

In 2014, the author reported a relatively small multicenter series of 245 consecutive TP biopsies with a zero rate of sepsis. The accompanying literature review identified 16 reports comprising more than 6600 cases of TP biopsy with a total sepsis rate of 0.08%. The author has since reported updates of his own multicenter series,[38] more recently on nearly 1200 consecutive patients, finding the sepsis rate remaining at zero.[39] Importantly, the latter 60% of this cohort only received a single dose of cefazolin as prophylaxis. This antibiotic is now recommended for use in TP biopsy by Australia's Therapeutic Guidelines publication.[40]

Using TP biopsy, sepsis has been virtually eliminated from practice, and the unnecessary use of quinolones and other broad-spectrum antibiotics can be simultaneously avoided. This clearly benefits not only individual patients but also potentially the broader community as well.

TP biopsy under local anesthetic, using a template to take at least 20 cores, has been reported with acceptable pain scores.[41–43] However, to date, it has been typically performed under general anesthesia. TP biopsy has been slow to gain traction because of the consequent logistical issues.

This may be about to change however, if in the future only MRI-targeted biopsies are performed. If only 2 to 4 cores are taken transperineally in close proximity to each other under local anesthesia, this is likely to be far more acceptable to patients than the large number of widespread cores required for saturation biopsy. MRI-ultrasound fusion platforms initially built for TR biopsy have now adapted models to allow TP biopsy in anticipation of this (see later discussion).

MRI-Targeted Only Biopsy

When performing only targeted biopsies, as few as 2 cores may be taken. This can be the case regardless of targeted method, that is, in-bore MRI-guided biopsy or by TR ultrasound guidance with cognitive or software fusion; however, most literature on targeted-only biopsies is on in-bore biopsy.[6,44] In Borghesi and colleagues'[7] recent systematic review, the investigators query whether it is the limited number of cores taken by in-bore biopsy or the TP approach that affords a near-zero sepsis rate. However, only one study of a TR in-bore MRI-targeted series with 23 patients showing no sepsis is cited.[44] Other cited studies reported on the TP approach in up to 6000 patients,[45] where as many as 24 cores are routinely taken. It is therefore clear that in TP biopsy, regardless of the number of cores taken, the sepsis rate remains zero or near-zero. What remains unknown, given other studies published of small volume only,[46,47] is whether a low number of cores taken transrectally, afforded by a targeted-only technique, would result in low sepsis rates as well. However, as with any TR approach, broad-spectrum or targeted antibiotic prophylaxis with prior rectal swabs would still be required.

No Biopsy

The final method for avoiding sepsis and other complications of prostate biopsy is of course to not biopsy at all. This may be an option for some men with a negative MRI and is discussed elsewhere in this issue.[14]

DIAGNOSTIC ACCURACY

As mentioned earlier, it is difficult to make meaningful comparisons of diagnostic accuracy between biopsy techniques because of the multitude of definitions of SPC used in studies. Compounding this difficulty is the now wide array of biopsy options available to compare as well as the different clinical settings in which they are used, that is, initial biopsy, repeat biopsy following a negative biopsy, repeat biopsy in active surveillance.

The current range of prostate biopsy methods includes the following:

- TR versus TP
- Freehand[48] versus brachytherapy grid[49] versus robotic[19]
- Nontargeted (random) versus MRI-targeted versus combination of both

Options for nontargeted include the following:

- "Standard" random 10- to 12-core versus saturation/template

Options for MRI-targeted biopsy include the following:

- In-bore MRI-guided versus MRI-US software fusion versus MRI-US cognitive fusion

Which of all these methods might be the most accurate, or might some be equivalent?

Nontargeted: Transrectal Versus Transperineal

In the recent update on the European Association of Urology guidelines for PC, it stated that "when the same number of cores are taken, both TR and TP approaches have comparable detection rates."[2] A single randomized controlled trial[50,51] of 246 patients is cited comparing 12-core TR biopsy versus 12-core TP biopsy. Notwithstanding the limitation that there are no data or subanalysis on detection of SPC in this study, the results are not surprising. TR and TP biopsies are simply entering the prostate from 2 different directions, so the cancer detection rate when using the same number of cores is expected to be similar. This has also been shown in a study comparing the 2 approaches using 24 cores.[52]

Although some evidence does exist for superior detection of SPC anteriorly in TP biopsy,[53–55] particularly in the repeat biopsy setting, this is more likely due to the template used, rather than the approach, because TR cores should be able to reach just as anteriorly if the trocar is advanced far enough. Furthermore, in patients with a large gland and narrow pubic arch, the TP approach can sometimes even prevent access to the anterior gland.

The real advantage of the TP approach in the nontargeted setting is that a much more extensive sampling with more than 24 cores (template or saturation) can be undertaken without any increase in the near-zero rate of sepsis. Clinicians (and patients) would be understandably reluctant to perform such thorough sampling transrectally because of the risk of sepsis. As expected, performing an extensive biopsy with a high number of cores across all areas of the prostate results in a high detection rate of SPC of up to 47% in men undergoing an initial biopsy.[49,54,56]

MRI-Targeted Versus Random Transrectal Biopsy

TP template biopsy was introduced to simultaneously improve cancer detection rates and reduce infection risk. This occurred before the advent of MRI, when localized PC was not reliably visible on imaging. Now that MRI can identify the location of the vast majority of SPCs, biopsies can be performed that are targeted to the lesion, as occurs in all other solid organ cancers.

A meta-analysis by Schoots and colleagues[57] found that although MRI-targeted biopsy had a similar detection rate to traditional random TR biopsy of overall PC, of more importance was its higher detection rate of SPC and a lower rate of insignificant cancer in men undergoing a repeat biopsy. This has also been found in men undergoing initial biopsy in a randomized study.[58] Another randomized trial was reported as a negative study, showing no difference in detection of SPC between MRI-targeted biopsy and random TR biopsy.[59] However, targeted biopsies included

PIRADS 3 lesions, which are known to be equivocal for SPC. When comparing targeted biopsies of only PIRADS 4 and 5 lesions to random biopsies, targeted biopsies were superior. Most recently, the PROMIS trial of 576 men undergoing initial biopsy found that MRI-targeted biopsy diagnosed 18% more SPC than random TR biopsy; however, SPC was restrictively defined as Gleason score $\geq 4 + 3 = 7$ and cancer core length ≥ 6 mm.[14] Finally, Wegelin and colleagues'[11] recent meta-analysis found that, as per Schoots and colleagues, overall PC detection was similar between the 2 groups, but SPC detection, as defined in each study included, was significantly higher in the MRI-targeted biopsy group with a relative sensitivity of 1.16 (90% vs 79%). Stated differently, MRI-targeted biopsy missed 10%, whereas random TR biopsy missed 21%, of SPCs. Random TR biopsy also detected twice as many insignificant cancers.

Also included in Wegelin and colleagues' paper, but after their meta-analysis, Peltier and colleagues'[60] study showed significantly higher detection of SPC in initial biopsy patients by using MRI-targeted biopsy over random TR biopsy, and Siddiqui and colleagues'[61] findings concurred. In a large study of more than 1000 patients including men who had either initial biopsy, repeat biopsy for previous negative biopsy, or repeat biopsy in untreated cancer, they also found a significantly higher rate of detection (30%) of higher-risk (SPC) cancer by MRI-targeted biopsy over random TR biopsy, and significantly lower detection rate (17%) of low-risk cancer. Results were comparable across each subgroup.[62] In a degree of contrast, Quentin and colleagues,[63] in a study of 132 initial biopsy patients, did not find a significant difference in detection of SPC between in-bore MRI-targeted biopsy and random TR biopsy. However, this may be partly due to their more liberal definition of significant disease included Gleason 6 greater than 5 mm in total cancer length, as MRI less commonly detects low-grade disease. Furthermore, they did find that MRI-targeted cores required significantly fewer cores and contained significantly longer lengths of cancer per core.

The vast majority of current evidence informs us that MRI-targeted biopsy is superior to the traditional random TR biopsy for detection of SPC; however, it is defined.[11] It should also be remembered that although studies to date have typically been conducted at centers experienced in prostate MRI and biopsy, the evidence still represents only the beginning of the clinical experience in targeted prostate biopsy. It is likely that over time the gap between targeted and random biopsy will widen further.

The remaining questions are, which targeted biopsy method is best, and should template biopsy still be performed as well?

MRI-Targeted Biopsy: In-Bore Versus MRI-Ultrasound Software Fusion Versus MRI-Ultrasound Cognitive Fusion

MRI-targeted biopsy can be performed via either TR or TP approach in these 3 ways. In-bore biopsy is performed with the patient in the MRI scanner. Software fusion biopsy is performed using TR ultrasound with various software products available to fuse the prior MRI images onto real-time ultrasound images in either rigid or elastic conformation. In cognitive fusion biopsy, the clinician simply uses the prior MRI images to mentally estimate where to target when using real-time TR ultrasound images to perform the biopsy.

In Wegelin and colleagues'[11] recently reported systematic review and meta-analysis comparing these 3 methods of MRI-targeted biopsy, 43 studies were included in the meta-analysis. In-bore biopsy was superior to cognitive fusion biopsy in detection of overall PC. However, from the 11 studies identified to specifically compare detection of SPC between the 3 different techniques, pooled sensitivities for in-bore, software fusion, and cognitive fusion biopsy were 92%, 89%, and 86%, respectively. No significant difference was found.

The investigators note the limited number of studies that could be included in this analysis and commented on the lack of data in each study to make meaningful comparisons. For example, only 5% of the 43 studies included data on lesion size and only 58% used PIRADS classification. There was also a markedly heterogeneous threshold for targeted biopsy across the studies. Only 2 studies in the meta-analysis performed a direct comparison between techniques.

Wysock and colleagues[64] compared one of the available software fusion platforms to cognitive fusion using 2 TR cores per target for 172 targets in 125 men. They found no statistically significant difference in detection of SPC defined as Gleason score ≥ 7: 20.3% for software fusion biopsy versus 15.1% for cognitive fusion biopsy ($P = .0523$). However, there was a trend toward improved detection with software fusion biopsy in all subsets, suggesting the study was underpowered, and multivariate analysis showed significant superiority of detection by software fusion biopsy for smaller lesions. The 2 methods were compared with a standard of only a 12-core random TR biopsy in each patient rather than a more thorough template biopsy, and there was no comparison to whole gland specimens, so it is not possible to determine the true rate of SPC present. In addition, the cognitive fusion biopsies were performed by highly experienced clinicians, which may not reflect the broader urologic community, where a greater improvement by using software over cognitive fusion biopsy might be expected.

Puech and colleagues[17] also compared software fusion biopsy using another platform to cognitive fusion biopsy and measured it against a standard of random 12-core TR biopsy in 95 patients. They found targeted biopsy discovered longer core lengths of higher grades of cancer than random biopsy, but no difference between fusion techniques. However, only 68 men, giving 79 targets, underwent both fusion methods, and as per Wysock and colleagues's[65] study, the operators performing cognitive fusion biopsy were highly experienced.

The current evidence shows no difference between the 3 MRI-targeted biopsy methods. Further larger studies are required, including studies to compare head to head the different software fusion platforms, but it should be appreciated that cognitive fusion biopsy is highly accurate in experienced hands. Software fusion platforms may in the future be found to be more beneficial for inexperienced operators.

MRI-Targeted Plus Template Biopsies

When comparing against the highest Gleason pattern in whole-mount radical prostatectomy specimens, Le and colleagues[66] found that both MRI-targeted biopsy and template biopsy cores each detected the same Gleason pattern as the surgical specimens 54% of the time, but that this increased to 81% when combined. Radtke and colleagues[16] reported on 294 men who each underwent both TP template biopsy and MRI-targeted biopsy using software fusion. Of the 86 SPCs detected, template biopsy missed 21% and targeted biopsy missed 13%. Targeted biopsy did not detect 44% of the insignificant cancers found on template biopsy. They concluded that a combination of targeted and template cores should be performed at initial biopsy, recognizing the increased detection of insignificant cancer. Similarly, Siddiqui and colleagues[61] found maximal cancer detection by combining targeted with random biopsy, but noted that including random biopsy mainly added detection of low-risk disease (83%). Quentin and colleagues[63] also found highest detection of SPC when combining the 2 methods.

The highest detection rates of SPC are found by combining MRI-targeted cores with template cores in the one biopsy sitting. However, this comes at the cost of increased detection of insignificant cancer as well.

SUMMARY

The TP approach offers the safest method of prostate biopsy because it prevents sepsis risk and avoids the need for broad-spectrum antibiotics. Where unavailable, methods beyond standard antibiotic prophylaxis are required to reduce sepsis risk in TR biopsy. When MRIs are read by experienced clinicians, MRI-targeted biopsy is superior to nontargeted biopsy for diagnostic accuracy, with highest detection rates of SPC and lowest rates of insignificant cancer. MRI-targeted plus non-targeted biopsy provides the highest detection of SPC, at the cost of additional detection of insignificant disease.

Where feasible, MRI-targeted plus template biopsy, performed transperineally, provides the optimal combination for patients. As it remains unknown which method of MRI-targeted biopsy is most accurate for which clinical setting, further prospective study is required in this area.

We now have the technology to make an accurate diagnosis of SPC from the outset, and to do it safely. In today's era of patient-centered care, we should therefore no longer accept the diagnostic inaccuracy of traditional biopsy methods, or subject our patients to invasive procedures with unnecessary risk. Today's patients rightly demand nothing less.

REFERENCES

1. Carroll PR, Parsons JK, Andriole G, et al. NCCN guidelines insights: prostate cancer early detection, version 2.2016. J Natl Compr Canc Netw 2016; 14(5):509–19.
2. Mottet N, Bellmunt J, Bolla M, et al. EAU-ESTRO-SIOG guidelines on prostate cancer. Part 1: screening, diagnosis, and local treatment with curative intent. Eur Urol 2017;71(4):618–29.
3. Medd JC, Stockler MR, Collins R, et al. Measuring men's opinions of prostate needle biopsy. ANZ J Surg 2005;75(8):662–4.
4. Huang S, Pepdjonovic L, Konstantatos A, et al. Penthrox alone versus penthrox plus periprostatic infiltration of local analgesia for analgesia in transrectal ultrasound-guided prostate biopsy. ANZ J Surg 2016;86(3):139–42.
5. Lee C, Woo HH. Penthrox inhaler analgesia in transrectal ultrasound-guided prostate biopsy. ANZ J Surg 2015;85(6):433–7.
6. Pokorny MR, de Rooij M, Duncan E, et al. Prospective study of diagnostic accuracy comparing

prostate cancer detection by transrectal ultrasound-guided biopsy versus magnetic resonance (MR) imaging with subsequent MR-guided biopsy in men without previous prostate biopsies. Eur Urol 2014; 66(1):22–9.

7. Borghesi M, Ahmed H, Nam R, et al. Complications after systematic, random, and image-guided prostate biopsy. Eur Urol 2017;71(3):353–65.

8. Moyer VA. Screening for prostate cancer: U.S. Preventive Services Task Force recommendation statement. Ann Intern Med 2012;157(2):120–34.

9. Bell N, Gorber SC, Shane A, et al. Recommendations on screening for prostate cancer with the prostate-specific antigen test. CMAJ 2014;186(16): 1225–34.

10. Weinreb JC, Barentsz JO, Choyke PL, et al. PI-RADS prostate imaging - reporting and data system: 2015, Version 2. Eur Urol 2016;69(1):16–40.

11. Wegelin O, van Melick HH, Hooft L, et al. Comparing three different techniques for magnetic resonance imaging-targeted prostate biopsies: a systematic review of in-bore versus magnetic resonance imaging-transrectal ultrasound fusion versus cognitive registration. is there a preferred technique? Eur Urol 2017;71(4):517–31.

12. Graham J, Kirkbride P, Cann K, et al. Prostate cancer: summary of updated NICE guidance. BMJ 2014;348:f7524.

13. Thompson JE, Moses D, Shnier R, et al. Multiparametric magnetic resonance imaging guided diagnostic biopsy detects significant prostate cancer and could reduce unnecessary biopsies and over detection: a prospective study. J Urol 2014;192(1): 67–74.

14. Ahmed HU, El-Shater Bosaily A, Brown LC, et al. Diagnostic accuracy of multi-parametric MRI and TRUS biopsy in prostate cancer (PROMIS): a paired validating confirmatory study. Lancet 2017; 389(10071):815–22.

15. Eggener SE, Scardino PT, Walsh PC, et al. Predicting 15-year prostate cancer specific mortality after radical prostatectomy. J Urol 2011;185(3):869–75.

16. Radtke JP, Kuru TH, Boxler S, et al. Comparative analysis of transperineal template saturation prostate biopsy versus magnetic resonance imaging targeted biopsy with magnetic resonance imaging-ultrasound fusion guidance. J Urol 2015;193(1):87–94.

17. Puech P, Rouviere O, Renard-Penna R, et al. Prostate cancer diagnosis: multiparametric MR-targeted biopsy with cognitive and transrectal US-MR fusion guidance versus systematic biopsy–prospective multicenter study. Radiology 2013; 268(2):461–9.

18. Roberts MJ, Bennett HY, Harris PN, et al. Prostate biopsy-related infection: a systematic review of risk factors, prevention strategies, and management approaches. Urology 2017;104:11–21.

19. Kaufmann S, Mischinger J, Amend B, et al. First report of robot-assisted transperineal fusion versus off-target biopsy in patients undergoing repeat prostate biopsy. World J Urol 2017;35(7):1023–9.

20. Nam RK, Saskin R, Lee Y, et al. Increasing hospital admission rates for urological complications after transrectal ultrasound guided prostate biopsy. J Urol 2013;189(1 Suppl):S12–7 [discussion: S7–8].

21. Anastasiadis E, van der Meulen J, Emberton M. Hospital admissions after transrectal ultrasound-guided biopsy of the prostate in men diagnosed with prostate cancer: a database analysis in England. Int J Urol 2015;22(2):181–6.

22. Gershman B, Van Houten HK, Herrin J, et al. Impact of prostate-specific antigen (PSA) screening trials and revised PSA screening guidelines on rates of prostate biopsy and postbiopsy complications. Eur Urol 2017;71(1):55–65.

23. Jones TA, Radtke JP, Hadaschik B, et al. Optimizing safety and accuracy of prostate biopsy. Curr Opin Urol 2016;26(5):472–80.

24. FDA Drug Safety Communication: FDA updates warnings for oral and injectable fluoroquinolone antibiotics due to disabling side effects: U.S. Food and Drug Administration. 2016. Available at: http://www.fda.gov/Drugs/DrugSafety/ucm511530.htm. Accessed September 24, 2016.

25. Roberts MJ, Williamson DA, Hadway P, et al. Baseline prevalence of antimicrobial resistance and subsequent infection following prostate biopsy using empirical or altered prophylaxis: a bias-adjusted meta-analysis. Int J Antimicrob Agents 2014;43(4): 301–9.

26. Cussans A, Somani BK, Basarab A, et al. The role of targeted prophylactic antimicrobial therapy before transrectal ultrasonography-guided prostate biopsy in reducing infection rates: a systematic review. BJU Int 2016;117(5):725–31.

27. Womble PR, Linsell SM, Gao Y, et al. A statewide intervention to reduce hospitalizations after prostate biopsy. J Urol 2015;194(2):403–9.

28. Liss MA, Taylor SA, Batura D, et al. Fluoroquinolone resistant rectal colonization predicts risk of infectious complications after transrectal prostate biopsy. J Urol 2014;192(6):1673–8.

29. Antibiotic Resistance Threats in the Unites States, 2013. 2016. Available at: http://www.cdc.gov/drugresistance/threat-report-2013/pdf/ar-threats-2013-508.pdf. Accessed September 24, 2016.

30. Leahy OR, O'Reilly M, Dyer DR, et al. Transrectal ultrasound-guided biopsy sepsis and the rise in carbapenem antibiotic use. ANZ J Surg 2015;85(12): 931–5.

31. Losco G, Studd R, Blackmore T. Ertapenem prophylaxis reduces sepsis after transrectal biopsy of the prostate. BJU Int 2014;113(Suppl 2):69–72.

32. Zani EL, Clark OA, Rodrigues Netto N Jr. Antibiotic prophylaxis for transrectal prostate biopsy. Cochrane Database Syst Rev 2011;(5):CD006576.

33. Abughosh Z, Margolick J, Goldenberg SL, et al. A prospective randomized trial of povidone-iodine prophylactic cleansing of the rectum before transrectal ultrasound guided prostate biopsy. J Urol 2013;189(4):1326–31.

34. Pu C, Bai Y, Yuan H, et al. Reducing the risk of infection for transrectal prostate biopsy with povidone-iodine: a systematic review and meta-analysis. Int Urol Nephrol 2014;46(9):1691–8.

35. Issa MM, Al-Qassab UA, Hall J, et al. Formalin disinfection of biopsy needle minimizes the risk of sepsis following prostate biopsy. J Urol 2013;190(5):1769–75.

36. Singla N, Walker J, Woldu SL, et al. Formalin disinfection of prostate biopsy needles may reduce post-biopsy infectious complications. Prostate Cancer Prostatic Dis 2017;20(2):216–20.

37. Chan M. Combat drug resistance: no action today means no cure tomorrow. 2011. Available at: http://www.who.int/mediacentre/news/statements/2011/whd_20110407/en/. Accessed September 24, 2016.

38. Pepdjonovic L, Tan GH, Huang S, et al. Zero hospital admissions for infection after 577 transperineal prostate biopsies using single-dose cephazolin prophylaxis. World J Urol 2016. [Epub ahead of print].

39. Grummet J, Pepdjonovic L, Moon D, et al. Re: Marco Borghesi, Hashim Ahmed, Robert Nam, et al. Complications after systematic, random, and image-guided prostate biopsy. Eur Urol, in press. http://dx.doi.org/10.1016/j.eururo.2016.08.004. Eur Urol 2016.

40. Antibiotic: Transperineal prostatic biopsy: therapeutic guidelines. 2016. Available at: http://online.tg.org.au/ip/desktop/index.htm. Accessed October 3, 2016.

41. Smith JB, Popert R, Nuttall MC, et al. Transperineal sector prostate biopsies: a local anesthetic outpatient technique. Urology 2014;83(6):1344–9.

42. Kubo Y, Kawakami S, Numao N, et al. Simple and effective local anesthesia for transperineal extended prostate biopsy: application to three-dimensional 26-core biopsy. Int J Urol 2009;16(4):420–3.

43. Iremashvili VV, Chepurov AK, Kobaladze KM, et al. Periprostatic local anesthesia with pudendal block for transperineal ultrasound-guided prostate biopsy: a randomized trial. Urology 2010;75(5):1023–7.

44. Panebianco V, Barchetti F, Manenti G, et al. MR imaging-guided prostate biopsy: technical features and preliminary results. Radiol Med 2015;120(6):571–8.

45. Penzkofer T, Tuncali K, Fedorov A, et al. Transperineal in-bore 3-T MR imaging-guided prostate biopsy: a prospective clinical observational study. Radiology 2015;274(1):170–80.

46. Meier-Schroers M, Homsi R, Kukuk G, et al. In-bore transrectal MRI-guided prostate biopsies: are there risk factors for complications? Eur J Radiol 2016;85(12):2169–73.

47. Schiavina R, Vagnoni V, D'Agostino D, et al. "In-bore" MRI-guided prostate biopsy using an endorectal nonmagnetic device: a prospective study of 70 consecutive patients. Clin Genitourin Cancer 2017;15(3):417–27.

48. Dundee PE, Grummet JP, Murphy DG. Transperineal prostate biopsy: template-guided or freehand? BJU Int 2015;115(5):681–3.

49. Vyas L, Acher P, Kinsella J, et al. Indications, results and safety profile of transperineal sector biopsies (TPSB) of the prostate: a single centre experience of 634 cases. BJU Int 2014;114(1):32–7.

50. Hara R, Jo Y, Fujii T, et al. Optimal approach for prostate cancer detection as initial biopsy: prospective randomized study comparing transperineal versus transrectal systematic 12-core biopsy. Urology 2008;71(2):191–5.

51. Takenaka A, Hara R, Ishimura T, et al. A prospective randomized comparison of diagnostic efficacy between transperineal and transrectal 12-core prostate biopsy. Prostate Cancer Prostatic Dis 2008;11(2):134–8.

52. Abdollah F, Novara G, Briganti A, et al. Trans-rectal versus trans-perineal saturation rebiopsy of the prostate: is there a difference in cancer detection rate? Urology 2011;77(4):921–5.

53. Hossack T, Patel MI, Huo A, et al. Location and pathological characteristics of cancers in radical prostatectomy specimens identified by transperineal biopsy compared to transrectal biopsy. J Urol 2012;188(3):781–5.

54. Ong WL, Weerakoon M, Huang S, et al. Transperineal biopsy prostate cancer detection in first biopsy and repeat biopsy after negative transrectal ultrasound-guided biopsy: the Victorian Transperineal Biopsy Collaboration experience. BJU Int 2015;116(4):568–76.

55. Mabjeesh NJ, Lidawi G, Chen J, et al. High detection rate of significant prostate tumours in anterior zones using transperineal ultrasound-guided template saturation biopsy. BJU Int 2012;110(7):993–7.

56. Eldred-Evans D, Kasivisvanathan V, Khan F, et al. The use of transperineal sector biopsy as a first-line biopsy strategy: a multi-institutional analysis of clinical outcomes and complications. Urol J 2016;13(5):2849–55.

57. Schoots IG, Roobol MJ, Nieboer D, et al. Magnetic resonance imaging-targeted biopsy may enhance the diagnostic accuracy of significant prostate cancer detection compared to standard transrectal ultrasound-guided biopsy: a systematic review and meta-analysis. Eur Urol 2015;68(3):438–50.

58. Panebianco V, Barchetti F, Sciarra A, et al. Multiparametric magnetic resonance imaging vs. standard care in men being evaluated for prostate cancer: a randomized study. Urol Oncol 2015; 33(1):17.e1-7.

59. Baco E, Rud E, Eri LM, et al. A randomized controlled trial to assess and compare the outcomes of two-core prostate biopsy guided by fused magnetic resonance and transrectal ultrasound images and traditional 12-core systematic biopsy. Eur Urol 2016;69(1):149–56.

60. Peltier A, Aoun F, Lemort M, et al. MRI-targeted biopsies versus systematic transrectal ultrasound guided biopsies for the diagnosis of localized prostate cancer in biopsy naive men. Biomed Res Int 2015;2015:571708.

61. Siddiqui MM, Rais-Bahrami S, Turkbey B, et al. Comparison of MR/ultrasound fusion-guided biopsy with ultrasound-guided biopsy for the diagnosis of prostate cancer. JAMA 2015;313(4): 390–7.

62. Taneja SS. Re: comparison of MR/ultrasound fusion-guided biopsy with ultrasound-guided biopsy for the diagnosis of prostate cancer. J Urol 2015;194(1): 112–5.

63. Quentin M, Blondin D, Arsov C, et al. Prospective evaluation of magnetic resonance imaging guided in-bore prostate biopsy versus systematic transrectal ultrasound guided prostate biopsy in biopsy naive men with elevated prostate specific antigen. J Urol 2014;192(5):1374–9.

64. Wysock JS, Rosenkrantz AB, Huang WC, et al. A prospective, blinded comparison of magnetic resonance (MR) imaging-ultrasound fusion and visual estimation in the performance of MR-targeted prostate biopsy: the PROFUS trial. Eur Urol 2014; 66(2):343–51.

65. Taneja SS. Re: prostate cancer diagnosis: multiparametric MR-targeted biopsy with cognitive and transrectal US-MR fusion guidance versus systematic biopsy–prospective multicenter study. J Urol 2013; 190(5):1765.

66. Le JD, Stephenson S, Brugger M, et al. Magnetic resonance imaging-ultrasound fusion biopsy for prediction of final prostate pathology. J Urol 2014; 192(5):1367–73.

Prediagnostic Risk Assessment with Prostate MRI and MRI-Targeted Biopsy

Marc A. Bjurlin, DO, MSc[a], Samir S. Taneja, MD[b],*

KEYWORDS

- Prebiopsy • MRI • MRI-ultrasonography fusion • Risk assessment • Targeted biopsy

KEY POINTS

- Prebiopsy MRI allows localization of occult missed cancers, improved risk stratification through targeted biopsy sampling, and noninvasive risk assessment using suspicion score and quantitative MRI metrics.
- MRI-ultrasonography fusion biopsy results in an increased detection of clinically significant disease and reduction in the detection of indolent disease, and allows tumor localization during targeted biopsy.
- MRI tumor visibility, PI-RADS (Prostate Imaging Reporting and Data System), and quantitative MRI metrics, such as apparent diffusion coefficient, correlate with Gleason score, progression on active surveillance, prediction of adverse pathology on targeted biopsy and radical prostatectomy, and biochemical relapse after treatment.
- The performance characteristics, and relative benefit, of prebiopsy MRI and MRI-ultrasonography fusion–targeted biopsy seem to vary between men with no prior biopsy, those who have had a previous negative biopsy, and men with previous biopsy showing cancer.

INTRODUCTION

Prostate MRI is increasingly used in the diagnostic pathway for prostate cancer (PCa).[1,2] MRI may add value as both a prebiopsy risk assessment tool, influencing the decision whether to perform biopsy, as well as a minimally invasive method for tumor localization to direct targeted biopsy.[2] Incorporating MRI with MRI-ultrasonography (US) fusion–targeted biopsy has improved the detection of high-grade PCa and reduced the detection of clinically insignificant, indolent disease.[3,4] This article presents the role of prostate MRI in prediagnostic risk assessment and image-guided biopsy, highlighting its utility along with our institutional, as well as global, outcomes.

EVOLUTION OF MRI IN THE PREDIAGNOSTIC SPACE

Traditional prebiopsy risk stratification among men presenting with suspicion for PCa is based on a combination of clinical parameters known to predict the likelihood of cancer based on historical data. These data include patient age, prostate-specific antigen (PSA), digital rectal examination, and family history. Based on these characteristics, men meeting a subjectively sufficient level of clinical suspicion are offered biopsy, resulting in an estimated 1 million biopsies performed each year in the United States.[5] Using the standard 10-core to 12-core transrectal ultrasonography (TRUS)–guided systematic biopsy strategy nearly 50% of

[a] Department of Urology, New York University Langone Hospital - Brooklyn, 150 55th Street, Brooklyn, NY 11220, USA; [b] Division of Urologic Oncology, Department of Urology, New York University Langone Medical Center, 135 East 31st Street, 2nd Floor, New York, NY 10016 USA
* Corresponding author.
E-mail address: Samir.taneja@nyumc.org

Urol Clin N Am 44 (2017) 535–546
http://dx.doi.org/10.1016/j.ucl.2017.07.012
0094-0143/17/© 2017 Elsevier Inc. All rights reserved.

clinically significant cancers are missed or under-estimated (cancers are frequently missed on initial biopsy and are mischaracterized in terms of size, location, and grade), resulting in inappropriate risk stratification.[6] Men with continued suspicion for PCa commonly undergo repeat prostate biopsy[7] with diminishing returns in terms of cancer detection but consistent attendant risks.[8]

Prostate MRI in the prediagnostic space offers advantages of improved prebiopsy risk stratification through 3 means: (1) localizing occult missed disease, (2) improved risk stratifications through targeted biopsy sampling, and (3) noninvasive risk assessment using suspicion score and quantitative MRI metrics. MRI has been shown to identify areas suspicious for PCa that have been missed on prior biopsy or would be missed using the standard systematic TRUS-guided biopsy strategy. Functional sequences used in multiparametric (mp) prostate MRI, particularly diffusion-weighted imaging (DWI) and its quantitative metric, apparent diffusion coefficient (ADC), improve diagnostic accuracy. Importantly, DWI is based on the molecular diffusion of water molecules in biological tissues, whereas the ADC value is a quantitative parameter of DWI representing water diffusion in extracellular and extravascular space and capillary perfusion. Several studies show that ADC measurement on DWI can localize PCa.[9–11] In general, the use of mp sequences enhances the localization and detection of peripheral zone tumors.[12] The ability to identify suspicious areas within the prostate using MRI greatly facilitates targeted sampling. In a study of 24 men who underwent T2-weighted and dynamic contrast-enhanced (DCE) MRI before radical prostatectomy, Villers and colleagues[13] reported 77% and 90% sensitivity of MRI to detect 0.2 cm^3 and 0.5 cm^3 tumors, respectively, with associated negative predictive values of 85% and 95%, respectively.

Investigation into the utility of prostate MRI before biopsy has shown the examination's potential for improved individualized risk stratification. For example, several clinical outcomes studies have shown an association between the level of suspicion on prebiopsy MRI and outcomes of biopsy.[14–16] In particular, MRI suspicion score has consistently served as a strong predictor of the likelihood of significant PCa on subsequent biopsy, even in the context of other clinical risk factors. A recent pooled data meta-analysis assessing the performance of prostate MRI in PCa detection showed a specificity of 88%, sensitivity of 74%, with a negative predictive value of 65% to 94%.[17] A separate study showed the PI-RADS (Prostate Imaging Reporting and Data System, Version 2) score to be highly associated with tumor significance.[18]

ROLE OF MULTIPARAMETRIC SEQUENCES AND RELATIONSHIP TO GLEASON SCORE AND DISEASE MORPHOLOGY

Although individual imaging sequences have utility in the detection of PCa, results are optimized by mp-MRI, which combines all of the sequences in an integrated fashion to improve specificity. mp-MRI offers superior diagnostic accuracy for PCa detection compared with T2-weighted images alone, and can assist risk stratification based on lesion size, morphology, extent, and ADC value.[19] In one study, mp-MRI sensitivity exceeded 80% for detecting 0.2 cm^3 of Gleason 4 + 3 or greater and 0.5 cm^3 of greater than or equal to Gleason 3 + 4.[13] Adding DCE and/or DWI to T2-weighted MRI has been shown to significantly improve sensitivity from 63% to 79% to 81% in the peripheral zone, while maintaining a stable specificity.[20] Prostate tumors generally show increased signal on high b value DWI as well as decreased ADC given the association between tumor cellularity and restricted diffusion. DWI provides information that significantly correlates with PCa aggressiveness.[21] ADC values of PCa may help differentiate between low-risk (Gleason, 6) and intermediate-risk (Gleason score 7) disease and between low-risk and high-risk (Gleason>7) disease.[22] Lower ADC values are associated with a higher percentage of cancer on core biopsy and higher Gleason score. ADC values are also inversely correlated with the Gleason score of cancer foci on surgical pathology[23]; however, the confidence intervals are widely overlapping, limiting the ability to use ADC as a surrogate for the Gleason score. DCE-MRI is based on the permeability of blood vessels and extravasation of contrast agent into the surrounding tissue. In PCa, fast angiogenesis results in the formation of leaky endothelia with a higher permeability than normal vessels. When a contrast agent is administered into the vessels it leaks out of the capillaries into tissue, where it temporarily changes the T1 relaxation time. DCE-MRI has the potential to assess the aggressiveness of PCa in the peripheral zone[24] and may correlate with additional risk stratification factors in PCa, including PSA and maximum tumor diameter.[25]

CORRELATION OF MRI-VISIBILITY/PROSTATE IMAGING REPORTING AND DATA SYSTEM WITH CLINICAL OUTCOMES

The lesion observed on MRI as defined by PI-RADS, or MRI suspicion score before the advent of PI-RADS, along with the ADC has been shown to correlate with clinical outcomes (**Table 1**).[23,26–40]

Table 1
Clinical observations regarding Prostate Imaging Reporting and Data System and/or apparent diffusion coefficient in predicting clinical outcomes

Author, Year	Setting	Clinical Outcome	Sample Size	MRI Metric
Tamada et al,[27] 2017	AS	Three-dimensional whole-lesion ADC analysis is associated with tumor growth and Gleason ≥3 + 4 on follow-up biopsy	72	ADC 0–10th percentile
Henderson et al,[28] 2016	AS	ADC predicts time to treatment, time to adverse histology	86	ADC median
van As et al,[29] 2009	AS	ADC predicts adverse repeat biopsy findings and time to radical treatment	86	ADC value
Giles et al,[26] 2011	AS	ADC is an independent predictor of histologic progression on AS	81	ADC (all), ADC (fast), and ADC (slow)
De Cobelli et al,[23] 2015	RP	ADC predicts harboring poorly differentiated cancer on RP	72	ADC mean
Lee et al,[40] 2016	RP	Adverse findings on preoperative mp-MRI are significantly related to worse postoperative pathologic outcomes as well as postoperative biochemical recurrence	1045	mpMRI sequences
Borofsky et al,[41] 2013	RP	Tumor suspicion on T2-WI/DWI is an independent predictor of aggressive disease: Gleason ≥4– on RP	154	T2-WI/DWI
Park et al,[36] 2016	BCR after RP	PI-RADS >4 predicts BCR	158	PI-RADS
Park et al,[30] 2014	BCR after RP	ADC predicts BCR	282	T2WI, DWI, and DCE-MRI
Yoon et al,[34] 2017	BCR after RP	ADC associated with BCR-free survival after RP	157	ADC values <746 × 10⁻⁶ mm²/s
Rosenkrantz et al,[35] 2015	BCR after RP	ADC predicts BCR better than standard pathologic features alone	193	Mean of the bottom 10th percentile ADC, and entropy ADC
Westphalen et al,[32] 2011	BCR after RT	Imaging data improve nomogram prediction of BCR after RT	99	MRI and MR spectroscopy
Riaz et al,[37] 2012	BCR after RT	Imaging features predict BCR after combined RT + brachytherapy	279	mpMRI sequences
Fuchsjager et al,[38] 2010	BCR after RT	MRI ECE predicts BCR after RT	224	MRI ECE
Yamaguchi et al,[39] 2016	BCR after RT	ADC ratio is an independent prognostic factor for BCR after IMRT	101	ADC ratios

The metric in the Yoon row: ADC values $<746 \times 10^{-6}$ mm²/s

Abbreviations: AS, active surveillance; BCR, biochemical recurrence; ECE, extracapsular extension; IMRT, intensity-modulated radiation therapy; RP, radical prostatectomy; RT, radiation therapy; T2-WI, T2-weighted imaging.

Recent data have explored the value of MRI in monitoring tumors in patients on an active surveillance (AS) protocol. In patients with low-risk, localized disease, tumor ADC on DWI may be a useful marker of PCa progression and may help to identify patients who stand to benefit from radical treatment.[26] In a study of 72 men on AS, ADC 0 to 10th percentile achieved highest performance for predicting the strongest association with lesion growth on follow-up MRI.[27] Henderson and colleagues[28] evaluated 86 men on AS, and, at a median of 9.5 years of follow-up, men with baseline ADC values less than the median had a significantly shorter time to adverse pathology and time to treatment, indicating they likely harbored aggressive disease all along. The investigators hypothesized that baseline diffusion-weighted MRI may be a more appropriate measure of candidate selection than biopsy. Tumor ADC has been shown to be a significant predictor of both adverse repeat biopsy findings ($P<.0001$; hazard ratio [HR], 1.3; 95% confidence interval [CI], 1.1–1.6), and time to radical treatment ($P<.0001$; HR, 1.5; 95% CI, 1.2–1.8).[29] Receiver operating characteristic curves for ADC showed an area under the curve (AUC) of 0.7 for prediction of adverse repeat biopsy findings and an AUC of 0.83 for prediction of radical treatment.[29]

As a preoperative imaging tool, tumor ADC and PI-RADS may be useful to predict biochemical recurrence (BCR) after radical prostatectomy and radiation therapy.[30–32] In a study of 158 men, no subject with a PI-RADS score less than 4 had BCR. PI-RADS was the only independent parameter for BCR in multivariate analysis.[36] Park and colleagues[33] reported that the tumor ADC is an independent predictor of BCR following radical prostatectomy; a lower tumor ADC is correlated with a higher probability of BCR. In patients with high-risk PCa, Yoon and colleagues[34] found that ADC value was significantly associated with BCR-free survival after radical prostatectomy, suggesting that the ADC value is a useful tool for predicting the prognoses of these high-risk patients. A model integrating whole-lesion ADC metrics in men who had radical prostatectomy showed significantly higher performance for prediction of BCR than did standard pathologic features alone and may help guide postoperative prognostic assessments and decisions regarding adjuvant therapy.[35]

MRI data improve the prediction of biochemical failure with nomograms after external-beam radiation therapy.[32] Pretreatment MRI findings have also been found to predict for BCR in intermediate-risk and high-risk patients with PCa treated with combination brachytherapy and external-beam radiotherapy.[37]

OUTCOMES OF MRI-TARGETED BIOPSY/FUSION AS IT RELATES TO MRI FINDINGS: CORRELATION OF PROSTATE IMAGING REPORTING AND DATA SYSTEM AND FUSION BIOPSY OUTCOMES; THE GLOBAL EXPERIENCE

Clinical outcomes of prebiopsy MRI followed by MRI-targeted biopsy suggest the potential to improve detection of clinically significant cancer and avoid detection of low-grade, clinically indolent disease (**Table 2**).

In a recent study of 1042 men who underwent MRI and targeted and systematic biopsies, the addition of systematic biopsy to targeted biopsy found 7% (60/825) additional clinically significant cancer.[56] Men with very-high-suspicion (suspicion score, 5) regions of interest (ROIs) had 9 times the odds of having clinically significant PCa compared with men with intermediate suspicion (suspicion score, 3) ROI. The combination of targeted and systematic treatment resulted in the detection of more clinically significant PCa cases than the use of either method alone. Siddiqui and colleagues[2] reported on 1003 men at risk for PCa in whom targeted MRI-US fusion biopsy, compared with standard extended TRUS-guided biopsy, was associated with increased detection of high-risk PCa and decreased detection of low-risk PCa. In a recent retrospective review of 601 men who underwent both MRI-US fusion–targeted biopsy and systematic biopsy, targeted MRI-US fusion biopsy detected fewer cases of Gleason score 6 PCa (75 vs 121; $P<.001$) and more Gleason score greater than or equal to 7 PCa (158 vs 117; $P<.001$) compared with systemic biopsy.[48] A meta-analysis of 21 studies showed that MRI-US fusion biopsy detected more clinically significant cancers than standard biopsy (relative risk = 1.22; $P <.01$).[57]

In general, higher PI-RADS scores correlate with higher overall cancer detection rates and clinically significant cancer rates, with the highest cancer detection rates found in PI-RADS 5 ROI (**Table 3**).[16,58–62]

Mertan and colleagues[63] prospectively evaluated 116 lesions in 62 patients who underwent MRI-US fusion–guided biopsy and systematic biopsy. Histopathology revealed 55 of 116 (47.4%) cancers. Based on targeted biopsy on a per-lesion basis, the overall cancer detection rates of PI-RADS 2, 3, 4, and 5 scores for all tumors was 22.2%, 15.8%, 29.8%, and 78.1%, respectively. The cancer detection rate of PI-RADS 2, 3, 4, and 5 scores for Gleason 3 + 4 or greater tumors were 5.6%, 0%, 21.3%, and 75%, respectively. In a study of 155 men who underwent MRI-guided biopsy, Osses and colleagues[64] found an overall 65% cancer detection rate.[64] No biopsy of

Table 2
Overall and clinically significant cancer detection rates in men with a prior negative biopsy and no prior biopsy

Reference	Patients (N)	Patients: Prior Negative Biopsy Only (N)	Overall Cancer Detection (%)		Clinically Significant Cancer Detection (%)	
			TB + SB	SB	TB + SB	SB
Abdi et al,[42] 2015	172	172	42	22	35	16
Brock et al,[43] 2015	121	121	52	46	44	34
Filson et al,[56] 2016	1024	324	38	23	23	23
Mariotti et al,[44] 2016	389	143	51	41	27	13
Martorana et al,[18] 2016	157	157	50	23	NR	NR
Maxeiner et al,[45] 2015	169	169	42	NR	NR	NR
Mendhiratta et al,[46] 2015	161	161	29	19	16	9
Salami et al,[47] 2015	140	140	52	49	48	31
Siddiqui et al,[2] 2015	1003	432	NR	NR	NR	NR
Sonn et al,[48] 2014	94	94	22	27	20	14
Truong et al,[49]	113	113	52	42	42	26
Volkin et al,[50] 2014	162	92	NR	NR	NR	NR

Reference	Patients (N)	Patients: No Prior Biopsy Only (N)	Overall Cancer Detection (%)		Clinically Significant Cancer Detection (%)	
			TB	SB	TB	SB
Baco et al,[51] 2016	175	175	59	54	44	49
Filson et al	1024	328	44	54	30	29
Meng et al,[3] 2016	601	81	39	40	26	19
Mendhiratta et al,[52] 2015	382	382	24	18	16	9
Mozer et al,[53] 2015	152	152	54	57	43	37
Pokorny et al,[54] 2014	223	223	70	57	65	36
Porpiglia et al,[4] 2016	212	212	51	30	44	18
Siddiqui et al,[2] 2015	1003	199	46	47	17	12
Wysock et al,[55] 2014	125	43	36	NR	23	NR
No prior biopsy	NR	NR	NR	NR	NR	NR

Abbreviations: NR, not reported; SB, systematic biopsy; TB, targeted biopsy.

Table 3
Cancer detection rates for all disease and clinically significant disease stratified by MRI suspicion score/Prostate Imaging Reporting and Data System

MRI Suspicion Score[a]/ PI-RADS	NYU Experience (TB)		Mertan et al,[63] 2016 (SB + TB)		Osses et al,[64] 2017 (TB)		Tan et al,[58] 2017 (TB)		Mehralivand et al,[60] 2017 (SB + TB)		Venderink et al,[61] 2017 (TB)		Filson et al,[56] 2016	NiMhurchu et al,[16] 2016 (SB + TB)	Ukimur et al,[62] 2015 (SB + TB)	Pinto et al,[59] 2011 (SB + TB)
	Overall	CS	Overall	CS	Overall	CS	Overall	CS	Overall	CS	Overall	CS	CS	Overall	Overall	Overall
1	NA	NA	—	—	—	—	—	—	25	0	—	—	—	—	—	—
2	17	5	22	6	0	0	13	—	20	10	—	—	—	—	—	—
3	34	14	16	0	10	3	20	11	25	12	35	17	24	11	—	—
4	68	49	30	21	77	45	78	44	39	22	60	34	37	44	—	—
5	91	82	78	75	89	67	83	100	87	72	91	67	80	100	—	—
Low/unlikely	—	—	—	—	—	—	—	—	—	—	—	—	—	—	0	28
Intermediate/ likely	—	—	—	—	—	—	—	—	—	—	—	—	—	—	45	67
High/highly suspicious	—	—	—	—	—	—	—	—	—	—	—	—	—	—	92	90

Abbreviations: CS, clinically significant cancer; NYU, New York University.

[a] 5 point liker scale or PI-RADS.

PI-RADS 2 ROI was positive for cancer. PI-RADS 3 and 4 ROI were, respectively, PCa positive in 10% and 77%. Biopsies of PI-RADS 5 ROI were positive in 89% of cases. Most of the detected cancers (63%) were Gleason score 7 or greater, and this number increased to 75% in positive PI-RADS 5 ROI.

OUTCOMES OF MRI-TARGETED BIOPSY/FUSION AS IT RELATES TO MRI FINDINGS: CORRELATION OF PROSTATE IMAGING REPORTING AND DATA SYSTEM AND FUSION BIOPSY OUTCOMES; THE NEW YORK UNIVERSITY EXPERIENCE

The authors have previously reported the outcomes of our institution's first 800 MRI-US fusion–targeted biopsies and our results are in concordance with the global experience.[3] After exclusions, 601 men were included in the analysis. MRI-US fusion–targeted biopsies detected fewer cases of Gleason score 6 PCa (75 vs 121; P<.001) and more cases of Gleason score greater than or equal to 7 PCa (158 vs 117; P<.001) than systematic biopsy. Higher MRI suspicion scores were associated with higher detection of Gleason score greater than or equal to 7 PCa (P<.001) but was not correlated with detection of Gleason score 6 PCa. Prediction of Gleason score greater than or equal to 7 disease by MRI suspicion score varied according to biopsy indication. Compared with systematic biopsy, MRI-US fusion–targeted biopsies identified more Gleason score greater than or equal to 7 PCa in men with no prior biopsy (88 vs 72; P = .012), in men with a prior negative biopsy (28 vs 16; P = .010), and in men with a prior cancer diagnosis (42 vs 29; P = .043). MRI-US fusion–targeted biopsies detected fewer cases of Gleason score 6 PCa in men with no prior biopsy (32 vs 60; P<.001) and men with prior cancer (30 vs 46; P = .034).

Our institutional experience is in line with the global literature correlating higher PI-RADS scores with higher overall and clinically significant cancer detection rates.[3] Of 1243 men who underwent combined MRI-US fusion–targeted biopsy and systematic biopsy, including those who were biopsy naive, had a prior negative biopsy, and those with known cancer, the authors found the overall targeted biopsy cancer detection rates for PI-RADS 2 to 5 to be 17%, 34%, 68%, and 91% respectively, with clinically significant cancer (Gleason score ≥7) found in 5%, 14%, 49%, and 82% of men with PI-RADS 2 to 5 ROI, respectively. Similar trends were observed in subset analysis of each biopsy indication as well as in detection rates of targeted biopsy only.

INFORMING PRACTICE USING MRI IN THE PREBIOPSY SETTING
Men with Previous Biopsy

In order to address the utility of MRI-US fusion biopsy in men with a previous negative biopsy, the authors evaluated 210 men presenting to our institution for prostate biopsy with greater than or equal to 1 prior negative biopsy, who underwent MRI followed by MRI-US fusion–targeted biopsy and systematic biopsy.[46] Forty-seven (29%) of 161 men meeting inclusion criteria were found to have PCa. MRI-US fusion–targeted biopsy and systematic biopsy had overall cancer detection rates of 21.7% and 18.6% (P = .36), respectively, and cancer detection rates for Gleason score greater than or equal to 7 disease of 14.9% and 9.3% (P = .02), respectively. Of 26 men with Gleason score greater than or equal to 7 disease, MRI-US fusion–targeted biopsy detected 24 cases (92.3%), whereas systematic biopsy detected 15 cases (57.7%; P<.01). Using UCSF-CAPRA (University of California-San Francisco–Cancer of the Prostate Risk Assessment) criteria, only 1 man was restratified from low risk to higher risk based on systematic results compared with MRI-US fusion–targeted biopsy alone. Among men with MRI suspicion score less than 4, 72% of detected cancers were low risk by UCSF-CAPRA criteria.

Men Who Are Biopsy Naive

In order to investigate the clinical outcomes of those men with no previous biopsy, the authors reviewed 452 consecutive men who underwent prebiopsy MRI followed by MRI-US fusion–targeted biopsy and systematic biopsy at our institution between June 2012 and June 2015.[52] PCa was detected in 207 of 382 men (54.2%). The cancer detection rates of systematic biopsy and MRI-US fusion–targeted biopsy were 49.2% and 43.5%, respectively (P = .006). MRI-US fusion–targeted biopsy detected more Gleason score 7 or greater cancers than systematic biopsy (117 of 132 or 88.6% vs 102 of 132 or 77.3%; P = .037). Of 41 cancers detected by systematic biopsy but not by MRI-US fusion–targeted biopsy 34 (82.9%) showed Gleason 6 disease, and 26 (63.4%) and 34 (82.9%) were clinically insignificant by Epstein criteria and a UCSF-CAPRA score of 2 or less, respectively.

Candidates for Active Surveillance

MRI may be a tool for better baseline risk stratification, resulting secondarily in better selection of candidates for surveillance, ultimately requiring fewer follow-up biopsies. In a prospective multi-institutional study, Hoeks and colleagues[65] found that men on AS with a PI-RADS score of 1 or 2 had a negative predictive value of 84% (38 of 45) for detection of any PCa and 100% (45 of 45) for detection of a Gleason pattern 4 or 5–containing cancer on MRI-targeted biopsy, respectively. These results are comparable with those of Vargas and colleagues,[66] who reported a negative predictive value of 96% to 100% and a sensitivity of 87% to 96% for biopsy upgrading in cases of a predefined MR imaging score of 2 or less and 5 or higher for cancer presence. Similar studies have shown a role of MRI to improve patient section for AS, ultimately reducing the number of biopsies as well as informing the decision to biopsy during the monitoring period.[67–69]

WHEN CAN BIOPSY BE DEFERRED?

In those men with no abnormalities on the mp-MRI sequences, biopsy can possibly be avoided. The authors have previously determined the rates of disease detection on systematic biopsy with a negative MRI, which could enhance decision-making capability for men considering prostate biopsy.[70] In our cohort of 75 patients, men with no previous biopsy, men with previously negative biopsy, and men enrolled in AS protocols, the overall cancer detection rates were 18.7%, 13.8%, 8.0%, and 38.1%, respectively, and the detection rates for cancer with Gleason score greater than or equal to 7 were 1.3%, 0%, 4.0%, and 0%, respectively. A negative prebiopsy MRI conferred an overall negative predictive value of 82% on 12-core biopsy for all cancer and 98% for Gleason score greater than or equal to 7 cancer.[70] In a similar study, Lu and colleagues[71] found an overall cancer detection of 27% in 100 men who had a negative MRI. PCa was detected in 26.3% of patients who were biopsy naive, 12.1% of patients who had a prior negative biopsy, and in 44.8% of patients previously on AS; Gleason grade greater than or equal to 7 was detected in 3% of patients overall. The negative predictive value of a negative MRI was 73% for all PCa and 97% for Gleason greater than or equal to 7 PCa.

IMPROVING THE PARADIGM: BIOMARKERS TO FURTHER REFINE RISK

New blood biomarkers, such as kallikrein panels (4K Score and Prostate Health Index) and urine biomarkers (PCA3 and TMPRSS2-ERG), may improve further on existing PCa screening, detection, and risk assessment tools. The implementation of these biomarkers as secondary tools in conjunction with MRI could improve specificity

markedly, sparing as many as half of men with increased PSA levels the need to undergo biopsy. In a study evaluating whether a combination of PCA3 and MRI suspicion score could further optimize detection of PCa on MRI fusion–targeted biopsy among men with no history of biopsy, Fenstermaker and colleagues[72] found that PCA3 less than 35 shows a high negative predictive value among MRI suspicion score 2 to 3. However, in the case of high-suspicion MRI, PCA3 was not associated with cancer detection on MRF-targeted biopsy, adding little to cancer diagnosis. By performing biopsy in men with an MRI suspicion score of 4 to 5 and obtaining PCA3 on men with an MRI suspicion score of 2 to 3, followed by biopsy only in men with PCA3 score greater than or equal to 35, 36% of biopsies would be avoided, and 5% of Gleason score greater than or equal to 3 + 4 cancers would have been missed. When obtaining a PCA3 first, 51% of biopsies would be avoided; however, 33% of Gleason score greater than or equal to 3 + 4 cancers would have been missed. Similar results were found using PCA3 in the rebiopsy setting, in which the diagnostic uncertainty in the PI-RADS intermediate group can potentially be ameliorated by the addition of PCA3 to avoid potential unnecessary biopsies.[73,74] Additional studies suggest that management of early-stage PCa may also benefit by performing MRI-targeted biopsy coupled with molecular analysis.[75] The emergence of PET/MRI may ultimately allow both staging and guidance for prostate biopsy in a single imaging session.[76]

SUMMARY

Prostate MRI is now commonly used in the detection of PCa with the goals of reducing the detection of clinically insignificant disease; maximizing the detection of clinically significant cancer; along with better assessment of disease size, grade, and location. MRI may add usefulness as both a prebiopsy risk assessment tool that may influence the decision whether to perform biopsy as well as a minimally invasive method for determining both treatment outcomes and progression on AS. Furthermore, prebiopsy risk stratification among men presenting with increased serum PSA levels may allow an opportunity to reduce PCa overdiagnosis through selective avoidance of biopsy in some men, and avoidance of systematic sampling in men undergoing biopsy. The clinical utility of MRI seems to apply to men with no prior biopsy, who have had a previous negative biopsy, and men who are candidate for AS. MRI, in conjunction with traditional clinical parameters and secondary biomarkers, may allow more accurate risk stratification and assessment of need for prostate biopsy.

REFERENCES

1. Bjurlin MA, Meng X, Le Nobin J, et al. Optimization of prostate biopsy: the role of magnetic resonance imaging targeted biopsy in detection, localization and risk assessment. J Urol 2014;192:648–58.

2. Siddiqui MM, Rais-Bahrami S, Turkbey B, et al. Comparison of MR/ultrasound fusion-guided biopsy with ultrasound-guided biopsy for the diagnosis of prostate cancer. JAMA 2015;313:390–7.

3. Meng X, Rosenkrantz AB, Mendhiratta N, et al. Relationship between prebiopsy multiparametric magnetic resonance imaging (MRI), biopsy indication, and MRI-ultrasound fusion-targeted prostate biopsy outcomes. Eur Urol 2016;69:512–7.

4. Porpiglia F, Manfredi M, Mele F, et al. Diagnostic pathway with multiparametric magnetic resonance imaging versus standard pathway: results from a randomized prospective study in biopsy-naive patients with suspected prostate cancer. Eur Urol 2016;72(2):282–8.

5. Loeb S, Carter HB, Berndt SI, et al. Complications after prostate biopsy: data from SEER-Medicare. J Urol 2011;186:1830–4.

6. Ahmed HU, El-Shater Bosaily A, Brown LC, et al. Diagnostic accuracy of multi-parametric MRI and TRUS biopsy in prostate cancer (PROMIS): a paired validating confirmatory study. Lancet 2017;389: 815–22.

7. Abraham NE, Mendhiratta N, Taneja SS. Patterns of repeat prostate biopsy in contemporary clinical practice. J Urol 2015;193:1178–84.

8. Loeb S, Carter HB, Berndt SI, et al. Is repeat prostate biopsy associated with a greater risk of hospitalization? Data from SEER-Medicare. J Urol 2013;189: 867–70.

9. Watanabe Y, Nagayama M, Araki T, et al. Targeted biopsy based on ADC map in the detection and localization of prostate cancer: a feasibility study. J Magn Reson Imaging 2013;37:1168–77.

10. Watanabe Y, Terai A, Araki T, et al. Detection and localization of prostate cancer with the targeted biopsy strategy based on ADC map: a prospective large-scale cohort study. J Magn Reson Imaging 2012;35:1414–21.

11. Shah V, Turkbey B, Mani H, et al. Decision support system for localizing prostate cancer based on multiparametric magnetic resonance imaging. Med Phys 2012;39:4093–103.

12. Rosenkrantz AB, Mannelli L, Kong X, et al. Prostate cancer: utility of fusion of T2-weighted and high b-value diffusion-weighted images for peripheral zone tumor detection and localization. J Magn Reson Imaging 2011;34:95–100.

13. Villers A, Puech P, Mouton D, et al. Dynamic contrast enhanced, pelvic phased array magnetic resonance imaging of localized prostate cancer for predicting tumor volume: correlation with radical prostatectomy findings. J Urol 2006;176:2432–7.

14. Liddell H, Jyoti R, Haxhimolla HZ. mp-MRI prostate characterised PIRADS 3 lesions are associated with a low risk of clinically significant prostate cancer - a retrospective review of 92 biopsied PIRADS 3 lesions. Curr Urol 2015;8:96–100.

15. Kuru TH, Roethke MC, Rieker P, et al. Histology core-specific evaluation of the European Society of Urogenital Radiology (ESUR) standardised scoring system of multiparametric magnetic resonance imaging (mpMRI) of the prostate. BJU Int 2013;112: 1080–7.

16. NiMhurchu E, O'Kelly F, Murphy IG, et al. Predictive value of PI-RADS classification in MRI-directed transrectal ultrasound guided prostate biopsy. Clin Radiol 2016;71:375–80.

17. de Rooij M, Hamoen EH, Futterer JJ, et al. Accuracy of multiparametric MRI for prostate cancer detection: a meta-analysis. AJR Am J Roentgenol 2014; 202:343–51.

18. Martorana E, Pirola GM, Scialpi M, et al. Lesion volume predicts prostate cancer risk and aggressiveness: validation of its value alone and matched with prostate imaging reporting and data system score. BJU Int 2016;120(1):92–103.

19. Turkbey B, Choyke PL. Multiparametric MRI and prostate cancer diagnosis and risk stratification. Curr Opin Urol 2012;22:310–5.

20. Delongchamps NB, Rouanne M, Flam T, et al. Multiparametric magnetic resonance imaging for the detection and localization of prostate cancer: combination of T2-weighted, dynamic contrast-enhanced and diffusion-weighted imaging. BJU Int 2011;107: 1411–8.

21. Vargas HA, Akin O, Franiel T, et al. Diffusion-weighted endorectal MR imaging at 3 T for prostate cancer: tumor detection and assessment of aggressiveness. Radiology 2011;259:775–84.

22. Rosenkrantz AB, Meng X, Ream JM, et al. Likert score 3 prostate lesions: association between whole-lesion ADC metrics and pathologic findings at MRI/ultrasound fusion targeted biopsy. J Magn Reson Imaging 2016;43:325–32.

23. De Cobelli F, Ravelli S, Esposito A, et al. Apparent diffusion coefficient value and ratio as noninvasive potential biomarkers to predict prostate cancer grading: comparison with prostate biopsy and radical prostatectomy specimen. AJR Am J Roentgenol 2015;204:550–7.

24. Vos EK, Litjens GJ, Kobus T, et al. Assessment of prostate cancer aggressiveness using dynamic contrast-enhanced magnetic resonance imaging at 3 T. Eur Urol 2013;64:448–55.

25. Chung MP, Margolis D, Mesko S, et al. Correlation of quantitative diffusion-weighted and dynamic contrast-enhanced MRI parameters with prognostic factors in prostate cancer. J Med Imaging Radiat Oncol 2014;58:588–94.

26. Giles SL, Morgan VA, Riches SF, et al. Apparent diffusion coefficient as a predictive biomarker of prostate cancer progression: value of fast and slow diffusion components. AJR Am J Roentgenol 2011;196:586–91.

27. Tamada T, Dani H, Taneja SS, et al. The role of whole-lesion apparent diffusion coefficient analysis for predicting outcomes of prostate cancer patients on active surveillance. Abdom Radiol (NY) 2017. [Epub ahead of print].

28. Henderson DR, de Souza NM, Thomas K, et al. Nine-year follow-up for a study of diffusion-weighted magnetic resonance imaging in a prospective prostate cancer active surveillance cohort. Eur Urol 2016;69:1028–33.

29. van As NJ, de Souza NM, Riches SF, et al. A study of diffusion-weighted magnetic resonance imaging in men with untreated localised prostate cancer on active surveillance. Eur Urol 2009;56:981–7.

30. Park JJ, Kim CK, Park SY, et al. Prostate cancer: role of pretreatment multiparametric 3-T MRI in predicting biochemical recurrence after radical prostatectomy. AJR Am J Roentgenol 2014;202:W459–65.

31. Ho R, Siddiqui MM, George AK, et al. Preoperative multiparametric magnetic resonance imaging predicts biochemical recurrence in prostate cancer after radical prostatectomy. PLoS One 2016;11: e0157313.

32. Westphalen AC, Koff WJ, Coakley FV, et al. Prostate cancer: prediction of biochemical failure after external-beam radiation therapy–Kattan nomogram and endorectal MR imaging estimation of tumor volume. Radiology 2011;261:477–86.

33. Park SY, Kim CK, Park BK, et al. Prediction of biochemical recurrence following radical prostatectomy in men with prostate cancer by diffusion-weighted magnetic resonance imaging: initial results. Eur Radiol 2011;21:1111–8.

34. Yoon MY, Park J, Cho JY, et al. Predicting biochemical recurrence in patients with high-risk prostate cancer using the apparent diffusion coefficient of magnetic resonance imaging. Investig Clin Urol 2017;58:12–9.

35. Rosenkrantz AB, Ream JM, Nolan P, et al. Prostate cancer: utility of whole-lesion apparent diffusion coefficient metrics for prediction of biochemical recurrence after radical prostatectomy. AJR Am J Roentgenol 2015;205:1208–14.

36. Park SY, Oh YT, Jung DC, et al. Prediction of biochemical recurrence after radical prostatectomy with PI-RADS version 2 in prostate cancers: initial results. Eur Radiol 2016;26:2502–9.

37. Riaz N, Afaq A, Akin O, et al. Pretreatment endorectal coil magnetic resonance imaging findings predict biochemical tumor control in prostate cancer patients treated with combination brachytherapy and external-beam radiotherapy. Int J Radiat Oncol Biol Phys 2012;84:707–11.

38. Fuchsjager MH, Pucar D, Zelefsky MJ, et al. Predicting post-external beam radiation therapy PSA relapse of prostate cancer using pretreatment MRI. Int J Radiat Oncol Biol Phys 2010;78:743–50.

39. Yamaguchi H, Hori M, Suzuki O, et al. Clinical significance of the apparent diffusion coefficient ratio in prostate cancer treatment with intensity-modulated radiotherapy. Anticancer Res 2016;36: 6551–6.

40. Lee H, Kim CK, Park BK, et al. Accuracy of preoperative multiparametric magnetic resonance imaging for prediction of unfavorable pathology in patients with localized prostate cancer undergoing radical prostatectomy. World J Urol 2016;35:929–34.

41. Borofsky MS, Rosenkrantz AB, Abraham N, et al. Does suspicion of prostate cancer on integrated T2 and diffusion-weighted MRI predict more adverse pathology on radical prostatectomy? Urology 2013;81:1279–83.

42. Abdi H, Zargar H, Goldenberg SL, et al. Multiparametric magnetic resonance imaging-targeted biopsy for the detection of prostate cancer in patients with prior negative biopsy results. Urol Oncol 2015;33: 165.e1-7.

43. Brock M, Loppenberg B, Roghmann F, et al. Impact of real-time elastography on magnetic resonance imaging/ultrasound fusion guided biopsy in patients with prior negative prostate biopsies. J Urol 2015; 193:1191–7.

44. Mariotti GC, Costa DN, Pedrosa I, et al. Magnetic resonance/transrectal ultrasound fusion biopsy of the prostate compared to systematic 12-core biopsy for the diagnosis and characterization of prostate cancer: multi-institutional retrospective analysis of 389 patients. Urol Oncol 2016;34:416.e9-14.

45. Maxeiner A, Stephan C, Durmus T, et al. Added value of multiparametric ultrasonography in magnetic resonance imaging and ultrasonography fusion-guided biopsy of the prostate in patients with suspicion for prostate cancer. Urology 2015; 86:108–14.

46. Mendhiratta N, Meng X, Rosenkrantz AB, et al. Pre-biopsy MRI and MRI-ultrasound fusion-targeted prostate biopsy in men with previous negative biopsies: impact on repeat biopsy strategies. Urology 2015;86:1192–8.

47. Salami SS, Ben-Levi E, Yaskiv O, et al. In patients with a previous negative prostate biopsy and a suspicious lesion on magnetic resonance imaging, is a 12-core biopsy still necessary in addition to a targeted biopsy? BJU Int 2015;115:562–70.

48. Sonn GA, Chang E, Natarajan S, et al. Value of targeted prostate biopsy using magnetic resonance-ultrasound fusion in men with prior negative biopsy and elevated prostate-specific antigen. Eur Urol 2014;65:809–15.

49. Truong M WE, Holleberg G, Borch M, et al. Institutional learning curve associated with implementation of a MR/US fusion biopsy program using PI-RADS Version 2: factors that influence success. Urology Practice 2016. http://dx.doi.org/10.1016/j.urpr.2016.1011.1007.

50. Volkin D, Turkbey B, Hoang AN, et al. Multiparametric magnetic resonance imaging (MRI) and subsequent MRI/ultrasonography fusion-guided biopsy increase the detection of anteriorly located prostate cancers. BJU Int 2014;114:E43–9.

51. Baco E, Rud E, Eri LM, et al. A randomized controlled trial to assess and compare the outcomes of two-core prostate biopsy guided by fused magnetic resonance and transrectal ultrasound images and traditional 12-core systematic biopsy. Eur Urol 2016;69:149–56.

52. Mendhiratta N, Rosenkrantz AB, Meng X, et al. MRI-ultrasound fusion-targeted prostate biopsy in a consecutive cohort of men with no previous biopsy: reduction of over-detection through improved risk stratification. J Urol 2015;194(6):1601–6.

53. Mozer P, Rouprêt M, Le Cossec C, et al. First round of targeted biopsies using magnetic resonance imaging/ultrasonography fusion compared with conventional transrectal ultrasonography-guided biopsies for the diagnosis of localised prostate cancer. BJU Int 2015;115:50–7.

54. Pokorny MR, de Rooij M, Duncan E, et al. Prospective study of diagnostic accuracy comparing prostate cancer detection by transrectal ultrasound-guided biopsy versus magnetic resonance (MR) imaging with subsequent MR-guided biopsy in men without previous prostate biopsies. Eur Urol 2014;66:22–9.

55. Wysock JS, Rosenkrantz AB, Huang WC, et al. A prospective, blinded comparison of magnetic resonance (MR) imaging-ultrasound fusion and visual estimation in the performance of MR-targeted prostate biopsy: the PROFUS trial. Eur Urol 2014;66:343–51.

56. Filson CP, Natarajan S, Margolis DJ, et al. Prostate cancer detection with magnetic resonance-ultrasound fusion biopsy: The role of systematic and targeted biopsies. Cancer 2016;122:884–92.

57. Jiang X, Zhang J, Tang J, et al. Magnetic resonance imaging - ultrasound fusion targeted biopsy outperforms standard approaches in detecting prostate cancer: a meta-analysis. Mol Clin Oncol 2016;5:301–9.

58. Tan N, Lin WC, Khoshnoodi P, et al. In-bore 3-T MR-guided transrectal targeted prostate biopsy: Prostate Imaging Reporting and Data System Version 2-based diagnostic performance for detection of prostate cancer. Radiology 2017;283:130–9.

59. Pinto PA, Chung PH, Rastinehad AR, et al. Magnetic resonance imaging/ultrasound fusion guided prostate biopsy improves cancer detection following transrectal ultrasound biopsy and correlates with multiparametric magnetic resonance imaging. J Urol 2011;186:1281–5.

60. Mehralivand S, Bednarova S, Shih JH, et al. Prospective evaluation of Prostate Imaging-Reporting and Data System Version 2 using the International Society of Urological Pathology Prostate Cancer Grade Group system. J Urol 2017. [Epub ahead of print].

61. Venderink W, van Luijtelaar A, Bomers JG, et al. Results of targeted biopsy in men with magnetic resonance imaging lesions classified equivocal, likely or highly likely to be clinically significant prostate cancer. Eur Urol 2017. [Epub ahead of print].

62. Ukimura O, Marien A, Palmer S, et al. Trans-rectal ultrasound visibility of prostate lesions identified by magnetic resonance imaging increases accuracy of image-fusion targeted biopsies. World J Urol 2015;33:1669–76.

63. Mertan FV, Greer MD, Shih JH, et al. Prospective evaluation of the prostate imaging reporting and data system version 2 for prostate cancer detection. J Urol 2016;196:690–6.

64. Osses DF, van Asten JJ, Kieft GJ, et al. Prostate cancer detection rates of magnetic resonance imaging-guided prostate biopsy related to Prostate Imaging Reporting and Data System score. World J Urol 2017;35:207–12.

65. Hoeks CM, Somford DM, van Oort IM, et al. Value of 3-T multiparametric magnetic resonance imaging and magnetic resonance-guided biopsy for early risk restratification in active surveillance of low-risk prostate cancer: a prospective multicenter cohort study. Invest Radiol 2014;49:165–72.

66. Vargas HA, Akin O, Afaq A, et al. Magnetic resonance imaging for predicting prostate biopsy findings in patients considered for active surveillance of clinically low risk prostate cancer. J Urol 2012;188:1732–8.

67. Tay KJ, Gupta RT, Holtz J, et al. Does mpMRI improve clinical criteria in selecting men with prostate cancer for active surveillance? Prostate Cancer Prostatic Dis 2017. [Epub ahead of print].

68. Lai WS, Gordetsky JB, Thomas JV, et al. Factors predicting prostate cancer upgrading on magnetic resonance imaging-targeted biopsy in an active surveillance population. Cancer 2017;123:1941–8.

69. Tran GN, Leapman MS, Nguyen HG, et al. Magnetic resonance imaging-ultrasound fusion biopsy during prostate cancer active surveillance. Eur Urol 2016;72(2):275–81.

70. Wysock JS, Mendhiratta N, Zattoni F, et al. Predictive value of negative 3T multiparametric magnetic resonance imaging of the prostate on 12-core biopsy results. BJU Int 2016;118:515–20.

71. Lu AJ, Syed JS, Nguyen KA, et al. Negative multiparametric magnetic resonance imaging of the prostate predicts absence of clinically significant prostate cancer on 12-core template prostate biopsy. Urology 2017;105:118–22.

72. Fenstermaker M, Mendhiratta N, Bjurlin MA, et al. Risk stratification by urinary prostate cancer gene 3 testing before magnetic resonance imaging-ultrasound fusion-targeted prostate biopsy among men with no history of biopsy. Urology 2017;99: 174–9.

73. Kaufmann S, Bedke J, Gatidis S, et al. Prostate cancer gene 3 (PCA3) is of additional predictive value in patients with PI-RADS grade III (intermediate) lesions in the MR-guided re-biopsy setting for prostate cancer. World J Urol 2016;34:509–15.

74. De Luca S, Passera R, Cattaneo G, et al. High prostate cancer gene 3 (PCA3) scores are associated with elevated Prostate Imaging Reporting and Data System (PI-RADS) grade and biopsy Gleason score, at magnetic resonance imaging/ultrasonography fusion software-based targeted prostate biopsy after a previous negative standard biopsy. BJU Int 2016;118:723–30.

75. Renard-Penna R, Cancel-Tassin G, Comperat E, et al. Multiparametric magnetic resonance imaging predicts postoperative pathology but misses aggressive prostate cancers as assessed by cell cycle progression score. J Urol 2015;194:1617–23.

76. Lindenberg L, Ahlman M, Turkbey B, et al. Evaluation of prostate cancer with PET/MRI. J Nucl Med 2016;57:111S–6S.

Whom to Treat
Postdiagnostic Risk Assessment with Gleason Score, Risk Models, and Genomic Classifier

Annika Herlemann, MD[a,b], Samuel L. Washington III, MD[a],
Renu S. Eapen, MD[a], Matthew R. Cooperberg, MD, MPH[a,c],*

KEYWORDS

- Prostate cancer • Risk assessment • Treatment • Gleason score • Risk models • Nomograms
- Genomic assays

KEY POINTS

- Accurate risk stratification at time of diagnosis is crucial to providing the best treatment recommendation for each patient diagnosed with prostate cancer.
- Traditional risk grouping by the D'Amico classification or its extensions (eg, NCCN or American Urological Association risk groups) is still widely used; however, this approach has multiple, major limitations and is not adequate for contemporary practice.
- Multivariable nomograms and risk scores using clinical characteristics at time of diagnosis have been developed to predict outcomes and to stratify patients more accurately.
- Genomic assays, novel imaging, and other biomarkers may complement current risk assessment tools in men with newly diagnosed prostate cancer, but must be shown to improve on a multivariable clinical risk assessment.

INTRODUCTION

With the implementation of prostate-specific antigen (PSA) screening in current clinical practice, the incidence of prostate cancer (PCa) increased substantially.[1,2] However, the lack of specificity of PSA for PCa may lead to unnecessary biopsies and overdiagnosis of indolent disease. Once diagnosed, management of patients with PCa must be individualized based on the variable and usually prolonged natural history of this disease. Accurate risk stratification at the time of diagnosis is therefore the cornerstone for clinical decision-making and optimal management for each patient.

Clinicians use various clinical parameters, such as PSA level, biopsy Gleason grade, and clinical T stage, to estimate PCa aggressiveness. In more recent years, prognostic scores and nomograms based on these variables have been validated to risk-stratify patients with good accuracy. With the advent of genomic analysis, genome data may now be incorporated into these prediction tools to improve accuracy. In this review

Disclosure Statement: Dr M.R. Cooperberg is consultant at Myriad and MDx Health; receives departmental research support from Genomic Health and GenomeDx.

[a] Department of Urology, University of California, San Francisco, Helen Diller Family Comprehensive Cancer Center, Box 0981, San Francisco, CA 94143-0981, USA; [b] Department of Urology, Ludwig-Maximilians-University of Munich, Marchioninistrasse 15, 81377 Munich, Germany; [c] Department of Epidemiology and Biostatistics, University of California, San Francisco, Helen Diller Family Comprehensive Cancer Center, 550 16th Street, San Francisco, CA 94143, USA
* Corresponding author. Department of Epidemiology and Biostatistics, University of California, San Francisco, 550 16th Street, Box 1695, San Francisco, CA 94143.
E-mail address: mcooperberg@urology.ucsf.edu

Urol Clin N Am 44 (2017) 547–555
http://dx.doi.org/10.1016/j.ucl.2017.07.003
0094-0143/17/

of the literature, we discuss established and novel concepts in risk stratification for men with confirmed PCa. The aim is to evaluate how these tools may guide treatment decisions and enable more accurate postdiagnosis risk stratification in men with PCa.

HISTOPATHOLOGIC GRADING OF PROSTATE CANCER
Gleason Grading

Since the introduction of the Gleason grading system 50 years ago, the two most prevalent patterns of glandular architecture, each scored from 1 to 5 during histologic review, are reported as the Gleason score (GS).[3,4] The GS at biopsy consists of the Gleason grade of the most extensive pattern plus the highest pattern, regardless of its extent.[5] At the consensus conference in 2005, the International Society of Urological Pathology (ISUP) updated the Gleason grading system. The ISUP changes were mainly aimed at limiting the scope of glandular architecture pattern 3 while widening the scope of pattern 4.[4,6,7] As a result, some cancers previously considered Gleason pattern 3 were subsequently reclassified as Gleason pattern 4. All cribriform cancers are also now considered pattern 4.[3,6] In radical prostatectomy specimens, a Gleason pattern comprising less than or equal to 5% of PCa volume is not incorporated in the GS but reported separately if tertiary grade 4 or 5 is noted.[5] Billis and colleagues[8] showed that the revised Gleason system better predicts biochemical-free progression after radical prostatectomy compared with the current system.

Recently, there has been increasing interest in histologic subtypes of Gleason pattern 4. Among the subtypes, a finding of cribriform architecture has been a new focus of interest. The finding of PCa glands with cribriform architecture has been associated with more aggressive disease, compared with poorly formed or fused glands. Recent literature has also shown it to be associated with extraprostatic extension, positive surgical margins, distant metastases, and cancer-specific mortality.[9–12]

Limitations of Gleason grading may include intraobserver and interobserver variability. In the study of McKenney and coworkers,[13] interobserver reproducibility among genitourinary subspecialist pathologists for classic Gleason patterns was substantial (κ 0.76). However, interobserver reproducibility for histopathologic distinction of tangentially sectioned Gleason pattern 3 from Gleason pattern 4 was only fair (κ 0.27).[13] Mean intraobserver reproducibility was 81.5% (range, 65%–100%).[13]

Grade Group System

To better predict clinical outcomes, Pierorazio and colleagues[14] recommended collapsing Gleason grades into prognostic grade groups (GG) that more accurately reflect prognosis while offering a simplified, intuitive classification system for physicians and patients. The authors proposed a modified PCa grading system using GG based on the likelihood of biochemical recurrence (BCR)[14]: GS less than or equal to 6 (GG 1), GS 3 + 4 = 7 (GG 2), GS 4 + 3 = 7 (GG 3), GS 4 + 4 = 8 (GG 4), and GS 9 to 10 (GG 5). The GG system was presented and accepted for use at the 2014 grading consensus of ISUP, initially to be used in conjunction with the Gleason system.[7,15]

This new GG system was validated in 2016 by Epstein and colleagues[16] with a multi-institutional study of BCR in more than 20,000 men treated by radical prostatectomy and more than 5000 men who underwent radiotherapy. In the surgical cohort, Gleason 3 + 4 versus 4 + 3 and Gleason 8 versus 9 differed significantly in rates of BCR. Relative to GS 6, each increasing score was associated with higher risk of BCR (hazard ratio [HR], 1.9 [95% confidence interval (CI), 1.7–2.2] for Gleason 3 + 4; HR, 5.1 [95% CI, 4.4–6.0] for Gleason 4 + 3; HR, 8.0 [95% CI, 6.7–9.5] for Gleason 8; and HR, 11.7 [95% CI, 9.9–13.8] for Gleason 9 to 10).[16] These differences were also observed in the radiotherapy arm.[16] In a national population-based cohort, the new five-tier GG system demonstrated a predictive accuracy similar to that of the current three- and four-tier classifications.[17] The new GG system did not improve prediction of clinical recurrence in radical prostatectomy patients.[18] However, other studies have demonstrated that the GGs correlated well with metastasis and PCa-specific death.[19,20]

To be clear, the new GGs represent a renaming of the primary + secondary grading convention, not a new grading system. The advantages include clear distinction between GS 3 + 4 (GG 2) and GS 4 + 3 (GG 3), and better clinical interpretation for patients (ie, the lowest GG is 1 rather than the lowest GS being 3 + 3 = 6). The new groups, however, have not been shown to be more accurate than the old naming convention, and still do not constitute a linear scale, requiring modeling as an ordinal variable in prediction studies.

Quantitative Gleason Score

Gleason 3 + 4 implies a relative proportion of high-grade disease ranging from 5% to 49%, and risk heterogeneity certainly exists along this continuum. Multiple groups have therefore extensions to the GS that quantify the extent of higher grades. The quantitative GS, for example, is based on the weighted average of Gleason patterns present in the pathology specimen.[21–23] Compared with traditional Gleason scoring, the quantitative GS resulted in improvement in the concordance between biopsy and pathologic GS (area under the receiver operating characteristic curve, 0.79 vs 0.71) and the prediction of BCR after radical prostatectomy.[21] Deng and colleagues[22] confirmed that quantitative measures of Gleason pattern 4 predict BCR better than the traditional GS. Sauter and colleagues[23] defined an integrated quantitative GS, which combines quantitative Gleason grading and tertiary Gleason grades in one highly prognostic numerical score.

RISK MODELS

Risk stratification models are increasingly used to guide management in men with newly diagnosed PCa. Clinicopathologic characteristics, such as PSA, tumor grading, and extent of biopsy involvement, independently predict oncologic outcomes. The incorporation of these parameters into multivariable models offers an improved accuracy of risk assessment for clinical progression, compared with traditional risk grouping systems. Many of these models have been presented as risk classifications or nomograms to predict oncologic outcomes.

Risk Groups

Based on the predictive value of initial PSA, biopsy GS, and clinical T stage, multiple postdiagnostic PCa risk classifications have been proposed. In 1998, D'Amico and colleagues[24,25] first proposed a three-group risk stratification system to predict biochemical failure after external-beam radiation therapy or radical prostatectomy. Patients with PCa are classified as low, intermediate, and high risk. Low-risk PCa was defined as PSA less than 10 ng/mL, GS less than or equal to 6, and cT1/T2a. Intermediate-risk PCa included a PSA 10 to 20 ng/mL, and/or GS 7, and/or cT2b disease. High-risk PCa was defined as PSA greater than 20 ng/mL, and/or GS greater than or equal to 8, and/or greater than or equal to cT2c disease.[25,26]

The D'Amico classification remains commonly used given its simplicity. However, it is marked by several notable limitations, and in 2017 can no longer be considered state of the art. First, it does not distinguish Gleason 3 + 4 (GG 2) from Gleason 4 + 3 (GG 3), cancer grades with notably divergent aggressiveness. Second,

it overemphasizes the importance of T stage, which tends to be inaccurately reported[27] and falls out of multivariable models including better estimates of tumor volume, such as extent of biopsy core involvement.[28] Most importantly, it is not a multivariable tool and does not account for multiple adverse parameters. For example, a man with a cT1c, PSA 4.2, Gleason 3 + 4 tumor in 1 of 12 cores is placed in the same "intermediate" group as one with a cT2b, PSA 18, Gleason 4 + 3 tumor in 8 of 12 cores, but these men clearly have different tumor biology and risk of progression.

The D'Amico classification has been adapted and extended by the National Comprehensive Cancer Network (NCCN), American Urological Association, European Association of Urology, and the National Institute for Health and Clinical Excellence (**Table 1**).[5,29–31] These extensions provide some additional granularity, but the definition of "very low-risk" disease, for example, is a somewhat arbitrary implementation of the Epstein criteria for indolent tumors, which are highly restrictive and difficult to implement in practice given the large number of parameters. The new American Urological Association guideline implements the same "very low-risk" definition, and subdivides the intermediate group into "favorable" and "unfavorable" subgroups. However, the new groups still do not constitute a multivariable model, and have not been prospectively validated in any study. Different variables (six per stratum) drive each of these new risk groups, they do not perform as a linear scale, and they are increasingly difficult to learn or to implement in research or clinical practice.

Nomograms

Risk prediction tools developed using a multivariable regression models offers much better precision and accuracy than risk groups, and furthermore are analyzed as linear, continuous variables. Nomograms (diagrams that allow determination of a risk score based on clinical values) are one way to express the results of these models ("nomogram" does not mean the risk model itself). Nomograms are evaluated for discriminatory accuracy, usually reflected in the concordance (c) index (ie, how often does the model correctly sort pairs of patients in terms of risk); and for calibration (eg, if a group of men is predicted by the nomogram to have an 85% risk of recurrence, how many in that group actually recurred).

Many such nomograms have been developed for PCa. Kattan and colleagues[32] were the first

Table 1
Risk group criteria for men

Risk Group	D'Amico	NCCN	EAU	AUA
Very low		PSA <10, PSAD <0.15, cT1c, GG1 ≤3 cores positive, ≤50% of any core positive		PSA <10, PSAD <0.15, cT1c, GG1, ≤3 cores positive, ≤50% of any core positive
Low	PSA <10, cT1/2a, GG1	PSA <10, cT1/2a, GG1	PSA <10, cT1/2a, GG1	PSA <10, cT1/2a, GG1
Favorable intermediate Unfavorable intermediate	PSA 10–20, cT2b, GG2-3	PSA 10–20, cT2b-c, GG2-3	PSA 10–20, cT2b, GG2-3	PSA 10 to <20 + GG1 or PSA <10 + GG2 GG2 + PSA 10 to <20/cT2b-c or PSA <20 + GG3
High	PSA >20, cT2c, GG 4–5	PSA >20, cT3a, GG 4–5	PSA >20, cT2c, GG 4–5 or any PSA, any GG, cT3-4, cN+	PSA >20, ≥cT3, GG 4–5
Very high		cT3b-4, ≥4 cores with GG 4–5 or primary Gleason pattern 5		

Abbreviations: AUA, American Urological Association; EAU, European Association of Urology; PSAD, PSA density.

group to report an approach that incorporates multiple risk variables in mathematical models to predict the likelihood of PCa recurrence or progression. After this initial discovery, many other important predictive models soon followed. The Kattan preoperative nomogram relates preoperative clinical characteristics with the 5-year probability of treatment failure among men with clinically localized PCa treated with radical prostatectomy[25,32] and has been externally validated.[33] Stephenson and colleagues[25,34] assessed PCa-specific mortality following radical prostatectomy in the PSA era. In addition, they developed and validated a preoperative nomogram to predict 15-year PCa-specific mortality using preoperative PSA, clinical stage, and GS in cohort of greater than 12,000 radical prostatectomy patients. The externally validated c index was 0.82.[34] A large variety of PCa nomograms have been introduced by other study groups.[35–41]

Despite their improved accuracy over risk groups, nomograms generally have not transformed clinical practice or PCa research. They tend to be cumbersome to use in practice, requiring either paper graphs or computer software, and because the regression equations underlying nomograms are rarely published, they are hard to validate or implement among large groups of patients. In fact, most nomograms are never validated, and the profusion of options among published nomograms in some cases creates more confusion than clarity.

University of California, San Francisco Cancer of the Prostate Risk Assessment Score

To combine the accuracy of a multivariable tool with the ease of calculation of risk groups, the University of California, San Francisco Cancer of the Prostate Risk Assessment (CAPRA) score was developed and initially published in 2005. It was originally based on a cohort of 1439 men diagnosed with PCa between 1992 and 2001, who had undergone radical prostatectomy and were followed in the Cancer of the Prostate Strategic Urologic Research Endeavor database.[42] The model includes patient age, PSA level, GS, percentage of biopsy core samples positive for cancer, and clinical stage.[42] It results in an easily calculable 0 to 10 point score (**Table 2**), which predicts relative rather than absolute risk for multiple oncologic outcomes including surgical pathology, BCR, metastasis, cancer-specific, and overall survival.[43] Every two-point increase in score represents an approximate doubling of risk. The CAPRA score is categorized into three risk strata: a score of 0 to 2 indicates low risk, 3 to 5 intermediate risk, and 6 to 10 high risk.[42] Following its initial publication, multiple external independent validations of the CAPRA score have been performed for various patient cohorts in academic and community-based settings on four continents.[43–45] The CAPRA score has also been successfully validated to predict PCa-specific mortality and other end points following other treatment modalities, such as radiation

Table 2
UCSF-CAPRA score (0–10 points)

Variable	Level	Points
PSA	2.1–6	0
	6.1–10	1
	10.1–20	2
	20.1–30	3
	>30	4
Gleason grade group	1	0
	2	1
	3–5	3
T stage	T1/T2	0
	T3a	1
% positive biopsy	<34	0
	≥34	1
Age	<50	0
	≥50	1

therapy, and androgen-deprivation therapy.[43–48] Validation studies showed superiority of the CAPRA score compared with D'Amico classification and equivalence to nomograms in terms of discrimination. With regard to calibration, most but not all studies demonstrated better calibration for the CAPRA score than for tested nomograms.[39,44,49,50]

GENOMIC ASSAYS

Both localized and advanced PCa are clinically heterogeneous diseases with varying oncologic outcomes, even among patients within the same risk group. Genomic sequencing has demonstrated the complexity of this tumor entity and its pathways.[51] In recent years, tissue-based genomic panels and biomarkers have been developed with the purpose of risk stratifying patients with PCa. There is a growing recognition that molecular biomarkers can complement conventional clinical and pathologic parameters to better personalize the care of patients with cancer and enable early, more accurate detection of lethal disease. An essential aspect of biomarker validation is to verify that the candidate marker can add independent prognostic information above and beyond a gold standard multivariable model. Simply substratifying the NCCN low-risk group, for example, is insufficient, because this can already be done with no additional effort or expense using one of the multivariable tools described previously. Although genomic assays show promising results, further studies are needed to quantify the actual benefit of these new technologies, and how they should be optimally implemented in routine practice.

Prolaris

Prolaris (Myriad Genetics, Salt Lake City, UT) is a prognostic gene assay, based on a panel of 46 genes. It quantifies the RNA expression of 31 cell-cycle progression (CCP) genes, normalized to 15 housekeeping genes.[52] One application of this test is to help better determine if immediate, definitive treatment (eg, radical prostatectomy, radiotherapy) or deferred treatment (active surveillance) may be beneficial for a man with low-risk PCa. Prolaris has shown advanced prognostic ability over baseline clinicopathologic characteristics, and is validated to evaluate outcomes for men who underwent a prostate biopsy.[53,54]

Cuzick and colleagues[55] evaluated the impact of CCP score on PCa-free survival in 349 biopsy samples of conservatively managed patients with PCa. In this study, CCP scores have demonstrated a strong correlation on univariate analysis with disease-specific death (HR, 2.02; 95% CI, 1.62–2.53). On multivariate analysis, the CCP score showed an HR of 1.65 (95% CI, 1.31–2.09), with GS and PSA being other significant additional factors. These findings were validated by the same group using a cohort of 585 men who underwent needle biopsy with disease-specific death as the outcome of interest. Similar HRs were found for each point increase in the CCP score and showed significance on multivariate analysis (HR, 1.76; 95% CI, 1.44–2.14).[53] Bishoff and colleagues[56] analyzed 582 patients who underwent prostate biopsy and had CCP scoring on biopsy samples before progressing to radical prostatectomy. In their analysis, higher CCP scores were associated with increased risk for BCR and metastatic disease after surgery. The association remained significant after adjusting for other clinical parameters. Oderda and colleagues[57] retrospectively evaluated the CCP score at biopsy in 52 patients with newly diagnosed PCa who underwent radical prostatectomy. The overall accuracy in assessing the correct risk class was good; however, seven high-risk and 13 intermediate-risk patients were misclassified by Prolaris test. The mean CCP score significantly differed across different risk classes based on histopathologic findings (−1.2 in low risk, −0.444 in intermediate risk, 0.208 in high risk). The CCP score was a significant predictor of high-risk PCa, after adjusting for clinical variables. Additionally, on univariate analysis CCP score was a significant predictor of BCR. Furthermore, CCP score improved the accuracy of European Association of Urology clinical risk score by approximately 10%, and that of CAPRA risk score by 7%.

Oncotype DX Genomic Prostate Score

Oncotype DX Genomic Prostate Score (GPS; Genomic Health Inc, Redwood City, CA) also generates RNA expression data from fixed paraffin-embedded prostate biopsy tissue. Seventeen genes are combined to calculate the GPS, ranging from 0 to 100.[58] Higher scores correlate with a higher probability of harboring adverse pathology (high grade and/or nonorgan-confined disease) at radical prostatectomy.[58,59] This assay is intended to aid in counseling men on the optimal management (active surveillance vs immediate treatment) in newly diagnosed early stage PCa.[58,59]

In their validation study, Klein and colleagues[60] evaluated 395 men with low- to intermediate-risk PCa who underwent radical prostatectomy. In multivariable analyses adjusting for significant clinical covariates, the GPS was a consistent predictor of high-grade and/or pT3 disease. The odds ratio for each 20-point increase in GPS was 2.1 (95% CI, 1.4–3.2) after adjusting for CAPRA score, and 1.9 (95% CI, 1.2–2.8) after adjusting for age, PSA, clinical stage, and biopsy GS.[60] In another study among 402 cases, Cullen and colleagues[61] found independent association of GPS with multiple clinical end points including BCR and metastatic recurrence. GPS predicted time to BCR (HR, 2.7 per 20 GPS unit increase; 95% CI, 1.8–4.0). GPS also predicted time to metastases (HR, 3.8 per 20 GPS unit increase; 95% CI, 1.1–12.6), although the event rate was low. GPS was strongly associated with adverse pathology (odds ratio, 2.7 per 20 GPS unit increase; 95% CI, 1.8–4.4).[61]

Decipher Genomic Classifier

Decipher, a validated genomic classifier, uses oligonucleotide microarrays to measure 22 RNA expression biomarkers, which relate to cell proliferation and differentiation, androgen signaling, motility, and immune modulation. The genomic classifier outputs a score between 0 and 1 at increments of 0.1 that predicts risk of metastatic progression after radical prostatectomy.[62–65]

Klein and colleagues[66] evaluated the ability of Decipher to predict metastasis using a cohort of 57 patients with available biopsy specimens who underwent radical prostatectomy. In this study, Decipher plus NCCN model had an improved c index of 0.88 (95% CI, 0.77–0.96) compared with NCCN alone (c index, 0.75; 95% CI, 0.64–0.87). Decipher was the only significant predictor of metastasis when adjusting for age, preoperative PSA, and biopsy GS (Decipher HR per 10% increase, 1.72; 95% CI, 1.07–2.81; $P = .02$).[66] In another study including 33 patients, Decipher scores showed a positive correlation ($r = 0.70$;

$P<.001$) between biopsy samples and radical prostatectomy specimens.[62]

International guidelines have begun to integrate genomic assays into their PCa guidelines recommendations. The NCCN endorses the use of Prolaris and Oncotype DX GPS for men diagnosed with very low- and low-risk PCa at biopsy in the post-biopsy period with a life expectancy of more than 10 years.[67]

SUMMARY

In an era of medicine increasingly driven toward individualized treatment, postdiagnostic risk stratification of men with PCa has become highly important and more complex because of the variable dynamics of this disease.[4,43] The limitations of traditional risk group assignment based on PSA, GS, and clinical stage are increasingly apparent.[4] Both clinical care and research should be driven by use of true multivariable models, which would likely lead to more accurate risk stratification and improve decision-making at time of diagnosis. The development of genomic assays and biomarkers offers further potential for improved personalized risk prediction; however, prospective studies and further refinement are required to determine the optimal use for these markers, and their cost-effectiveness, in contemporary clinical practice.

REFERENCES

1. Potosky AL, Miller BA, Albertsen PC, et al. The role of increasing detection in the rising incidence of prostate cancer. JAMA 1995;273(7):548–52.
2. Siegel RL, Miller KD, Jemal A. Cancer statistics, 2017. CA Cancer J Clin 2017;67(1):7–30.
3. Epstein JI. An update of the Gleason grading system. J Urol 2010;183(2):433–40.
4. Patel KM, Gnanapragasam VJ. Novel concepts for risk stratification in prostate cancer. J Clin Urol 2016;9(2 Suppl):18–23.
5. Mottet N, Bellmunt J, Bolla M, et al. EAU-ESTRO-SIOG guidelines on prostate cancer. Part 1: screening, diagnosis, and local treatment with curative intent. Eur Urol 2017;71(4):618–29.
6. Epstein JI, Allsbrook WC Jr, Amin MB, et al. The 2005 International Society of Urological Pathology (ISUP) consensus conference on Gleason grading of prostatic carcinoma. Am J Surg Pathol 2005; 29(9):1228–42.
7. Kryvenko ON, Epstein JI. Improving the evaluation and diagnosis of clinically significant prostate cancer. Curr Opin Urol 2017;27(3):191–7.
8. Billis A, Guimaraes MS, Freitas LL, et al. The impact of the 2005 International Society of Urological

Pathology consensus conference on standard Gleason grading of prostatic carcinoma in needle biopsies. J Urol 2008;180(2):548–52 [discussion: 52–3].

9. Keefe DT, Schieda N, El Hallani S, et al. Cribriform morphology predicts upstaging after radical prostatectomy in patients with Gleason score 3 + 4 = 7 prostate cancer at transrectal ultrasound (TRUS)-guided needle biopsy. Virchows Arch 2015;467(4): 437–42.

10. Kweldam CF, Kummerlin IP, Nieboer D, et al. Disease-specific survival of patients with invasive cribriform and intraductal prostate cancer at diagnostic biopsy. Mod Pathol 2016;29(6):630–6.

11. Kir G, Sarbay BC, Gumus E, et al. The association of the cribriform pattern with outcome for prostatic adenocarcinomas. Pathol Res Pract 2014;210(10): 640–4.

12. Choy B, Pearce SM, Anderson BB, et al. Prognostic significance of percentage and architectural types of contemporary Gleason pattern 4 prostate cancer in radical prostatectomy. Am J Surg Pathol 2016; 40(10):1400–6.

13. McKenney JK, Simko J, Bonham M, et al. The potential impact of reproducibility of Gleason grading in men with early stage prostate cancer managed by active surveillance: a multi-institutional study. J Urol 2011;186(2):465–9.

14. Pierorazio PM, Walsh PC, Partin AW, et al. Prognostic Gleason grade grouping: data based on the modified Gleason scoring system. BJU Int 2013; 111(5):753–60.

15. Epstein JI, Egevad L, Amin MB, et al. The 2014 International Society of Urological Pathology (ISUP) consensus conference on Gleason grading of prostatic carcinoma: definition of grading patterns and proposal for a new grading system. Am J Surg Pathol 2016;40(2):244–52.

16. Epstein JI, Zelefsky MJ, Sjoberg DD, et al. A contemporary prostate cancer grading system: a validated alternative to the Gleason score. Eur Urol 2016;69(3):428–35.

17. Loeb S, Folkvaljon Y, Robinson D, et al. Evaluation of the 2015 Gleason grade groups in a nationwide population-based cohort. Eur Urol 2016;69(6): 1135–41.

18. Dell'Oglio P, Karnes RJ, Gandaglia G, et al. The new prostate cancer grading system does not improve prediction of clinical recurrence after radical prostatectomy: results of a large, two-center validation study. Prostate 2017;77(3):263–73.

19. Berney DM, Beltran L, Fisher G, et al. Validation of a contemporary prostate cancer grading system using prostate cancer death as outcome. Br J Cancer 2016;114(10):1078–83.

20. Leapman MS, Cowan JE, Simko J, et al. Application of a prognostic Gleason grade grouping system to assess distant prostate cancer outcomes. Eur Urol 2017;71(5):750–9.

21. Reese AC, Cowan JE, Brajtbord JS, et al. The quantitative Gleason score improves prostate cancer risk assessment. Cancer 2012;118(24):6046–54.

22. Deng FM, Donin NM, Pe Benito R, et al. Size-adjusted quantitative Gleason score as a predictor of biochemical recurrence after radical prostatectomy. Eur Urol 2016;70(2):248–53.

23. Sauter G, Clauditz T, Steurer S, et al. Integrating tertiary Gleason 5 patterns into quantitative Gleason grading in prostate biopsies and prostatectomy specimens. Eur Urol 2017. [Epub ahead of print].

24. D'Amico AV, Whittington R, Malkowicz SB, et al. Biochemical outcome after radical prostatectomy, external beam radiation therapy, or interstitial radiation therapy for clinically localized prostate cancer. JAMA 1998;280(11):969–74.

25. Rodrigues G, Warde P, Pickles T, et al. Pre-treatment risk stratification of prostate cancer patients: a critical review. Can Urol Assoc J 2012;6(2):121–7.

26. D'Amico AV, Whittington R, Malkowicz SB, et al. Pre-treatment nomogram for prostate-specific antigen recurrence after radical prostatectomy or external-beam radiation therapy for clinically localized prostate cancer. J Clin Oncol 1999;17(1):168–72.

27. Reese AC, Sadetsky N, Carroll PR, et al. Inaccuracies in assignment of clinical stage for localized prostate cancer. Cancer 2011;117(2):283–9.

28. Reese AC, Cooperberg MR, Carroll PR. Minimal impact of clinical stage on prostate cancer prognosis among contemporary patients with clinically localized disease. J Urol 2010;184(1):114–9.

29. Graham J, Kirkbride P, Cann K, et al. Prostate cancer: summary of updated NICE guidance. BMJ 2014;348:f7524.

30. Mohler J, Bahnson RR, Boston B, et al. NCCN clinical practice guidelines in oncology: prostate cancer. J Natl Compr Canc Netw 2010;8(2):162–200.

31. Thompson I, Thrasher JB, Aus G, et al. Guideline for the management of clinically localized prostate cancer: 2007 update. J Urol 2007;177(6):2106–31.

32. Kattan MW, Eastham JA, Stapleton AM, et al. A preoperative nomogram for disease recurrence following radical prostatectomy for prostate cancer. J Natl Cancer Inst 1998;90(10):766–71.

33. Ondracek RP, Kattan MW, Murekeyisoni C, et al. Validation of the Kattan nomogram for prostate cancer recurrence after radical prostatectomy. J Natl Compr Canc Netw 2016;14(11):1395–401.

34. Stephenson AJ, Kattan MW, Eastham JA, et al. Prostate cancer-specific mortality after radical prostatectomy for patients treated in the prostate-specific antigen era. J Clin Oncol 2009;27(26):4300–5.

35. Kim TH, Jeon HG, Jeong BC, et al. Development of a new nomogram to predict insignificant prostate

cancer in patients undergoing radical prostatectomy. Scand J Urol 2017;51(1):27–32.

36. Dell'Oglio P, Suardi N, Boorjian SA, et al. Predicting survival of men with recurrent prostate cancer after radical prostatectomy. Eur J Cancer 2016;54: 27–34.

37. Iremashvili V, Manoharan M, Pelaez L, et al. Clinically significant Gleason sum upgrade: external validation and head-to-head comparison of the existing nomograms. Cancer 2012;118(2):378–85.

38. Kutikov A, Cooperberg MR, Paciorek AT, et al. Evaluating prostate cancer mortality and competing risks of death in patients with localized prostate cancer using a comprehensive nomogram. Prostate Cancer Prostatic Dis 2012;15(4):374–9.

39. Lughezzani G, Budaus L, Isbarn H, et al. Head-to-head comparison of the three most commonly used preoperative models for prediction of biochemical recurrence after radical prostatectomy. Eur Urol 2010;57(4):562–8.

40. Shariat SF, Karakiewicz PI, Roehrborn CG, et al. An updated catalog of prostate cancer predictive tools. Cancer 2008;113(11):3075–99.

41. Shariat SF, Karakiewicz PI, Suardi N, et al. Comparison of nomograms with other methods for predicting outcomes in prostate cancer: a critical analysis of the literature. Clin Cancer Res 2008;14(14): 4400–7.

42. Cooperberg MR, Pasta DJ, Elkin EP, et al. The University of California, San Francisco Cancer of the Prostate Risk Assessment score: a straightforward and reliable preoperative predictor of disease recurrence after radical prostatectomy. J Urol 2005; 173(6):1938–42.

43. Brajtbord JS, Leapman MS, Cooperberg MR. The CAPRA score at 10 years: contemporary perspectives and analysis of supporting studies. Eur Urol 2017;71(5):705–9.

44. Cooperberg MR, Freedland SJ, Pasta DJ, et al. Multiinstitutional validation of the UCSF cancer of the prostate risk assessment for prediction of recurrence after radical prostatectomy. Cancer 2006; 107(10):2384–91.

45. Halverson S, Schipper M, Blas K, et al. The cancer of the prostate risk assessment (CAPRA) in patients treated with external beam radiation therapy: evaluation and optimization in patients at higher risk of relapse. Radiother Oncol 2011;101(3):513–20.

46. Delouya G, Krishnan V, Bahary JP, et al. Analysis of the cancer of the prostate risk assessment to predict for biochemical failure after external beam radiotherapy or prostate seed brachytherapy. Urology 2014;84(3):629–33.

47. Krishnan V, Delouya G, Bahary JP, et al. The cancer of the prostate risk assessment (CAPRA) score predicts biochemical recurrence in intermediate-risk prostate cancer treated with external beam

radiotherapy (EBRT) dose escalation or low-dose rate (LDR) brachytherapy. BJU Int 2014;114(6): 865–71.

48. Vainshtein JM, Schipper M, Vance S, et al. Limitations of the cancer of the prostate risk assessment (CAPRA) prognostic tool for prediction of metastases and prostate cancer-specific mortality in patients treated with external beam radiation therapy. Am J Clin Oncol 2016;39(2):173–80.

49. Ishizaki F, Hoque MA, Nishiyama T, et al. External validation of the UCSF-CAPRA (University of California, San Francisco, Cancer of the Prostate Risk Assessment) in Japanese patients receiving radical prostatectomy. Jpn J Clin Oncol 2011; 41(11):1259–64.

50. Tamblyn DJ, Chopra S, Yu C, et al. Comparative analysis of three risk assessment tools in Australian patients with prostate cancer. BJU Int 2011; 108(Suppl 2):51–6.

51. Fraser M, Sabelnykova VY, Yamaguchi TN, et al. Genomic hallmarks of localized, non-indolent prostate cancer. Nature 2017;541(7637):359–64.

52. Cuzick J, Swanson GP, Fisher G, et al. Prognostic value of an RNA expression signature derived from cell cycle proliferation genes in patients with prostate cancer: a retrospective study. Lancet Oncol 2011;12(3):245–55.

53. Cuzick J, Stone S, Fisher G, et al. Validation of an RNA cell cycle progression score for predicting death from prostate cancer in a conservatively managed needle biopsy cohort. Br J Cancer 2015; 113(3):382–9.

54. Spahn M, Boxler S, Joniau S, et al. What is the need for prostatic biomarkers in prostate cancer management? Curr Urol Rep 2015;16(10):70.

55. Cuzick J, Berney DM, Fisher G, et al. Prognostic value of a cell cycle progression signature for prostate cancer death in a conservatively managed needle biopsy cohort. Br J Cancer 2012;106(6):1095–9.

56. Bishoff JT, Freedland SJ, Gerber L, et al. Prognostic utility of the cell cycle progression score generated from biopsy in men treated with prostatectomy. J Urol 2014;192(2):409–14.

57. Oderda M, Cozzi G, Daniele L, et al. Cell-cycle progression-score might improve the current risk assessment in newly diagnosed prostate cancer patients. Urology 2017;102:73–8.

58. Knezevic D, Goddard AD, Natraj N, et al. Analytical validation of the oncotype DX prostate cancer assay: a clinical RT-PCR assay optimized for prostate needle biopsies. BMC Genomics 2013;14:690.

59. Moschini M, Spahn M, Mattei A, et al. Incorporation of tissue-based genomic biomarkers into localized prostate cancer clinics. BMC Med 2016;14:67.

60. Klein EA, Cooperberg MR, Magi-Galluzzi C, et al. A 17-gene assay to predict prostate cancer aggressiveness in the context of Gleason grade

heterogeneity, tumor multifocality, and biopsy under-sampling. Eur Urol 2014;66(3):550–60.

61. Cullen J, Rosner IL, Brand TC, et al. A biopsy-based 17-gene genomic prostate score predicts recurrence after radical prostatectomy and adverse surgical pathology in a racially diverse population of men with clinically low- and intermediate-risk prostate cancer. Eur Urol 2015;68(1):123–31.

62. Knudsen BS, Kim HL, Erho N, et al. Application of a clinical whole-transcriptome assay for staging and prognosis of prostate cancer diagnosed in needle core biopsy specimens. J Mol Diagn 2016;18(3):395–406.

63. Ross AE, Feng FY, Ghadessi M, et al. A genomic classifier predicting metastatic disease progression in men with biochemical recurrence after prostatectomy. Prostate Cancer Prostatic Dis 2014;17(1):64–9.

64. Erho N, Crisan A, Vergara IA, et al. Discovery and validation of a prostate cancer genomic classifier that predicts early metastasis following radical prostatectomy. PLoS One 2013;8(6):e66855.

65. Karnes RJ, Bergstralh EJ, Davicioni E, et al. Validation of a genomic classifier that predicts metastasis following radical prostatectomy in an at risk patient population. J Urol 2013;190(6):2047–53.

66. Klein EA, Haddad Z, Yousefi K, et al. Decipher genomic classifier measured on prostate biopsy predicts metastasis risk. Urology 2016;90:148–52.

67. Mohler JL, Armstrong AJ, Bahnson RR, et al. Prostate cancer, version 1.2016. J Natl Compr Canc Netw 2016;14(1):19–30.

68Gallium–Prostate-Specific Membrane Antigen PET/Computed Tomography for Primary and Secondary Staging in Prostate Cancer

Michael Chaloupka, MD[a],*, Annika Herlemann, MD[a],
Melvin D'Anastasi, MD[b], Clemens C. Cyran, MD[b], Harun Ilhan, MD[c],
Christian Gratzke, MD[a,d], Christian G. Stief, MD[a,d]

KEYWORDS

- Prostate cancer staging • PSMA • PET/CT • Biochemical recurrence

KEY POINTS

- Preoperative staging is a generally recommended tool for risk stratification of intermediate- to high-risk prostate cancer.
- So far, staging of patients with prostate cancer relies mostly on morphologic imaging. Prostate-specific membrane antigen (PSMA) PET has shown to be able to contribute molecular information on distribution of the disease.
- Studies have shown that PSMA PET combined with conventional imaging offers similar or higher detection rates in primary staging.
- In patients with biochemical recurrence of prostate cancer, PSMA imaging is able to distinguish between local recurrence or lymph node metastases even at very low prostate-specific antigen levels, thus, guiding treatment decisions.

INTRODUCTION

Preoperative imaging is important to accurately risk classify oncologic patients and to guide treatment decisions. Patients diagnosed with intermediate-risk (predominant Gleason pattern 4) or high-risk prostate cancer (PCa) should undergo clinical staging before curative therapy.[1]

Several imaging techniques are used to evaluate local extension, nodal involvement, or bone metastasis. Common methods, such as computed tomography (CT) or MRI, rely on morphologic patterns, such as size, shape, or increased contrast enhancement of tumor lesions. During the past 2 decades, the combination of CT or

Disclosure statement: The authors have nothing to disclose.
[a] Department of Urology, Ludwig-Maximilians-University Munich, Marchioninistraße 15, Munich 81377, Germany; [b] Institute for Clinical Radiology, Ludwig-Maximilians-University Munich, Marchioninistraße 15, Munich 81377, Germany; [c] Department of Nuclear Medicine, Ludwig-Maximilian-University Munich, March-ioninistraße 15, Munich 81377, Germany; [d] Comprehensive Cancer Center, Ludwig-Maximilians-University Munich, Marchioninistraße 15, Munich 81377, Germany
* Corresponding author. Department of Urology, Ludwig-Maximilians-University Munich, Marchioninistraße 15, Munich 81377, Germany.
E-mail address: Michael.chaloupka@med.uni-muenchen.de

Urol Clin N Am 44 (2017) 557–563
http://dx.doi.org/10.1016/j.ucl.2017.07.004

MRI with PET improved our knowledge about the extent of the disease. In contrast to CT or MRI, PET scans visualize biochemical and molecular characteristics of suspect lesions. So far, ^{18}F-fluorodeoxyglucose (^{18}F-FDG) is the most commonly used radiotracer in oncology. However, its ability to detect PCa in primary and secondary staging is limited to patients with poorly differentiated cancer,[2] most likely because of a low level of metabolic activity in differentiated PCa cells.[3,4] Choline-based tracers, which are more frequently used in patients with PCa, are also of limited sensitivity.[5] However, new radiotracers targeting the prostate-specific membrane antigen (PSMA) have shown promising results in the evaluation of primary and recurrent disease and in monitoring treatment response.

PROSTATE-SPECIFIC MEMBRANE ANTIGEN

PSMA is a 750-amino-acid type II transmembrane protein located within the apical epithelium of the secretory ducts of noncancerous prostate tissue. Several functions have been described for this protein, including enzyme activity in nutrient uptake, cell migration, signal transduction, and receptor activity for yet mostly unidentified physiologic ligands.[6] After binding to PSMA, the physiologic or artificial ligand is taken up into endosomal compartments or the cytoplasm of the cell via an internalization motif. During neoplastic transformation, PSMA transforms from the apical membrane to the luminal surface of the ducts.[7] PSMA expression is elevated in malignant prostate tissue, in contrast to benign prostatic hyperplasia specimens, in which no elevated expression was observed.[8] Studies have shown that PSMA expression positively correlates with Gleason score and prostate-specific antigen (PSA) level and is largely expressed in hormone-refractory PCa.[9] These features make PSMA an ideal target for diagnosis and treatment of PCa. Antibodies as well as synthetic small molecules are currently being used to target PSMA. However, antibodies lack diagnostic efficacy because of poor tumor penetrability, long circulating half-life, and high unspecific background activity.[10] The small molecule PSMA-inhibitor[11] radiolabeled with [68]gallium (^{68}Ga) is the most common agent for PET imaging to date. After ligation, the inhibitor is internalized into the malignant cell and cleared rapidly from nontarget tissue, resulting in a beneficial target to background ratio. Still, PSMA is not entirely prostate specific; there is physiologic uptake in the kidneys, parotid and submandibular glands, small intestines, spleen, and liver.[12,13] It is also expressed in tumor-associated neoangiogenesis and has, therefore, been described in other tumor entities, such as gastric, colorectal, breast cancer, and renal cell carcinoma.[14–17]

PRIMARY PROSTATE CANCER STAGING

For local staging, MRI of the prostate has a high diagnostic value for the detection of suspicious lesions within the prostate and for the evaluation of capsule penetration and invasion of adjacent structures due to excellent soft tissue resolution and comprehensive multi-parametric assessment.[18,19] It can also facilitate diagnostic yield after negative standardized biopsy and persistent clinical suspicion of PCa by the use of MRI–transrectal ultrasound fused biopsy or cognitive targeting.[20] However, accuracy of MRI of the prostate may be hindered by diagnostic challenges, such as benign changes mimicking malignancy, or technical issues considering acquisition. Differences in imaging interpretation due to interobserver variability may also lead to decreased sensitivity in tumor detection.[21] PET scans have been evaluated to address some of these limitations but performed generally poorly. PET alone cannot offer the necessary spatial resolution to detect small tumors within the organ. In combination with conventional imaging, PET/MRI is considered to be superior to PET/CT for the evaluation of local infiltration. Several studies have shown positive correlation between morphologic lesion plus increased uptake of choline-based tracers and postoperative pathologic finding, thus, offering beneficial diagnostic value compared with MRI alone.[22] PSMA ligands outperformed other radiotracers in detection rates. Tumor lesions were detected in PET/MRI with a specificity of 97% compared with 78% when using different radiotracers. However, sensitivity was similar with both techniques (76% vs 79%).[23]

In intermediate- to high-risk PCa, the current standard of care for preoperative evaluation of lymphatic spread and visceral or bone metastases includes MRI/CT and bone scintigraphy. Thus, for detection of suspect lymph nodes, the current standard of care relies solely on morphologic factors, whereas lymph nodes are considered likely to be tumor infiltrated if larger than 8 mm in diameter. However, many lymph node metastases are too small to be classified as positive by either CT or MRI. Both methods do not differ in accuracy to identify lymphatic spread with a sensitivity of 42% and 39% and a specificity of 82% and 82% for CT and MRI, respectively.[24] By providing additional molecular information, combination of conventional imaging

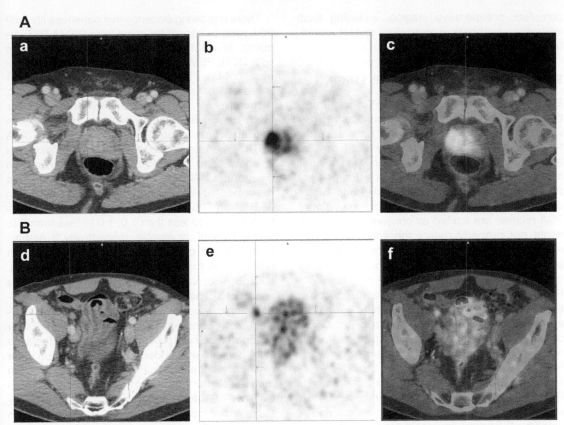

Fig. 1. (*A*) ^{68}Ga PSMA PET/CT of a 71-year-old patient with PCa and preoperative PSA of 7.67 ng/mL. Contrast-enhanced CT image (a) shows mild increased enhancement of the right prostatic lobe. Attenuation-corrected (b) and fused PET/CT image (c) show intense pathologic tracer uptake in the right prostatic lobe und to a lesser extent in the left prostatic lobe. (*B*) ^{68}Ga PSMA PET/CT of a 71-year-old patient with PCa and preoperative PSA of 7.67 ng/mL. A right iliac lymph node anterior to the external iliac artery with a short axis diameter of 7 mm is shown on the contrast-enhanced CT image (d). Attenuation-corrected image (e) and fused PET/CT image (f) show a pathologic tracer uptake in this lymph node. A radical prostatectomy with pelvic lymph node dissection was performed. Histopathology confirmed a pT3b PCa involving both lobes of the prostate with a Gleason score of 4 + 5 = 9 and a singular right external iliac lymph node metastasis.

with PSMA PET has enhanced the diagnostic yield (**Fig. 1**). Herlemann and colleagues[25] evaluated the diagnostic performance of PSMA PET as the primary imaging technique for lymph node staging in 20 patients and correlated findings with histopathology. They reported a region-based sensitivity and specificity of 86% and 88%, respectively. Forty percent of PET true positive lymph nodes were 5 mm or less and, therefore, would have not been recognized by CT alone. Budäus and colleagues[26] retrospectively evaluated 30 patients in a similar setting, reporting a fairly low sensitivity of 33% but 100% specificity for PSMA PET/CT. The largest cohort so far (130 patients) was retrospectively analyzed by Maurer and colleagues,[27] who observed a sensitivity and specificity of 65.9% and 98.9%, respectively, for PSMA PET/MRI. These detections rates are superior to those reported for

PET/CT with choline-based tracers.[28] Although a high specificity for PSMA PET combined with either CT or MRI has been confirmed by most studies so far, sensitivity differs considerably. Published data on this issue are still rare, and there is need for further research before drawing final conclusions.

For the detection of bone metastasis, bone scintigraphy with radiolabeled phosphates, for example, ^{99m}technetium methylene diphosphonate (^{99m}Tc-MDP) is still considered standard of care. ^{99m}Tc-MDP indicates osteoblastic activity nonspecifically as it appears in PCa metastasis. However, it also accumulates in degenerative joint disease, inflammation, and fractures resulting in a low specificity for the detection of PCa metastases.[29] Studies have shown that PSMA PET outperforms bone scintigraphy in the detection of bone metastasis, hereby offering the chance of a complete preoperative staging, including local infiltration, lymphatic spread, and distant metastasis in a single examination.[30]

SECONDARY PROSTATE CANCER STAGING

Biochemical recurrence (BCR) of PCa after curative treatment is defined as 2 consecutive PSA values greater than 0.2 ng/mL after radical prostatectomy and as any PSA increase of 2 ng/mL or greater higher than the PSA nadir value after radiotherapy, respectively.[31] PSA after primary therapy for PCa correlates directly with tumor burden. Therapeutic options at this early point of PSA relapse are limited as conventional imaging might not properly detect the source of recurrence. In absence of skeletal symptoms, bone scintigraphy is unlikely to detect bone metastases with a serum PSA level less than 7 ng/mL.[32] With PSA levels less than 10 ng/mL and a PSA doubling time greater than 6 months, there is hardly any chance of positive findings in pelvic CT to detect local recurrence or suspicious lymph nodes.[33,34] Therefore, the current guidelines from the European Association of Urology guidelines only recommend imaging for patients with PSA values greater than 10 ng/mL, high PSA kinetics (PSA doubling time <6 months or PSA velocity >0.5 ng/mL/mo), or in patients with symptoms of bone metastasis.[31]

However, precise knowledge about local recurrence, extent of lymphatic spread, and metastatic burden is crucial to plan further disease management. Patients with low PSA values in combination with local recurrence represent good candidates for salvage interventions. In case of local recurrence, salvage radiotherapy should be initiated as soon as possible and is most effective at PSA values less than 0.5 ng/mL.[35] For these patients, the 6-year estimated progression-free survival rate is 48%, compared with 26% for patients with higher preradiation PSA.[36] If isolated nodal recurrence is confirmed, salvage lymph node dissection may represent a therapeutic option. In patients presenting with lymph node metastases after definitive treatment, several studies have reported a biochemical response up to 67% after salvage lymph node dissection with an 8-year BCR-free and clinical recurrence-free survival rate of 23% and 38%, respectively.[37–39] Here, preoperative staging was performed by choline PET/CT or ^{18}F-FDG PET/CT at mean PSA values of 3.95 ng/mL or 9.8 ng/mL, respectively. Accurate staging in patients with early BCR is mandatory in order to offer new options of salvage treatments or to delay androgen deprivation therapy in case of clinical recurrence.

There is growing evidence that patients with early PSA relapse benefit the most from PSMA PET imaging. In a retrospective study of 155 patients with BCR, PSMA PET/CT identified recurrent disease in 44%, 79%, and 89% of patients with PSA levels of 1 or less, 1 to 2, and 2 ng/mL or greater, respectively.[40] Another evaluation with a similar study design including 70 patients confirms these findings. Here, a detection rate of 85% for PSMA PET/CT was described, with PSA levels less than 2 ng/mL and a PSA doubling time less than 6.5 months.[41] A retrospective study of 248 patients described detection rates of 57.9%, 72.7%, 93.0%, and 96.8% for PSA values of 0.2 to less than 0.5, 0.5 to less than 1.0, 1.0 to less than 2.0, and 2.0 ng/mL or greater, respectively.[42] Afshar-Oromieh and colleagues[43] reported a detection rate of 50% for PSA values less than 0.5 ng/mL and 58% for values 0.5 to 1.0 ng/mL in a large cohort of 319 patients. Yet, most studies lack histopathological confirmation. Herlemann and colleagues[25] observed a sensitivity of 83% for histopathologically proven lymph node metastases in 14 patients who underwent salvage lymph node dissection after radical prostatectomy. These data are similar to a recent study reporting a sensitivity of 77.9% for histopathologically proven metastatic lymph nodes in 48 cases of salvage lymph node dissection with preoperative PSMA PET/CT or PSMA PET/MRI. The median PSA value was 1.31 ng/mL at the time PSMA imaging was performed.[44] Morphologic imaging, such as CT or MRI alone, showed a limited sensitivity of 26.9% at this early stage of BCR. These detection rates are superior to PET techniques using choline-based tracers. In direct comparison, PSMA PET has shown a significantly higher detection rate compared with choline-based PET tracers.[45,46] In a study performed on 125 patients with BCR and negative ^{18}F-choline PET/CT, an additionally performed PSMA PET/CT detected sites of clinical recurrence in 43.8% (14 of 32 patients).[47]

Generally, most recent studies have shown that PSMA PET scan is superior to other available imaging techniques at the early point of BCR, which has a major influence on therapeutic decisions (**Fig. 2**). Clinical parameters, indicating the optimal time point to conduct PSMA imaging at most efficacy, are still subject to current research. Ceci and colleagues[41] suggested a PSA cutoff value of 0.83 ng/mL or greater, resulting in a detection rate of 85.7%. Furthermore, they reported a PSA doubling time of less than 6.5 versus 6.5 months or greater being the optimal cutoff value, with detection rates of 93.0% versus 34.8%, respectively. A recent large meta-analysis demonstrated detection rates of 58% and 76% for PSA values

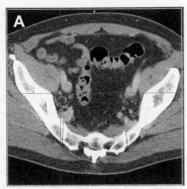
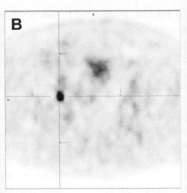
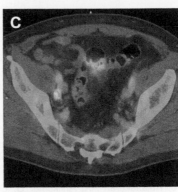

Fig. 2. ^{68}Ga PSMA PET/CT of a 67-year-old patient after radical prostatectomy (pT3b, Gleason 7, R0, pNX, PSA 9 ng/mL) and salvage radiotherapy a year later due to PSA recurrence (PSA 0.2 ng/mL). PSA was 1.5 ng/mL at the time of imaging, 8 months following salvage radiotherapy. Contrast-enhanced CT image (*A*) shows a small lymph node posterolateral to the right external iliac vein with a short axis diameter of 0.4 cm and with a fatty hilum. Attenuation-corrected PET image (*B*) and fused PET/CT image (*C*) show a pathologic PSMA uptake corresponding to the location of this node. Histopathology confirmed metastatic involvement.

of 0.2 to 0.99 and 1.00 to 1.99 ng/mL, respectively, indicating a PSA threshold of 1 ng/mL.[48]

DRAWBACKS AND OUTLOOK

Even though PSMA PET seems to have surpassed conventional imaging methods in the detection of PCa in primary and secondary staging, some limitations need to be addressed. A large meta-analysis of 16 studies involving 1309 patients found a high heterogeneity regarding the sensitivity and specificity profile of PSMA imaging, making it hard to conclude recommendations for the treating physician.[48] Notably, this sensitivity and specificity profile is additionally dampened by the existence of PSMA-negative PCa.[49] Maurer and colleagues[27] reported 3 false-negative PSMA PET results with existing lymph node involvement due to a PSMA-negative primary tumor. Another challenge to any imaging technique is the detection of micrometastases. All present PSMA PET studies with subsequent histopathological verification showed cases of micrometastases in false-negative findings.[25–27]

Furthermore, considering aspects such as availability, costs, and therapeutic consequence, the optimal time point of PSMA PET scan is still to be determined. So far, PSMA PET scans are only available in a few centers within Europe, South America, Asia, and Australia.[10] In the United States, PSMA-linked imaging is mostly available within clinical trials.

With PSMA being expressed exclusively in most PCa cells, this target can also be used for radionuclide imaging and therapy at the same time (theranostics). Linking PSMA antibodies to radioligands offers the chance of selective radiation. The

internalization motif of PSMA leads to endocytosis of bound proteins and, thus, to concentration of radioisotopes within the cell. Several studies showed a therapeutic benefit of PSMA-lutetium-177 (^{177}Lu) radionuclide therapy in metastatic castrate-resistant PCa (mCRPC).[50–54] Retrospective and mostly single arm studies evaluating a small number of patients with mCRPC treated with ^{177}Lu-conjugated PSMA-ligands showed a PSA response up to 80% and stable disease in up to 52% of patients.

About 10% to 30% of patients did not respond to PSMA-radioligand therapy, likely because of a heterogeneous expression pattern of PSMA among patients.

SUMMARY

PSMA PET/CT has become an essential part of staging in patients with PCa. In primary staging, PSMA imaging has shown to be as efficient as conventional imaging. In patients with BCR, PSMA PET detects clinical recurrence even at very low PSA levels and in lymph nodes too small to be detected by conventional imaging. This ability can be considered a breakthrough in distinguishing local recurrence from metastatic disease at the time of BCR and, thus, may guide treatment decisions.

REFERENCES

1. Mottet N, Bellmunt J, Bolla M, et al. EAU-ESTRO-SIOG guidelines on prostate cancer. part 1: screening, diagnosis, and local treatment with curative intent. Eur Urol 2017;71(4):618–29.

2. Minamimoto R, Uemura H, Sano F, et al. The potential of FDG-PET/CT for detecting prostate cancer in patients with an elevated serum PSA level. Ann Nucl Med 2011;25(1):21–7.

3. Sanz G, Robles JE, Gimenez M, et al. Positron emission tomography with 18fluorine-labelled deoxyglucose: utility in localized and advanced prostate cancer. BJU Int 1999;84(9):1028–31.

4. Jadvar H. Is there use for FDG-PET in prostate cancer? Semin Nucl Med 2016;46(6):502–6.

5. Evangelista L, Guttilla A, Zattoni F, et al. Utility of choline positron emission tomography/computed tomography for lymph node involvement identification in intermediate- to high-risk prostate cancer: a systematic literature review and meta-analysis. Eur Urol 2013;63(6):1040–8.

6. Rajasekaran AK, Anilkumar G, Christiansen JJ. Is prostate-specific membrane antigen a multifunctional protein? Am J Physiol Cell Physiol 2005; 288(5):C975–81.

7. Santoni M, Scarpelli M, Mazzucchelli R, et al. Targeting prostate-specific membrane antigen for personalized therapies in prostate cancer: morphologic and molecular backgrounds and future promises. J Biol Regul Homeost Agents 2014;28(4):555–63.

8. Lapidus RG, Tiffany CW, Isaacs JT, et al. Prostate-specific membrane antigen (PSMA) enzyme activity is elevated in prostate cancer cells. Prostate 2000; 45(4):350–4.

9. Ross JS, Sheehan CE, Fisher HA, et al. Correlation of primary tumor prostate-specific membrane antigen expression with disease recurrence in prostate cancer. Clin Cancer Res 2003;9(17):6357–62.

10. Maurer T, Eiber M, Schwaiger M, et al. Current use of PSMA-PET in prostate cancer management. Nat Rev Urol 2016;13(4):226–35.

11. Eder M, Schafer M, Bauder-Wust U, et al. 68Ga-complex lipophilicity and the targeting property of a urea-based PSMA inhibitor for PET imaging. Bioconjug Chem 2012;23(4):688–97.

12. Demirci E, Sahin OE, Ocak M, et al. Normal distribution pattern and physiological variants of 68Ga-PSMA-11 PET/CT imaging. Nucl Med Commun 2016;37(11):1169–79.

13. Minamimoto R, Hancock S, Schneider B, et al. Pilot comparison of (6)(8)Ga-RM2 PET and (6)(8)Ga-PSMA-11 PET in patients with biochemically recurrent prostate cancer. J Nucl Med 2016;57(4):557–62.

14. Haffner MC, Kronberger IE, Ross JS, et al. Prostate-specific membrane antigen expression in the neovasculature of gastric and colorectal cancers. Hum Pathol 2009;40(12):1754–61.

15. Milowsky MI, Nanus DM, Kostakoglu L, et al. Vascular targeted therapy with anti-prostate- specific membrane antigen monoclonal antibody J591 in advanced solid tumors. J Clin Oncol 2007;25(5): 540–7.

16. Chang SS, O'Keefe DS, Bacich DJ, et al. Prostate-specific membrane antigen is produced in tumor-associated neovasculature. Clin Cancer Res 1999; 5(10):2674–81.

17. Siva S, Callahan J, Pryor D, et al. Utility of 68 Ga prostate specific membrane antigen - positron emission tomography in diagnosis and response assessment of recurrent renal cell carcinoma. J Med Imaging Radiat Oncol 2017;61(3):372–8.

18. NiMhurchu E, O'Kelly F, Murphy IG, et al. Predictive value of PI-RADS classification in MRI- directed transrectal ultrasound guided prostate biopsy. Clin Radiol 2016;71(4):375–80.

19. Tewes S, Hueper K, Hartung D, et al. Targeted MRI/TRUS fusion-guided biopsy in men with previous prostate biopsies using a novel registration software and multiparametric MRI PI- RADS scores: first results. World J Urol 2015;33(11):1707–14.

20. Verma S, Rosenkrantz AB, Choyke P, et al. Commentary regarding a recent collaborative consensus statement addressing prostate MRI and MRI-targeted biopsy in patients with a prior negative prostate biopsy. Abdom Radiol 2017;42(2):346–9.

21. Rosenkrantz AB, Taneja SS. Radiologist, be aware: ten pitfalls that confound the interpretation of multiparametric prostate MRI. Am J Roentgenol 2014; 202(1):109–20.

22. Rosenkrantz AB, Friedman K, Chandarana H, et al. Current status of Hybrid PET/MRI in oncologic imaging. Am J Roentgenol 2016;206(1):162–72.

23. Eiber M, Weirich G, Holzapfel K, et al. Simultaneous 68Ga-PSMA HBED-CC PET/MRI improves the localization of primary prostate cancer. Eur Urol 2016; 70(5):829–36.

24. Hovels AM, Heesakkers RA, Adang EM, et al. The diagnostic accuracy of CT and MRI in the staging of pelvic lymph nodes in patients with prostate cancer: a meta-analysis. Clin Radiol 2008;63(4):387–95.

25. Herlemann A, Wenter V, Kretschmer A, et al. 68Ga-PSMA positron emission tomography/computed tomography provides accurate staging of lymph node regions prior to lymph node dissection in patients with prostate cancer. Eur Urol 2016;70(4):553–7.

26. Budäus L, Leyh-Bannurah SR, Salomon G, et al. Initial experience of (68)Ga-PSMA PET/CT imaging in high-risk prostate cancer patients prior to radical prostatectomy. Eur Urol 2016;69(3):393–6.

27. Maurer T, Gschwend JE, Rauscher I, et al. Diagnostic efficacy of (68)gallium-psma positron emission tomography compared to conventional imaging for lymph node staging of 130 consecutive patients with intermediate to high risk prostate cancer. J Urol 2016;195(5):1436–43.

28. Beheshti M, Imamovic L, Broinger G, et al. 18F choline PET/CT in the preoperative staging of prostate cancer in patients with intermediate or high risk of extracapsular disease: a prospective study of 130 patients. Radiology 2010;254(3):925–33.

29. Tombal B, Lecouvet F. Modern detection of prostate cancer's bone metastasis: is the bone scan era over? Adv Urol 2012;2012:893193.

30. Pyka T, Okamoto S, Dahlbender M, et al. Comparison of bone scintigraphy and 68Ga-PSMA PET for skeletal staging in prostate cancer. Eur J Nucl Med Mol Imaging 2016;43(12):2114–21.

31. Cornford P, Bellmunt J, Bolla M, et al. EAU-ESTRO-SIOG guidelines on prostate cancer. part II: treatment of relapsing, metastatic, and castration-resistant prostate cancer. Eur Urol 2017;71(4):630–42.

32. Gomez P, Manoharan M, Kim SS, et al. Radionuclide bone scintigraphy in patients with biochemical recurrence after radical prostatectomy: when is it indicated? BJU Int 2004;94(3):299–302.

33. Kane CJ, Amling CL, Johnstone PA, et al. Limited value of bone scintigraphy and computed tomography in assessing biochemical failure after radical prostatectomy. Urology 2003;61(3):607–11.

34. Okotie OT, Aronson WJ, Wieder JA, et al. Predictors of metastatic disease in men with biochemical failure following radical prostatectomy. J Urol 2004; 171(6 Pt 1):2260–4.

35. King CR. The timing of salvage radiotherapy after radical prostatectomy: a systematic review. Int J Radiat Oncol Biol Phys 2012;84(1):104–11.

36. Stephenson AJ, Scardino PT, Kattan MW, et al. Predicting the outcome of salvage radiation therapy for recurrent prostate cancer after radical prostatectomy. J Clin Oncol 2007;25(15):2035–41.

37. Tilki D, Mandel P, Seeliger F, et al. Salvage lymph node dissection for nodal recurrence of prostate cancer after radical prostatectomy. J Urol 2015; 193(2):484–90.

38. Suardi N, Gandaglia G, Gallina A, et al. Long-term outcomes of salvage lymph node dissection for clinically recurrent prostate cancer: results of a single-institution series with a minimum follow-up of 5 years. Eur Urol 2015;67(2):299–309.

39. Claeys T, Van Praet C, Lumen N, et al. Salvage pelvic lymph node dissection in recurrent prostate cancer: surgical and early oncological outcome. Biomed Res Int 2015;2015:198543.

40. Verburg FA, Pfister D, Heidenreich A, et al. Extent of disease in recurrent prostate cancer determined by [(68)Ga]PSMA-HBED-CC PET/CT in relation to PSA levels, PSA doubling time and Gleason score. Eur J Nucl Med Mol Imaging 2016;43(3):397–403.

41. Ceci F, Uprimny C, Nilica B, et al. (68)Ga-PSMA PET/CT for restaging recurrent prostate cancer: which factors are associated with PET/CT detection rate? Eur J Nucl Med Mol Imaging 2015;42(8):1284–94.

42. Eiber M, Maurer T, Souvatzoglou M, et al. Evaluation of hybrid (6)(8)Ga-PSMA ligand PET/CT in 248 patients with biochemical recurrence after radical prostatectomy. J Nucl Med 2015;56(5):668–74.

43. Afshar-Oromieh A, Avtzi E, Giesel FL, et al. The diagnostic value of PET/CT imaging with the (68)Ga-labelled PSMA ligand HBED-CC in the diagnosis of recurrent prostate cancer. Eur J Nucl Med Mol Imaging 2015;42(2):197–209.

44. Rauscher I, Maurer T, Beer AJ, et al. Value of 68Ga-PSMA HBED-CC PET for the assessment of lymph node metastases in prostate cancer patients with biochemical recurrence: comparison with histopathology after salvage lymphadenectomy. J Nucl Med 2016;57(11):1713–9.

45. Afshar-Oromieh A, Zechmann CM, Malcher A, et al. Comparison of PET imaging with a (68)Ga-labelled PSMA ligand and (18)F-choline-based PET/CT for the diagnosis of recurrent prostate cancer. Eur J Nucl Med Mol Imaging 2014;41(1):11–20.

46. Pfister D, Porres D, Heidenreich A, et al. Detection of recurrent prostate cancer lesions before salvage lymphadenectomy is more accurate with (68)Ga-PSMA-HBED-CC than with (18)F-fluoroethylcholine PET/CT. Eur J Nucl Med Mol Imaging 2016;43(8):1410–7.

47. Bluemel C, Krebs M, Polat B, et al. 68Ga-PSMA-PET/CT in patients with biochemical prostate cancer recurrence and negative 18F-choline-PET/CT. Clin Nucl Med 2016;41(7):515–21.

48. Perera M, Papa N, Christidis D, et al. Sensitivity, specificity, and predictors of positive 68Ga-prostate-specific membrane antigen positron emission tomography in advanced prostate cancer: a systematic review and meta-analysis. Eur Urol 2016;70(6):926–37.

49. Wright GL Jr, Haley C, Beckett ML, et al. Expression of prostate-specific membrane antigen in normal, benign, and malignant prostate tissues. Urol Oncol 1995;1(1):18–28.

50. Baum RP, Kulkarni HR, Schuchardt C, et al. 177Lu-labeled prostate-specific membrane antigen radioligand therapy of metastatic castration-resistant prostate cancer: safety and efficacy. J Nucl Med 2016;57(7):1006–13.

51. Rahbar K, Schmidt M, Heinzel A, et al. Response and tolerability of a single dose of 177Lu- PSMA-617 in patients with metastatic castration-resistant prostate cancer: a multicenter retrospective analysis. J Nucl Med 2016;57(9):1334–8.

52. Tagawa ST, Milowsky MI, Morris M, et al. Phase II study of lutetium-177-labeled anti- prostate-specific membrane antigen monoclonal antibody J591 for metastatic castration- resistant prostate cancer. Clin Cancer Res 2013;19(18):5182–91.

53. Kratochwil C, Giesel FL, Stefanova M, et al. PSMA-targeted radionuclide therapy of metastatic castration-resistant prostate cancer with 177Lu-labeled PSMA-617. J Nucl Med 2016;57(8):1170–6.

54. Ahmadzadehfar H, Eppard E, Kurpig S, et al. Therapeutic response and side effects of repeated radioligand therapy with 177Lu-PSMA-DKFZ-617 of castrate-resistant metastatic prostate cancer. Oncotarget 2016;7(11):12477–88.

Contemporary Active Surveillance
Candidate Selection, Follow-up Tools, and Expected Outcomes

Laurence Klotz, MD, FRCSC

KEYWORDS

- Active surveillance • Prostate cancer • Risk stratification • MRI • Biomarkers

KEY POINTS

- The molecular genetics of Gleason pattern 3 resemble normal cells in most cases. In contrast, pattern 4 harbors numerous genetic abnormalities involving most oncogenic pathways.
- Gleason pattern 3 has no metastatic potential. Case series involving tens of thousands of cases have demonstrated no metastases when the presence of occult higher grade cancer is excluded.
- The main significant of higher volume Gleason pattern 3 is its association with a higher risk of co-existent occult higher grade cancer. This is reflected in a higher PSA density, cancer core volume, and number of cores involved. Higher volume pattern 3 should prompt a more aggressive search for occult cancer (MRI, repeat biopsy), not treatment.
- MRI and biomarkers are complementary, and clearly enhance the diagnostic pathway. Current guidelines vary in their recommendation regarding the role of MRI (from selective to routine) and biomarkers (from investigational only to selective use).

INTRODUCTION

About half of men diagnosed with prostate cancer by systematic biopsy are found to have low-risk disease, also called Gleason 6 prostate cancer, or grade group 1. The 2011 US Preventive Services Task Force's (USPSTF) recommendation against prostate-specific antigen (PSA) screening, owing to the risks of overdiagnosis and overtreatment,[1] reflected a compelling concern about overtreatment of low-risk disease. Since then there has been an emerging consensus that most men with low-risk prostate cancer do not derive any meaningful benefit from radical treatment, and an initial conservative approach is warranted. Importantly, this shift to expectant management has resulted in the USPSTF proposing to revise their recommendation regarding screening from D in 2011 to a C (neutral) in 2017.[2]

Prostate cancer develops in most aging men. In Caucasian men, the likelihood of harboring prostate cancer is approximately one's age as a percentage, beginning in the 30s.[3] This trend has been confirmed in many autopsy studies of Caucasians, Asians, and other ethnic groups. These lesions are usually small (<1 mm³) and low grade. In an autopsy study in Japanese and Russian men who died of other causes, about 35% of both groups harbored prostate cancer, and 50% of the Japanese men older than 70 years had a Gleason score of 7 or higher.[4] Although the prevalence of histologic prostate cancer was lower in Japanese men between 30 and 60 years of age, there was essentially no difference in men older than 60 years.

Division of Urology, Sunnybrook Health Sciences Centre, University of Toronto, 2075 Bay view Ave MG 408, Toronto, Ontario M4N3M5, Canada
E-mail address: Laurence.klotz@sunnybrook.ca

Urol Clin N Am 44 (2017) 565–574
http://dx.doi.org/10.1016/j.ucl.2017.07.005

MOLECULAR HALLMARKS OF PROSTATE CANCER

This disparity between the prevalence of histologic prostate cancer and the lifetime risk of mortality from prostate cancer (3% in North America before the advent of screening and approximately 2% more recently) emphasizes the risks of overdiagnosis and the value of conservative therapy for low-risk patients. Molecular and genetic analyses have shown that the hallmarks of cancer differ profoundly between the two most common patterns of disease, Gleason 3 and Gleason 4. These hallmarks are a useful structure for determining the degree to which low-grade prostate cancer (Gleason pattern 3) looks like a true malignancy.[5,6]

In most cases, the molecular abnormalities associated with these characteristics are absent in Gleason pattern 3 and present in Gleason pattern 4 (**Table 1**). The differences are both qualitative and quantitative. It is remarkable how well the Gleason scoring system disaggregates prostate cancer between genetically normal and abnormal cells. According to those who knew him personally, Don Gleason himself thought that Gleason pattern 3 or less should not be called cancer.

Genetic aberrations are uncommon in Gleason pattern 3 and common in patterns 4 and 5. This finding is particularly true of genes regulating key oncogenic pathways. Genes involved in proliferation, including AKT and HER2, are expressed normally in Gleason 3 and abnormally expressed in Gleason 4 (see **Table 1**). Genes involved in cellular invasion and metastasis and genes regulating the cell cycle transition are not overexpressed in Gleason 3 but are in Gleason 4. Genes associated with resistance to apoptosis, angiogenesis, and the development of other proangiogenic factors, and genes involved in regulating cellular metabolism tend to be abnormally expressed in Gleason 4 but not in Gleason 3.[7–20]

Recent studies have indicated that the progression to higher-grade cancer is characterized by both qualitative and quantitative genetic differences. For example, about 10% of Gleason pattern 3 cancers have a PTEN deletion. This deletion is found much more commonly in Gleason 3 pattern cells in men with coexistent Gleason pattern 4, that is, Gleason score 7 cancers.[21] This may indicate that a field defect is present or that Gleason 3 cells harboring the PTEN deletion rapidly dedifferentiate to a higher Gleason pattern. An alternative explanation is that the deleterious genetic alterations present in the higher-grade cancers are transferred by exosomes into the lower-grade cancers.[22] This phenomenon of intertumoral and intratumoral communication and influence through extracellular circulating exosomes may explain several otherwise hard-to-understand observations in the field, for example, the effect of treatment of the primary in patients with metastatic disease.

POTENTIAL FOR METASTASIS

The data are very compelling that Gleason 6 cancer has little or no metastatic potential. One study of 14,000 men with pathologically confirmed Gleason pattern 6 identified only 22 cases with lymph node metastases.[23] All 22 men had higher-grade cancer on reexamination of the tissue. Thus, the rate of lymph node metastases in men whose prostate tissue contained no higher-grade cancer was zero. Another study of 12,000 men treated with radical prostatectomy whose specimen had

Table 1
Gleason 3 versus 4 and hallmarks of cancer

Pathway	Gleason 3	Gleason 4
EGF, EGFR[8]	No	Overexpressed
AKT, MAP2 kinase[7]	No	Aberrant
HER2neu[8]	No	Amplified
Insensitivity to growth inhibitory signals (cyclin D2, and so forth)[9–11]	Expressed	Absent
Resisting apoptosis, BCL2[13]	Negative	Strong expression
Absence of senescence, TMPRSS2-ERG[16–18]	ERG normal	Increased
VEGF, microvessel density, other proangiogenic factors[19,20]	Low expression	Increased
PTEN[21]	Present in 90%	Deleted in 70%–90%
Markers of tissue invasion and metastasis[14,15]	Normal	Overexpressed
Clinical evidence of metastasis/PCa mortality[23,24]	Virtually absent	Present

Abbreviation: PCa, prostate cancer.

only Gleason 6 cancer[24] found the prostate cancer mortality was 0.2% at 20 years. The few patients who had metastases had evidence of higher-grade cancer on rereview. This low level of metastasis is remarkable given the imprecision and between observer variation in the assignment of Gleason score.

Although coexistent higher-grade cancer is common, spontaneous grade progression (from Gleason 3–4 or 5) is uncommon. This progression has been modeled by several groups; the estimate is that 1% to 2% of patients per year will undergo grade progression. In most cases, this occurs in high-volume Gleason 6 cancers.[25]

PATIENT SELECTION FOR ACTIVE SURVEILLANCE

Based on these concepts, active surveillance (AS) should be offered to most men with grade group 1 (Gleason 6) prostate cancer. The Achilles heel of this approach is misattribution of grade, that is, that 25% to 30% of these men diagnosed from a systematic biopsy actually harbor higher-grade cancer. Although most of these misattributed cancers are grade group 2 (Gleason 3 + 4), and may still have a low metastatic potential, the presence of any Gleason 4 pattern cancer confers an increased risk of eventual metastasis. Thus, the mandate of managing men on surveillance is to evaluate patients further for the presence of coexistent high-grade cancer and, once higher-grade cancer is excluded, monitor them subsequently to ensure it does not develop.

The view that Gleason pattern 3 has little or no metastatic phenotype has had a significant impact on the management of patients with this cancer. Thus, there should be no lower age limit to entering patients on AS. The quality-of-life benefits of maintaining normal erectile function and voiding function are greater in young men. Prostate cancers are not rare in young men; microfocal low-grade cancer is found at autopsy in around 40% of men in their 40s.[26] Finding small amounts of Gleason 6 cancer on a transrectal ultrasound (TRUS)-guided biopsy cannot possibly mean that disease progression is inevitable. High-volume Gleason pattern 3 is important primarily as a marker for patients at higher risk for harboring higher-grade cancer. If higher-grade cancer can be excluded in patients with higher-volume Gleason 6 cancer (based on MRI, targeted/template biopsies, and/or biomarkers), such patients are unlikely to require treatment. In rare instances, men younger than 55 years present with extensive Gleason 6 cancer. In these unusual cases, radical intervention, such as surgery, may be appropriate.

ACTIVE SURVEILLANCE MANAGEMENT

The clinical management of men on AS is as follows: Eligible patients are those with Gleason 6 disease. Selected patients with Gleason 3 + 4 cancers with a low percentage of pattern 4 may also be candidates. Patients are followed with serial PSA assessments and repeat biopsies. An initial confirmatory biopsy should be performed within the first 6 to 12 months, targeting those zones of the prostate that tend to be underevaluated on the initial diagnostic biopsy. Because the lead time from diagnosis to clinical progression is usually long for low-risk disease, the concept is that delayed therapy at the first signs of risk reclassification will still be curative.

Following the initial assessment and confirmatory biopsy, patients should be followed with semiannual PSA, annual digital rectal examination (DRE), and repeat biopsy and/or imaging at 3- to 5-year intervals. This interval depends on patients' underlying risk factors and level of concern. Once patients' life expectancy is less than 5 to 7 years (around 80 years of age), in stable patients follow-up should be limited to annual PSA.

An additional consideration is patients in whom there may be a lower life expectancy, either because of age or comorbidities. An example might be patients with chronic obstructive pulmonary disease or other serious comorbidity, with a higher-volume Gleason 3 + 4 or a 4 + 3 tumor. Although there may be a greater risk of disease progression in such patients, in most cases progression (increasing PSA, for example) is not associated with any disease-related side effects. Consequential progression end points (pain, metastases, and death) are generally years away in such patients.

Toxicity of treatment is also relevant. For example, consider older patients with inflammatory bowel disease or another condition that could lead to severe side effects with radiation. If not a surgical candidate, the risk of disease progression and serious side effects of prostate cancer years later would need to be balanced against up-front serious consequences of radiotherapy; in such a situation, AS and delayed hormonal therapy (if necessary) may be a superior option.

MRI has recently been incorporated into many AS algorithms. Although most guidelines advocate selective use of MRI, the National Institute for Health and Care Excellence (NICE) guidelines from the United Kingdom mandate an MRI in all AS patients (**Table 2**). Clearly, MRI effectively identifies large high-grade cancers with high accuracy. These cancers are usually anterior and may be missed by conventional TRUS-guided biopsies.

Table 2
Summary of contemporary active surveillance guidelines

	Low-Risk Pca	Intermediate Risk	Tests	Other Tests	5 ARI
Cancer Care Ontario CUAJ 2015[57]	AS preferred management	Active treatment; AS for selected pts	PSA q 3–6 mo DRE q 1 y Systematic bx within 6–12 mo, then q 3–5 y	MRI when clinical and path findings discordant	May have a role
ASCO JCO 2016[58]	Same	Same	Same	Other tests remain investigational	No clear role
AUA 2017[60]	Same	AS for selected patients	Same	Same	
NICE 2016[59]	Same	Radical treatment of disease progression	PSA q 3–4 mo, monitor kinetics, otherwise same	MRI at enrollment	

Abbreviations: ARI, alpha reductase inhibitor; ASCO, American Society of Clinical Oncology; AUA, American Urological Association; bx, biopsy; CUAJ, *Canadian Urological Association Journal*; JCO, Journal of Clinical Oncology.

Thus, an MRI with targeted biopsies of any area of restricted diffusion is likely to significantly enhance the early identification of higher grade cancer.

A PiRads 4 to 5 lesion has been reported to have a 90% positive predictive value for high-grade cancer in an AS cohort.[26] This abnormality in patients on AS is very significant and should result in a targeted biopsy. A recent large study comparing multi-parametric MRI targeted biopsy to systematic biopsy reported 93% sensitivity for clinically significant cancer (compared with 48% with systematic biopsy).[27]

Can the biopsy be dispensed with if the MRI is normal? MRI is relatively ineffective at identifying small-volume high-grade cancers. The negative predictive value (NPV) of a normal MRI for Gleason 7 or higher cancer is approximately 85%, although this figure varies between studies (**Table 3**). This figure means that, in patients at risk, 15% of those with a negative MRI will still be found to have significant cancer on systematic or template biopsies. In some patients with a positive MRI, systematic biopsies are positive despite negative targeted biopsies.

Table 3
Results of mature active surveillance cohorts

Study	N	Median Follow-up (y)	Freedom from Treatment	bNED After Deferred Treatment	Prostate Cancer Mortality (%)	OS
UCSF[40]	321	3.6	67% at 5 y	1 recurrence at 3 y	0	0
University of Toronto[38]	993	8.5	70% at 5 y	5-y bNED: 47%	5% at 15 y	10-y OS: 68%
Multicenter PRIAS[41]	2494	1.6	77% at 2 y	No data	0	4-y OS: 87%
University of Miami[42]	230	2.6	85.7% at 5 y	No recurrences	0	No data
Johns Hopkins[43]	1298	5.0	59% at 5 y	90.6% recurrence free at 2 y	0.1% at 15 y	15 OS 69%
Royal Marsden[44]	471	5.7	70% at 5 y	85% PSA, failure free at 5 y	2% at 8 y	9% at 8 y

Abbreviations: bNED, No biochemical evidence of disease; OS, overall survival; PRIAS, Prostate Cancer Research International Active Surveillance; UCSF, University of California, San Francisco.

In the author's view, MRI should be viewed as a risk stratification parameter, much like PSA is today, but providing a much-enhanced risk adjustment. Nomograms incorporating MRI to predict clinically significant cancer are in development.[28] Thus, patients on surveillance with a low PSA density, low cancer volume on initial diagnostic biopsy, and no other risk factors, whose MRI is negative, has less than a 5% chance of significant cancer. In contrast, those with positive risk factors, that is, high PSA density, higher cancer volume, and so forth, should likely have systematic biopsies regardless of the MRI findings.

Biomarkers

Prospective AS cohorts now comprise greater than 10,000 patients, thousands of whom have been followed for greater than 10 years. Clinical parameters (PSA, PSA density, extent of disease on biopsy, race, T stage) allow for stratification for risk of coexistent higher-grade disease. Monitoring low-risk patients on surveillance is associated with a risk of clinical progression of 0.2% to 5.0% at 15 years. Therefore, the benefit to most patients of a biomarker to further stratify patients according to the risk of progression is modest.

However, selected patients, particularly those whose risk factors suggest they are at more than average risk for higher-grade disease, may benefit from genomic testing. There are 2 potential benefits: reassurance for those patients with a favorable genomic risk score that conservative management is likely to be safe and earlier identification of those at risk for disease progression on AS who could benefit from treatment. Clinical studies have demonstrated a greater utilization of conservative management in those who have access to genomic testing.

As of the publication of this document, 3 genetic tissue assays have been approved by the Food and Drug Administration for men with prostate cancer and are summarized as follows:

Genomic Classifier

This assay is a 22-marker genomic classifier (GC), based on RNA expression. GC had independent predictive value on multivariable analysis for predicting metastasis following prostatectomy, with a hazard ratio (HR) of 1.5 for each 10% increase in score[29]; these results were validated in 2 separate prostatectomy cohorts.[29,30] A high score is associated with an increased risk of prostate cancer–specific mortality and progressive disease following salvage radiation.

Genomic Prostate Score

This assay incorporates 12 cancer genes that represent 4 biological pathways of prostate cancer oncogenesis: the androgen receptor pathway, cellular organization, stromal response, and proliferation. A 20-point increase in the genomic prostate score is associated with a statistically significant increased risk of high-grade and/or non–organ-confined disease (odds ratio 1.9, 95% confidence interval 1.3–2.9).[31–34]

Cell Cycle Progression

This assay analyzes 31 cell cycle–related genes and 15 housekeeping genes by quantitative reverse transcription polymerase chain reaction.

The Transatlantic Prostate Group examined cell cycle progression (CCP) scores using needle biopsies of a conservatively managed prostate cancer cohort from Great Britain.[35] In this cohort, of 349 men managed without primary treatment, the cumulative incidence of death was increased among those with CCP scores greater than 2 (19% of the population) compared with those with lower CCP scores. Patient outcomes could not be differentiated in those with lower CCP scores. The HR of prostate cancer death was 1.7 per unit increase in CCP score to 10 or Cancer of the Prostate Risk Assessment high-risk disease.

A separate radical prostatectomy cohort demonstrated that CCP score was independently associated with biochemical PSA recurrence and metastasis (HR 1.47 and 4.19, respectively, per unit score increase, $P<.05$ for both) after surgery.[36,37]

There are 2 major limitations of tissue-based genomic testing. The first is genetic heterogeneity. A recent study performed exome-wide sequencing of individual prostate cancers microdissected from patients with multi-focality. The genes used in the GC, Cause specific survival, and CCP assays described earlier were then compared. Marked heterogeneity of the scores of all 3 tests between cancers from the same prostate was observed. The confounding problem of genetic heterogeneity of individual cancers in the same gland is considerable.

A second important consideration in the Gleason 6 population is the Bayesian problem, related to the low a priori risk. Thus, if patients with Gleason 6 cancer has a 3% chance of metastases at 15 years, and a genetic biomarker has a positive predictive value of 90% for significant cancer, the risk of overdiagnosis of significant cancer may be 3 times higher than the risk of metastases. Therefore, genetic testing of the tissue should be restricted to higher-risk patients. These patients include those with high cancer volume on biopsy, high PSA density, or Gleason 7 who are surveillance candidates.

EXPECTED OUTCOMES

Death in men on AS occurs most commonly from cardiovascular disease, and death from prostate cancer is rare. In the most mature cohort,[38] with a median follow-up of 9 years, the relative risk for non–prostate-cancer death was 10 times that for prostate cancer mortality. There is no evidence that adverse psychological effects are significant in men on AS. Anxiety accompanies a diagnosis of prostate cancer but seems to be influenced less by treatment. In the Scandinavian trial comparing radical prostatectomy with watchful waiting (without the option of definitive intervention), there was no difference in psychological functioning, anxiety, or depression between the two groups.[39]

Nine prospective studies of AS have included about 10,000 men.[38,40–48] The largest most mature studies are summarized in **Table 3**. The limitation of these studies is the length of follow-up. One key study that generated a great deal of concern about conservative management in young patients in Sweden reported that the HR for prostate cancer mortality in patients managed by watchful waiting was low for many years but tripled after 15 years of follow-up.[49] These patients did not have the benefit of selective intervention. It will be 5 to 7 years before the most mature AS cohorts have a median of 15 years of follow-up. However, collectively, experience with AS includes 200 patients followed for more than 15 years. A few of these patients have had late disease progression, but there is no evidence of a sharp increase in mortality after 15 years.

AS inclusion criteria have varied between groups. Two groups, Toronto and Hopkins, represent the two extremes of an inclusive and restrictive approach, respectively. Both groups have reported 15-year outcomes, and the comparison is instructive.

The Toronto group took an inclusive approach, including all low-risk and selected intermediate-risk (Gleason 7 or PSA >10) patients.[43] The actuarial 15-year prostate cancer mortality rate is 5%. Most of the metastatic cases were Gleason 7 at diagnosis. The HR for metastasis at 15 years was 3.75 times greater for intermediate- than low-risk patients. The Gleason 7 patients in particular were at risk; these patients had a 20% or greater metastasis rate at 15 years.[50,51] (Importantly, PSA >10 had very little correlation with likelihood of metastasis.)

In contrast, the Hopkins group took a restrictive approach, offering surveillance only to patients who fulfilled the Epstein criteria (Gleason 6 with no more than 2 positive cores, no core >50% involved, and PSA density <0.15). The benefit was a prostate cancer mortality rate of 0.5% at 15 years. The cost was that only about 20% of newly diagnosed patients were eligible (vs 50% in the Toronto cohort). Based on the data summarized in this article, there is an emerging consensus that the appropriate strategy lies between these 2 extremes. Most Gleason 6 patients are appropriately managed with surveillance (ie, not just those fulfilling Epstein criteria); surveillance should be offered only cautiously to Gleason 7 patients.

All of the mature surveillance cohorts reflect the pre-MRI/biomarker experience. Although favorable, it is very likely that the incorporation of these augmented strategies will broaden the indications for surveillance while further reducing the already low rate of metastasis.

The long-awaited Protect trial reported recently.[52] This randomized trial compared active monitoring, radical prostatectomy, and external-beam radiotherapy.[48] The primary end point was prostate cancer mortality at 10 years. A total of 1643 men identified in a screening trial agreed to undergo randomization between the 3 arms. There were 17 prostate cancer–specific deaths overall, and there was no difference between the 3 groups in Cause specific mortality or overall survival (OS). The active monitoring group had more metastases (33 men; 6.3 events per 1000 person-years) versus surgery (2.4 per 1000 person-years) or radiation (3.0 per 1000 person-years). The P value was .004 for the overall comparison.

A key fact in understanding the significance of this important trial is that 77% of the patients had low-grade cancer on biopsy at diagnosis. Patients with intermediate- and high-risk cancer were included in the active monitoring arm. Given the low rate of metastasis, a higher rate of progression in the 23% of patients in the intermediate- and high-risk groups is more than sufficient to explain the increase in metastasis rate. Further, active monitoring in the Protect trial did not mean AS as described earlier. Biopsies were not performed on an established schedule, and criteria for intervention were not clearly described. Quality of life on the active monitoring arm was the same or better in every domain measured.[53]

PROSTATE-SPECIFIC ANTIGEN KINETICS

The Prostate Cancer Research International Active Surveillance multi-institutional AS registry recently reported that 20% of men having intervention did so based on a PSA doubling time less than 3 years.[41] The problem is that the correlation between PSA kinetics and adverse disease characteristics is not sufficiently reliable (because of the lack of specificity) to be used as the basis for treatment decisions. An overview of this subject concluded that PSA kinetics did not add predictive value to absolute PSA concentration.[54] False-positive PSA triggers occurred in 50% of the patients with stable disease in the Toronto cohort at some point in time; this observation was noted a median of 3 times in these patients.[55] Thus, PSA kinetics are a useful guide for further evaluation but not as the only trigger for intervention.

Guidelines

Several groups have promoted guidelines for the use of AS. Recent guidelines from Cancer Care Ontario,[56] the American Society of Clinical Oncology,[57] NICE,[58] and the American Urological Association[59] are summarized in **Table 2**. Note that the basic approach is similar between groups. Differences exist regarding the use of MRI and biomarkers. Most groups, in 2017, advise that MRI be used selectively and biomarkers be considered investigational. It is reasonable to predict that, as data accumulate, both MRI and biomarkers will be increasingly used to enhance patient selection and outcomes.

The controversies and unanswered questions in this field have moved from concept to application. Given the enormous amount of data from randomized trials (Prostate Cancer Intervention Versus Observation Trial [PIVOT], Protect) and prospective series of conservative management reviewed in this book, no informed individual would argue that the principle of conservative management for low-risk disease is misplaced. The questions are now related to who, how, when, and what. The main areas of uncertainty are outlined next. They cover a broad swath of current research in prostate cancer.

1. What are the molecular events that signal progression of low-grade disease? For example, PTEN deletion has been identified as a key step in the progression of prostate cancer and is present in about 10% of Gleason 6 cancers. However, this deletion on its own may not be sufficient to induce a metastatic phenotype. We are just at the beginning of learning which genetic and epigenetic aberrations alter the behavior of prostate cancer cells. Many other tantalizing mechanisms have recently been identified, for example, the effect of circulating exosomes. Another priority is determining whether patients with certain known germline mutations, for example, BRCA1 or 2, are candidates for surveillance. We will learn much more about how these aberrant genetic pathways interact over the next decade.

2. How do we optimally identify the *wolves in sheep's clothing*. As described previously, the pitfall of AS is the misattribution of low risk in the 25% to 30% of patients who harbor a higher-grade cancer that was missed because of sampling. The increased use of MRI will address this substantially but not completely. We know much better today how to use baseline parameters to identify patients at risk (PSA density, extent of core involvement, race, and so forth). The use of MRI and molecular biomarkers is further refining this. Nomograms incorporating MRI and/or biomarker findings to predict the risk of coexistent higher-grade cancer are needed urgently. Sorting out how to use these tests optimally will require further research, for example, how to manage patients who have a Pirads 4 lesion whose targeted biopsy shows Gleason 6 cancer. Does the presence of restricted diffusion mean they have a biologically more aggressive cancer despite being Gleason 6; was a higher-grade cancer missed; or does it signify nothing? The role of a genetic biomarker in this setting seems obvious, but there are little data on this situation. Radiomics, that is, the molecular events associated with restricted diffusion and other MR abnormalities associated with cancer, is in its infancy. Similarly, what is the best strategy for patients with microfocal Gleason 6 cancer whose Prolaris or Oncotype Dx assay reveals a mildly elevated risk score? MRI with targeted biopsy also likely plays a role in this setting, but there are little data. How to integrate MRI and biomarkers into treatment decision-making is a major research priority.

3. Which intermediate-risk patients are candidates for surveillance? Recent data indicate that the approach to surveillance, based on PSA and serial biopsy, is imperfect for Gleason 7 patients. Despite close monitoring and selective delayed intervention, 20% or more of these patients progress to metastasis by 15 years. Yet the glass is also half full; 80% remained free of Metastases. Obviously, therefore, many intermediate-risk patients are candidates for surveillance; the key is to identify those with indolent disease accurately. Further studies using molecular biomarkers and MRI to select these patients are warranted.

Once patients have been selected for surveillance, a host of research questions present themselves.

4. What interventions (diet, exercise, micronutrients, pharmacologic agents) are warranted to reduce the risk of biological progression. This area is a fruitful and important area for research. Many studies are ongoing evaluating the role of exercise, dietary modification, and naturally occurring micronutrients in men on surveillance. These patients are followed for many years, and they are motivated; a great deal of evidence suggests that prostate cancer progression is amenable to modification by dietary or other influences. Specific questions include the role of exercise; weight loss; reduction of animal protein or carbohydrate in the diet; and the use of natural dietary micronutrients, including pomegranate, capsaicin, lycopene, and so forth. A host of other compounds have been suggested as being useful in the surveillance setting, so-called holistic surveillance.[60]

There is also a great deal of interest in the use of common drugs with metabolic or cardiovascular benefits, particularly statins and diabetic medications, that is, metformin. Clinical intervention trials testing these agents are warranted.

5. What is the most efficient and cost-effective way to follow patients longitudinally? Is serial biopsy still required and in whom? Can risk stratification allow some patients to minimize the burden of follow-up? This query is both a quality-of-life and economic question. An unmet need in the field is excessive reliance on serial biopsy. Can MRI, if negative, replace systematic biopsy; can targeted biopsy alone (ie, 2–4 cores) replace the 12 to 14 core systematic approach? Can patients with a negative molecular biomarker avoid or reduce the frequency of biopsies? Is the NPV of a negative MRI sufficiently high that a biopsy can be safely avoided; how does the NPV vary according to patient risk? Aside from discontinuing surveillance because of short life expectancy, are there patients whose disease is so predictably indolent that no further follow-up is required despite a 15- to 20-year life expectancy? How do we identify these?

Many national policy groups have recommended against PSA screening, largely because of the risks of overdetection and overtreatment. Can the widespread adoption of surveillance for low-risk disease rehabilitate prostate cancer screening and satisfy policy makers and methodologists that the benefits outweigh the risks at an acceptable cost? This question will require modeling studies based on recent data.

In summary, research is warranted at the molecular, epigenetic, epidemiologic, radiologic, and clinical trial levels.

SUMMARY

AS is an appealing approach for men diagnosed with low-risk prostate cancer and is a compelling antidote to the overtreatment problem. Multiparametric MRI and genetic biomarkers should reduce the need for serial systematic biopsies and improve the early identification of occult higher-risk disease and prediction of patients destined to have grade progression over time. All surveillance patients should have a confirmatory biopsy targeting the anterolateral horn and anterior prostate within 6 to 12 months. Subsequent biopsies should be done at 3- to 5-year intervals. Going forward, it is plausible that men with a negative MRI who are otherwise stable and at low risk for higher-grade disease may be followed safely with serial imaging in lieu of biopsy. Clinical trials evaluating this strategy are currently ongoing. PSA should be performed every 6 months until patients are no longer candidates for definitive therapy.

Approximately one-quarter of men will eventually be upgraded, and treatment should be offered for most patients with upgraded disease. The outcome in patients managed in this way is very favorable. The risk of prostate cancer mortality is approximately 3% at 15 years, and this should drop further with the incorporation of the enhanced detection techniques described in this article.

REFERENCES

1. Available at: http://www.uspreventiveservicestaskforce.org/uspstf12/prostate/prostateart.htm. Accessed August 29, 2017.
2. NEW USPSTF recommendation. Available at: https://www.uspreventiveservicestaskforce.org/Page/Document/RecommendationStatementFinal/prostate-cancer-screening. Accessed August 28, 2017.
3. Sakr WA, Grignon DJ, Crissman JD, et al. High grade prostatic intraepithelial neoplasia (HGPIN) and prostatic adenocarcinoma between the ages of 20-69: an autopsy study of 249 cases. In Vivo 1994;8(3):439–43.
4. Zlotta AR, Egawa S, Pushkar D, et al. Prevalence of prostate cancer on autopsy: cross-sectional study on unscreened Caucasian and Asian men. J Natl Cancer Inst 2013;105(14):1050–8.

5. Ahmed H, Emberton M. Do low-grade and low-volume prostate cancers bear the hallmarks of malignancy? Lancet Oncol 2012;13(11):e509–17. http://dx.doi.org/10.1016/S1470-2045(12)70388-1.

6. Hanahan D, Weinberg RA. Hallmarks of cancer: the next generation. Cell 2011;144(5):646–74.

7. Ross AE, Marchionni L, Vuica-Ross M, et al. Gene expression pathways of high grade localized prostate cancer. Prostate 2011;71:1568–77.

8. Skacel M, Ormsby AH, Pettay JD, et al. Aneusomy of chromosomes 7, 8, and 17 and amplification of HER-2/neu and epidermal growth factor receptor in Gleason score 7 prostate carcinoma: a differential fluorescent in situ hybridization study of Gleason pattern 3 and 4 using tissue microarray. Hum Pathol 2001;32:1392–7.

9. Susaki E, Nakayama KI. Multiple mechanisms for p27(Kip1) translocation and degradation. Cell Cycle 2007;6:3015–20.

10. Padar A, Sathyanarayana UG, Suzuki M, et al. Inactivation of cyclin D2 gene in prostate cancers by aberrant promoter methylation. Clin Cancer Res 2003;9:4730–4.

11. Guo Y, Sklar GN, Borkowski A, et al. Loss of the cyclin-dependent kinase inhibitor p27(Kip1) protein in human prostate cancer correlates with tumor grade. Clin Cancer Res 1997;3:2269–74.

12. True L, Coleman I, Hawley S, et al. A molecular correlate to the Gleason grading system for prostate adenocarcinoma. Proc Natl Acad Sci U S A 2006;103:10991–6.

13. Fleischmann A, Huland H, Mirlacher M, et al. Prognostic relevance of Bcl-2 overexpression in surgically treated prostate cancer is not caused by increased copy number or translocation of the gene. Prostate 2012;72:991–7.

14. Tomlins SA, Mehra R, Rhodes DR, et al. Integrative molecular concept modeling of prostate cancer progression. Nat Genet 2007;39:41–51.

15. Hendriksen PJ, Dits NF, Kokame K, et al. Evolution of the androgen receptor pathway during progression of prostate cancer. Cancer Res 2006;66:5012–20.

16. Bismar TA, Dolph M, Teng LH, et al. ERG protein expression reflects hormonal treatment response and is associated with Gleason score and prostate cancer specific mortality. Eur J Cancer 2012;48:538–46.

17. Furusato B, Gao CL, Ravindranath L, et al. Mapping of TMPRSS2-ERG fusions in the context of multifocal prostate cancer. Mod Pathol 2008;21:67–75.

18. Wang J, Cai Y, Ren C, et al. Expression of variant TMPRSS2/ERG fusion messenger RNAs is associated with aggressive prostate cancer. Cancer Res 2006;66:8347–51.

19. West AF, O'Donnell M, Charlton RG, et al. Correlation of vascular endothelial growth factor expression with fibroblast growth factor-8 expression and clinico-pathologic parameters in human prostate cancer. Br J Cancer 2001;85:576–83.

20. Erbersdobler A, Isbarn H, Dix K, et al. Prognostic value of microvessel density in prostate cancer: a tissue microarray study. World J Urol 2010;28:687–92.

21. Trock B, Fedor H, Gurel B, et al. PTEN loss and chromosome 8 alterations in Gleason grade 3 cores predicts the presence of un-sampled grade 4 tumor: implications for AS. Mod Pathol 2016;29(7):764–71.

22. Zomer A. Implications of extracellular vesicle (EV) transfer on cellular heterogeneity in cancer. Cancer Res 2016;76(8):2071–5.

23. Ross HM, Kryvenko ON, Cowan JE, et al. Do adenocarcinomas of the prostate with Gleason score (GS) ≤6 have the potential to metastasize to lymph nodes? Am J Surg Pathol 2012;36(9):1346–52.

24. Eggener S, Scardino P, Walsh P, et al. 20 year prostate cancer specific mortality after radical prostatectomy. J Urol 2011;185(3):869–75.

25. Inoue LY, Trock BJ, Partin AW, et al. Modeling grade progression in an active surveillance study. Stat Med 2014;33(6):930–9.

26. Vargas HA, Akin O, Afaq A, et al. Magnetic resonance imaging for predicting prostate biopsy findings in patients considered for active surveillance of clinically low risk prostate cancer. J Urol 2012;188(5):1732–8.

27. Ahmed HU, El-Shater Bosaily A, Brown LC, et al, PROMIS Study Group. Diagnostic accuracy of multi-parametric MRI and TRUS biopsy in prostate cancer (PROMIS): a paired validating confirmatory study. Lancet 2017;389(10071):815–22.

28. Simone G, Papalia R, Altobelli A, et al. MRI based nomogram predicting the probability of diagnosing a clinically significant prostate cancer with MRI-US fusion biopsy. J Urol 2017;197(4):e22–3.

29. Klein EA, Yousefi K, Haddad Z, et al. A genomic classifier improves prediction of metastatic disease within 5 years after surgery in node-negative high-risk prostate cancer patients managed by radical prostatectomy without adjuvant therapy. Eur Urol 2015;67:778.

30. Freedland SJ, Choeurng V, Howard L, et al. Utilization of a genomic classifier for prediction of metastasis following salvage radiation therapy after radical prostatectomy. Eur Urol 2016;70(4):588–96.

31. Klein EA, Cooperberg MR, Magi-Galluzzi C, et al. A 17-gene assay to predict prostate cancer aggressiveness in the context of Gleason grade heterogeneity, tumor multifocality, and biopsy undersampling. Eur Urol 2014;66:550.

32. Cullen J, Rosner IL, Brand TC, et al. A biopsy-based 17-gene genomic prostate score predicts recurrence after radical prostatectomy and adverse surgical pathology in a racially diverse population of

men with clinically low- and intermediate-risk prostate cancer. Eur Urol 2015;68:123.

33. Ross AE, Johnson MH, Yousefi K, et al. Tissue-based genomics augments post-prostatectomy risk stratification in a natural history cohort of intermediate- and high-risk men. Eur Urol 2016;69:157.

34. Brand TC, Zhang N, Crager MR, et al. Patient-specific meta-analysis of 2 clinical validation studies to predict pathologic outcomes in prostate cancer using the 17-gene genomic prostate score. Urology 2016;89:69.

35. Cuzick J, Berney DM, Fisher G, et al. Prognostic value of a cell cycle progression signature for prostate cancer death in a conservatively managed needle biopsy cohort. Br J Cancer 2012;106:1095.

36. Cuzick J, Stone S, Fisher G, et al. Validation of an RNA cell cycle progression score for predicting death from prostate cancer in a conservatively managed needle biopsy cohort. Br J Cancer 2015;113:382.

37. Bishoff JT, Freedland SJ, Gerber L, et al. Prognostic utility of the cell cycle progression score generated from biopsy in men treated with prostatectomy. J Urol 2014;192:409.

38. Klotz L, Vesprini D, Sethukavalan P, et al. Long-term follow-up of a large active surveillance cohort of patients with prostate cancer. J Clin Oncol 2015;33(3):272–7.

39. Steineck G, Helgesen F, Adolfsson J, et al, Scandinavian Prostatic Cancer Group Study Number 4. Quality of life after radical prostatectomy or watchful waiting. N Engl J Med 2002;347(11):790–6.

40. Dall'Era MA, Konety BR, Cowan JE, et al. Active surveillance for the management of prostate cancer in a contemporary cohort. Cancer 2008;112(12):2664–70.

41. Bul M, Zhu X, Valdagni R, et al. Active surveillance for low-risk prostate cancer worldwide: the PRIAS study. Eur Urol 2013;63:597.

42. Soloway MS, Soloway CT, Williams S, et al. Active surveillance; a reasonable management alternative for patients with prostate cancer: the Miami experience. BJU Int 2008;101(2):165–9.

43. Tosoian JJ, Mamawala M, Epstein JI, et al. Intermediate and longer-term outcomes from a prospective active-surveillance program for favorable-risk prostate cancer. J Clin Oncol 2015;33(30):3379–85.

44. Selvadurai ED, Singhera M, Thomas K, et al. Medium-term outcomes of active surveillance for localised prostate cancer. Eur Urol 2013;64(6):981–7.

45. Khatami A, Hugusson PSA. DT and surveillance. Int J Cancer 2006;120:170–4.

46. Roemeling S, Roobol MJ, de Vries SH, et al. Active surveillance for prostate cancers detected in three subsequent rounds of a screening trial: characteristics, PSA doubling times, and outcome. Eur Urol 2007;51(5):1244–50.

47. Patel MI, DeConcini DT, Lopez-Corona E, et al. An analysis of men with clinically localized prostate cancer who deferred definitive therapy. J Urol 2004;171(4):1520–4.

48. Kovac E, Lieser G, Elshafei A, et al. Outcomes of active surveillance after initial surveillance prostate biopsy. J Urol 2017;197(1):84–9.

49. Popiolek M, Rider JR, Andrén O, et al. Johansson JE natural history of early, localized prostate cancer: a final report from three decades of follow-up. Eur Urol 2013;63(3):428–35.

50. Yamamoto T, Musunuru B, Vesprini D, et al. Metastatic prostate cancer in men initially treated with active surveillance. J Urol 2016;195(5):1409–14.

51. Musunuru HB, Yamamoto T, Klotz L, et al. Active surveillance for intermediate risk prostate cancer: survival outcomes in the Sunnybrook experience. J Urol 2016;196(6):1651–8.

52. Hamdy FC, Donovan JL, Lane JA, ProtecTStudy Group. 10-year outcomes after monitoring, surgery, or radiotherapy for localized prostate cancer. N Engl J Med 2016;375(15):1415–24.

53. Donovan JL, Hamdy FC, Lane JA, et al, ProtecT Study Group. Patient-reported outcomes after monitoring, surgery, or radiotherapy for prostate cancer. N Engl J Med 2016;375(15):1425–37.

54. Vickers A. Systematic review of pretreatment PSA velocity and doubling time as PCA predictors. J Clin Oncol 2008;27:398–403.

55. Loblaw A, Zhang L, Lam A, et al. Comparing prostate specific antigen triggers for intervention in men with stable prostate cancer on active surveillance. J Urol 2010;184(5):1942–6.

56. Morash C, Tey R, Agbassi C, et al. Active surveillance for the management of localized prostate cancer: guideline recommendations. Can Urol Assoc J 2015;9(5–6):171–8.

57. Chen RC, Rumble RB, Loblaw DA, et al. Active surveillance for the management of localized prostate cancer (cancer care Ontario guideline): American Society of Clinical Oncology clinical practice guideline endorsement. J Clin Oncol 2016;34(18):2182–90.

58. NICE. National Collaborating Centre for Cancer. Prostate cancer: diagnosis and treatment. Clinical guideline. Available at: http://www.nice.org.uk.myaccess.library.utoronto.ca/nicemedia/live/14348/66232/66232.pdf. Accessed August 30, 2017.

59. Available at: http://www.auanet.org/guidelines/clinically-localized-prostate-cancer-new-(aua/astro/suo-guideline-2017).

60. Berg CJ, Habibian DJ, Katz AE, et al. Active 'holistic' surveillance. J Nutr Metab 2016;2016:2917065.

Focal Ablation of Early-Stage Prostate Cancer
Candidate Selection, Treatment Guidance, and Assessment of Outcome

Eric Edison, MA(Cantab), MBBS, MRCS[a],*,
Taimur Tariq Shah, MBBS, BSc, MRCS[b,c],
Hashim U. Ahmed, BM, BCh, MA, PhD, FRCS(Urol)[d,e]

KEYWORDS

- Prostate cancer • High-intensity focused ultrasound ablation • Cryotherapy • Laser therapy
- Photodynamic therapy

KEY POINTS

- Despite the multifocality of prostate cancer, there is evidence that lesions smaller than 0.5 m³, or Gleason pattern 3 or less, have a low potential for clinical progression.
- Clinically significant disease is, therefore, often limited to a single index lesion. Focal ablation offers the option to target this index lesion, maintain oncological control, and minimize complications by the preservation of the healthy gland.
- Candidates are selected using template mapping or multiparametric MRI targeted biopsies to identify appropriate index lesions.
- Multiple energy modalities have been tested, including high-intensity frequency ultrasound, cryoablation, laser ablation, photodynamic therapy, focal brachytherapy, radiofrequency ablation, and irreversible electroporation.
- Outcome is assessed by "for cause" biopsy of the ablated area, triggered by prostate-specific antigen measurements or MRI or performed per protocol at 12 months.

INTRODUCTION

Treatment of prostate cancer currently relies on either active surveillance in low-risk disease or strategies that target the whole gland, such as radical prostatectomy or radiotherapy in intermediate-risk to high-risk disease. A limitation of whole-gland treatments has been the risk of genitourinary adverse events related to neurovascular, external urinary sphincter, or bowel or bladder injury. Some have described this approach to be akin to "using a sledgehammer to kill a flea."[1] The necessity to treat the whole organ can be attributed to 2 main issues. First, diagnostic techniques have not previously been accurate enough to localize lesions. Random transrectal ultrasound biopsy techniques (TRUS) do not allow for reliable localization of lesions.[2] In

[a] Department of Urology, Kingston Hospital, Galsworthy Road, Kingston upon Thames, Surrey KT2 7QB, UK; [b] Division of Surgery and Interventional Science, University College London, 21 University Street, London WC1E 6AU, UK; [c] Department of Urology, Whittington Hospitals NHS Trust, Magdala Avenue, London N19 5NF, UK; [d] Division of Surgery, Department of Surgery and Cancer, Imperial College London, South Kensington Campus, London SW7 2AZ, UK; [e] Imperial Urology, Imperial College Healthcare NHS Trust, Fulham Palace Road, London W6 8RF, UK
* Corresponding author.
E-mail address: eric.edison@doctors.org.uk

Urol Clin N Am 44 (2017) 575–585
http://dx.doi.org/10.1016/j.ucl.2017.07.006
0094-0143/17/© 2017 Elsevier Inc. All rights reserved.

addition, imaging until recently had not been able to detect or localize significant lesions reliably.[3] Recent advances in diagnostics, however, with increased used of multiparametric (mp) MRI and targeted biopsies have allowed accurate localization of significant lesions. Second, a common criticism has been that prostate cancer is known to be a multifocal process.[4] It seems, however, that the multifocality is commonly related to secondary lesions that are small and low grade, particularly evident in postmortem studies, cystoprostatectomy, or prostatectomy series.[5] Within this multifocal landscape there is evidence that in many men an index lesion, the largest and highest grade, is the likely key driver of clinical disease progression. Thus, focal index lesion ablation can potentially halt or perhaps delay disease progression without the need for whole-gland treatment.[6] Third, there has been no widely accepted treatment modality that have been fully validated for focal ablation of prostate cancer. Multiple energy modalities have been tested including high-intensity frequency ultrasound (HIFU), cryoablation, interstitial laser ablation, photodynamic therapy (PDT), focal brachytherapy, radiofrequency ablation (RFA), and irreversible electroporation (IRE). With long-term data now available for large focal therapy series and prospective trials, including a randomized controlled trial (RCT),[7,8] there is now a large body of evidence supporting this treatment strategy.

The development of focal ablation has been driven by its significantly lower side-effect profile (erectile, urinary, and bowel dysfunction) compared with radical whole-gland surgery or radiation. In addition, it is a minimally invasive procedure performed in a day-case setting with many returning to normal activities within a few days rather than weeks during or after radical therapy.

CANDIDATE SELECTION

The basis for focal ablation relies on the following premises: candidates for focal ablation have a clinically significant index lesion; there may be other insignificant out-of-field lesions; tests can accurately identify the index lesion; and an appropriate energy modality is used to target and ablate the index lesion effectively and safely for a specific tumor in a particular individual.

The Index Lesion

There is growing acceptance of the index lesion theory of prostate cancer. Prostate specimens often demonstrate multifocal lesions[4] but there is evidence that small and low-grade lesions are clinically insignificant. In vitro studies demonstrate

that low-grade lesions (Gleason pattern 3) do not bear the hallmarks of malignancy: self-sufficiency in growth signals, insensitivity to antigrowth signals, resistance to apoptosis, unlimited replicative potential, sustained angiogenesis, and, most importantly, tissue invasion and metastasis.[9] This is borne out with clinical data from large series, which show that true Gleason score 6 (3 + 3) does not have metastatic potential, with lack of lymph node metastases in men with pure Gleason 6 disease on radical prostatectomy specimens[10] and a 0% mortality in 9772 patients 15 years after radical prostatectomy.[11]

Small lesions (<0.5 cm^3) are also common, can be considered incidental, and are unlikely to develop into significant disease. A cystoprostatectomy series performed for bladder cancer demonstrated incidental lesions in 30% of prostates, with multifocality in 60% of these. None of these lesions was grade 4 or 5, and 90% were less than 0.5 cm^3.[5] In a series of patients with radical prostatectomy performed for prostate cancer, the presence of tumors less than 0.5 cm^3 did not contribute to the rate of disease recurrence. The size and grade of the index tumor, however, did correlate significantly with the rate of recurrence.[12] Stamey and colleagues[13] demonstrated that all lesions that may have developed into clinically significant prostate cancer were greater than 0.5 cm^3. This gave rise to the Epstein criteria for clinically insignificant prostate cancer: an organ-confined (pT2) cancer, less than 0.5 cm^3, Gleason score less than or equal to 6, and lacking any Gleason grade 4 or 5 component.[14] A later study has suggested this cutoff may be too stringent. This suggests that a minimum threshold of 1.3 cm^3 can be taken, if stage and grade are taken into account.

Altogether, these data suggest that candidates for focal therapy and any active treatment should be selected with a minimum lesion size of 0.5 cm^3 and a Gleason score of greater than or equal to 7. There are less clear data to support a maximum size for lesions to be ablated, although a significant, functional proportion of tissue must remain for any therapy to be considered focal ablation. Early studies often used hemiablation, although this has been refined in many later studies.[7] An international task force review in 2007 recommended maximum lesion diameter of 12 mm.[15] The same task force also recommended no Gleason 4 or 5 disease should be treated with focal therapy. That recommendation is now 10 years old and may reflect a tentative approach to the early experimental status of ablative technology at that point. University of Chicago Medicine has extended the criteria to Gleason score 6 or 7.[16] This in the authors' opinion is also too conservative because results from the PROTECT and PIVOT studies show that low-risk Gleason 6 disease should not routinely be offered active treatment whether that be focal therapy or an alternative whole-gland treatment. Valerio and colleagues[7] argue a similar viewpoint, that to be of value, focal ablation should target clinically significant lesions only. Given these data, it could be suggested that the minimum criteria should be an index lesion greater than 0.5 cm^3 and Gleason grade 4 or more with clinically insignificant disease left untreated.

The boundaries could once again change. More recent data assessing the percentage pattern 4 component of cancerous lesions show that low-volume Gleason 4 disease may have a low rate of progression. The 5-year progression-free survival for lesions with 1% to 20% pattern 4 was 84% compared with 99% for Gleason 3 + 3 and between 32% and 66% for those with Gleason 4 component of greater than 50%. The data suggest that this cohort of low pattern 4 may be suitable for active surveillance.[17]

Diagnostic Strategies

With minimum criteria for focal ablation established, the next step is to delineate diagnostic strategies to select appropriate candidates. The somewhat random nature of conventional TRUS biopsy negates effective localization of lesions, which is one reason for the current reliance on therapies that destroy the whole gland.[9] TRUS biopsy has been shown to miss up to 50% of tumors and underestimate and under-stage disease in up to 70%. In contrast, template mapping biopsies (TPMs) detect 95% of tumors of 0.5 mL or greater compared with radical prostatectomy specimens.[18] Mapping biopsies are clearly not feasible in all and confer significant morbidity.

The development of mpMRI means that imaging can now be used in the noninvasive diagnosis of significant tumors. Although mpMRI detects only 70% of all tumors, not all of these are clinically significant.[3] Lesions greater than or equal to 0.5 cm^3 can be seen on mpMRI with a sensitivity of 90% and specificity of 88%,[19] and MRI is almost equivalent to transperineal saturation biopsies.[20] The index tumor, confirmed histologically on radical prostatectomy sections, is correctly identified in 92% of cases.[3] Data from the PROMIS (Prostate MRI Imaging Study), where 576 men underwent an mpMRI, TRUS, and 5-mm TPMs, found cancer in (71%) of 576 men on TPM, 56% of these clinically significant. For clinically significant cancer, mpMRI had a sensitivity of 93% compared with 48% for TRUS.[2] A subsequent meta-analysis by

Moldovan and colleagues[21] confirmed the utility of mpMRI with a negative predictive value (NPV) of 88.1% for clinically significant cancer. Furthermore, MRI can be augmented with MRI-TRUS fusion techniques.[22] Siddiqui and colleagues[23] performed transrectal MRI fusion biopsies in 1034 of 125 men assessed for possible prostate cancer and showed that targeted biopsy diagnosed 30% more high-risk and 17% less low-risk cancers compared with TRUS biopsy.

TPM or MRI-targeted biopsy is now recommended for all patients undergoing focal therapy by National Institute for Health and Clinical Excellence,[24] and the European Association of Urology.[25] An international consensus panel also deems mpMRI a satisfactory diagnostic tool for clinically significant focal prostate cancer, although it recognizes that studies to date are in experienced centers. To account for this, it is recommended that 2 experienced radiologists, separately and blinded, report on the images. To be experienced, they suggest a radiologist should have reported at least 50 MRIs under supervision, although they acknowledge this is somewhat arbitrary. Suspicious lesions seen on mpMRI must be biopsied.[26] A European consensus meeting suggests that mpMRI combined with intensive sampling results in an NPV of 90% to 95%.[27]

Contraindications to Focal Ablation

Appropriate candidates should have a clinically significant lesion and are selected using a combination of mpMRI and biopsy. In cases with discordance between mpMRI and biopsy results, image-directed therapy is inadequate for focal ablation.[16] Relative contraindications to focal ablation include any condition that would make accurate diagnosis or treatment delivery ineffective or unsafe. Patients with metalwork, including a pacemaker or MRI-unsafe surgical clips, are not able to undergo mpMRI. Furthermore, patients with conditions, such as significant kidney disease or allergy to contrast, are not able to tolerate the contrast required for the high-quality mpMRI. In these patients, focal ablation may be offered, however, require TPM.[28]

Focal ablation is also only appropriate when there is no ambiguity over the index lesion. A consensus conference organized by the International Society of Urological Pathology deems that the index tumor should be defined according to the following order of priority: extraprostatic extension, then Gleason score, then tumor volume.[29] Most of the time the index lesion is unambiguous, given that high-grade and large (>0.5 cm^3) satellite lesions are rare.[5] This definition of index lesion means, however, that occasionally a situation may arise when a smaller tumor with high Gleason score is defined as the index lesion or a situation where 2 distinct significant lesions are detected. Given that both lesions may be considered clinically significant, this constitutes true biologically relevant multifocal disease. This may occur in approximately 10% of patients: 1 series validating the use of mpMRI demonstrates that in 1 patient a secondary true-positive tumor was designated the index tumor, which would have misled focal therapy (**Figs. 1** and **2**[3]). The Gleason score of these tumors was always identical to those of the corresponding true index tumors. Thus, it is important to biopsy all possible significant lesions, and take into account both the imaging and the biopsy results to identify and exclude true multifocal disease. Unless the lesions are in proximity, focal ablation per se is not appropriate; however, in selected cases, bilateral focal ablation might be possible. mpMRI can also identify features of the index lesion that contraindicate focal treatment, including macroscopic extracapsular extension and extensive tumor involving more than half of the gland.[30] Traditionally clinical practice dictates that there may be little benefit in focal prostatic ablation in metastatic disease. There is a growing body of evidence, however, that treatment of the primary disease even in the presence of metastases may improve survival and focal ablation itself may also promote an antitumor immune response.[31–34] Such a strategy is under investigation.[35]

TREATMENT GUIDANCE

A majority of evidence for the 7 modalities of focal therapy consists of early-phase studies up to stage 2b[7] and more recently an RCT.[8] Many of the earlier studies and the RCT included patients with clinically insignificant disease with a focus on feasibility, safety, and functional outcomes. Given that high-quality evidence shows that early prostate cancer can be safely managed with active surveillance and that feasibility and safety has now been established, treatment should be offered to men with clinically significant disease. Future phase II/III trials should also target this population. There are well-established difficulties with performing and reporting interventional studies incorporating surgical procedures, especially RCTs.[36] In particular with regard to focal therapy, trials have failed at the recruitment stage because of a combination of a lack of clinician equipoise and lack of patient equipoise leading to an unwillingness to be randomised.[37] The Partial Prostate Ablation versus Radical Prostatectomy study is a feasibility study comparing focal ablation and radical prostatectomy in men with intermediate-risk unilateral prostate cancer.[38] Its main aim is to assess the feasibility of an RCT in this setting with the primary objective to recruit more than 50% eligible men. If this fails, novel approaches might be required. There are alternative approaches to randomization, such as a cohort-embedded multiple RCT or preference-based randomizations.[7,39] Equally, a pragmatic approach may be to consider other trial designs, such as

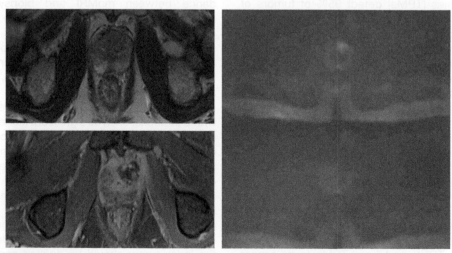

Fig. 1. Prefocal and postfocal cryotherapy mpMRI. A 64-year-old man, PSA = 6.12, anterior Gleason 3 + 4. (*Top left*) Preoperative T2-weighted image – low T2 signal in the left anterior region. (*Top right*) Preoperative B1400 diffusion-weighted image – restricted diffusion in the left anterior region. (*Bottom left*) One month postcryotherapy T1 dynamic contrast-enhanced image – left anterior focal necrosis can be seen. (*Bottom right*) One year postcryotherapy, B1400 diffusion-weighted image – showing resolution of the left anterior tumor.

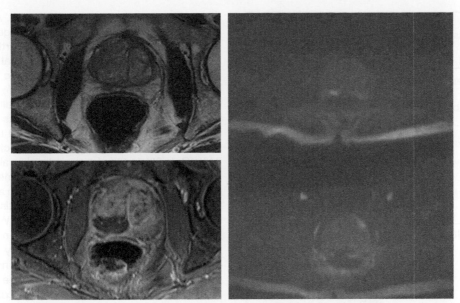

Fig. 2. Prefocal and postfocal HIFU mpMRI. A 76-year-old man, PSA = 6.67, posterior Gleason 4 + 3. (*Top left*) Preoperative T2-weighted image – low T2 signal in the right posterior peripheral zone. (*Top right*) Preoperative B1400 diffusion-weighted image – restricted diffusion in the right posterior peripheral zone. (*Bottom left*) One month post-HIFU T1 dynamic contrast-enhanced image – right posterior peripheral zone focal necrosis can be seen. (*Bottom right*) One year post-HIFU B1400 diffusion-weighted image – showing resolution of the right posterior peripheral zone.

patient preference trials and parallel prospective cohort studies.[40]

Treatment Modalities

All modalities can be delivered through transperineal needles, except HIFU, which is delivered though the urethra or rectum. Laser fibers can also be introduced transrectally. HIFU destroys tissue by heating it to over 60°C combined with cavitation effects. The transurethral approach uses in-bore guidance whereas the transrectal approach uses MRI–TRUS fusion. Cryotherapy induces extreme cold temperatures to less than −40° centigrade and below which causes ablation via several mechanisms that induce necrosis, apoptosis, and an immune response. Laser therapy is another form of direct thermal energy. In a phase I trial, magnetic resonance thermometry and secondary thermal probes positioned in the prostate were used to ensure that a dangerous amount of heat was not transmitted to surrounding areas.[41] PDT uses a drug activated by laser light to release a burst of reactive oxygen species to damage local tissue. The drug is administered intravenously and the laser fibers are inserted through the perineum.[8] Focal brachytherapy is an evolution of an already established therapy. The sealed seeds are inserted through the perineum, but only part of the prostate is irradiated, and no external beam radiation is used. Studies are ongoing in focal brachytherapy. IRE uses high-voltage electric current to create permanent nanopores in cells within a small, controlled radius. Electroneedles are inserted through the perineum.[42] RFA is another thermal modality, using alternating current. Only 1 phase I study in 15 men has been published to date for RFA, although others are in progress.

Technical refinement of modalities will progress with time. There are different patterns of ablation that can be used, such as hemiablation, hockey stick, zonal, and targeted focal (**Tables 1** and **2**). Many early studies used hemiablation but later studies have tended to target the index lesion more closely as centers develop more experience with modalities.[7] For example, recent work has described the physical effects of cryotherapy, enabling further refinement of technique. It has been demonstrated that cryoneedles develop a central core of less than or equal to 40°C to a radius of approximately 1 cm, necessitating placement between 1 cm and 1.5 cm apart to reliably maintain temperature less than or equal to 40°C.[43]

Clinical outcomes have been promising. Valerio and colleagues[7] reviewed 37 studies with 3230 patients undergoing focal therapy. The rate of significant cancer at control biopsy varied between

Table 1
Methods of focal ablation

Method	Diagram
Targetted focal ablation	
Hemiablation	
Posterior hockey stick	
Anterior hockey stick	

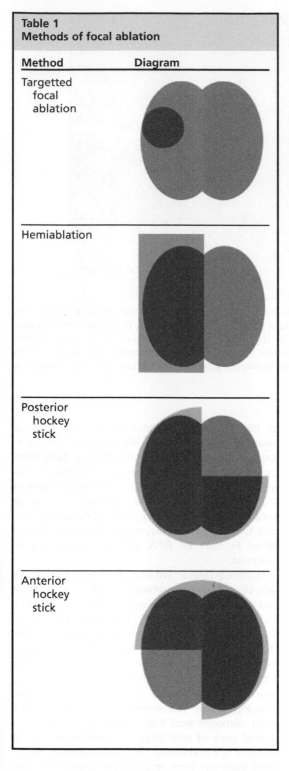

multiple centers in the United Kingdom. At a median follow-up of 56 (interquartile range 33–70) months, overall retreatment rate with further focal therapy was 20%, 7% transition to radical therapy, and 1% onto focal therapy to systemic therapy. The metastasis-free survival was 97%, cancer-specific survival was 100% and overall-survival was 99%. The rate of incontinence was 3% and erectile dysfunction 16% rate (any pad use) was 97% and preservation of erectile function was 84%. Only 2% to 3% developed a clinically significant recurrence outside of the treatment field, which adds credence to the index lesion and focal therapy strategy of leaving untreated tissue and cancers on surveillance.[44] Previously, Ward and Jones[45] had presented data on 1160 men from the US Cryo On-Line Database registry on focal cryotherapy. They also showed promising results with a 3-year biochemical disease-free survival rate of 75.7% at 3 years. The pad-free continence rate was 98.4% and there was preservation of erectile function in 58.1%. Rectourethral fistula occurred in only 1 patient.[45] The only RCT on focal therapy randomized 413 men with low-risk cancer to either active surveillance or focal vascular target PDT. After a median follow-up of 24 months, 58% of men had disease progression in the AS arm versus 28% in the vascular target PDT arm.[8] With the body of evidence now supporting active surveillance in low-risk disease, in the authors' opinion the cohort of presented in this study do not form ideal candidates for focal therapy. This limitation of the study can be attributed to the time period within which it was conceived and that patients were recruited between 2011 and 2013.

Further refinement of treatment may include the use of immunomodulatory adjuvants. The benefit conferred by focal ablation may come not only from the contemporaneous destruction of tissue but also by the activation of the immune system and ongoing effects once the energy source is removed. For example, antibodies may develop against the targeted tissue after cryotherapy.[31] Early work in animal models demonstrates that adjuncts, such as monoclonal antibodies, may boost this immune activation and may eventually be used in clinical practice.[32]

ASSESSMENT OF OUTCOME

The assessment of outcome in studies to date has been heterogeneous and inconsistent. A recent meta-analysis shows that studies to date measure outcome according to negative biopsy rate and/or avoidance of other local treatments.[7] Valerio and colleagues[7] point out the discordance in methods

0% and 13.4%. Incontinence rate was 0% to 16.7% and erectile dysfunction occurred in 0% to 18.5%. The authors' group recently presented data from 625 men undergoing focal HIFU largely for intermediate-risk disease (81%) across

Table 2
Summary of recommendations for diagnosis and follow-up

Diagnosis and candidate selection	A clinically significant index lesion is at least 0.5 cm³ (maximum cancer core length ≥6 mm) or any sized lesion that has Gleason pattern 4 or more. These should be targeted for focal ablation.
	mpMRI can be used to diagnose clinically significant focal prostate cancer. These must have 2 separated blinded reports from experience radiologists. Suspicious lesions on MRI must be biopsied.
	TPM or MRI-targeted biopsy is recommended for all patients undergoing focal therapy.
Treatment guidance	Targeted focal ablation, hemiablation, or hockey stick pattern ablation may be used.
	Smaller lesions are often present. Lesions that are not clinically significant should not be targeted.
Follow-up and assessment of outcomes	Disease recurrence is assessed with prostate biopsy, triggered by either a rising prostate-specific antigen, suspicious MRI, or performed at 1 year as part of an agreed protocol.
	Biopsy should use 4–6 targeted cores from the margins of the ablation zone, including at least 1 sample from within the area of ablated/fibrosed tissue.
	Follow-up MRI at 6–12 mo is recommended to identify failure or recurrence.
	Treatment strategies for patients with residual disease include active surveillance (low-volume low-risk), repeat focal therapy, or transition to whole-gland therapy.

to select and follow-up men may undermine the outcomes reported. For example, studies using systematic sampling at diagnosis may only use random sampling to diagnose local recurrence, which may lead to underdiagnosis. A recent international consensus meeting, however, has established a standard framework for the follow-up of focal ablation, which should enable more robust study design with less heterogeneous outcome measures.[46] The key outcomes are local treatment failure, which might be in-field or out-of-field. In-field treatment failure is the persistence of carcinoma in the treated area, detected on mpMRI and/or biopsy. Out-of-field disease denotes clinically significant cancer occurring anywhere in the gland outside of the original area and might be representative of progressive significant disease missed at baseline (staging error) or de no disease developing due to field effect changes in untreated tissues.[47] As with active surveillance in men diagnosed with low-risk disease, there is a need for stringent monitoring after focal ablation.

Biochemical Recurrence

Standard surveillance uses prostate-specific antigen (PSA) measurement. For example, successful radical prostatectomy is defined by PSA less than 0.2 ng/L. Successful radiotherapy cannot be reliably proved, however, with any specific nadir cutoff even though nadir level does correlate to outcomes.[48] Two criteria are validated to detect recurrence in radiation therapy. The Phoenix criteria rely on a rise of 2 ng/mL from the nadir.[49] The American Society for Radiation Oncology (ASTRO) criteria rely on 3 successive increases in PSA level to identify recurrence.[50] Many studies have used the Phoenix or ASTRO criteria to denote failure after focal therapy but it must be emphasized that these are not validated for modalities other than radiotherapy. Studies have demonstrated that when the Phoenix and ASTRO criteria are applied to the same series, different rates of recurrence are generated with Phoenix tending to generate a lower rate of recurrence.[51] The Phoenix criteria may be less sensitive in focal ablation because the nadir may have less relevance with the preservation of a large proportion of prostate tissue. Nevertheless, the index lesion does account for up to 80% of the PSA value.[52] One study demonstrated that the PSA nadir after whole-gland HIFU predicted biochemical recurrence, with 18.5% more patients having positive postprocedure biopsies when the PSA nadir was greater than 0.2.[53] However, this was not supported by Bahn and colleagues,[54] who showed a 70% drop in PSA, but did not find any difference in postprocedure recurrence. Similarly, there was no significant difference in PSA reduction between those with positive and negative follow-up biopsy after focal cryotherapy. In summary, PSA levels should be monitored as part of the follow-up after focal therapy but there is no consensus as to the expected drop after treatment and how specifically to diagnose recurrence. The different modalities may have different effects on the organ and, therefore, may have different patterns that need to be delineated with further research. In general a rising PSA should raise suspicions of recurrence and might guide the use of additional diagnostic tests.

Imaging

mpMRI should be used in follow-up as well as diagnosis. Specifically, dynamic contrast-enhanced MRI can reliably identify clinically significant lesions greater than 0.5 cm^3,[19] and it has similar sensitivity and specificity to serial PSA for detection of residual or recurrent disease.[55] An analysis of 118 pooled patient data from 3 prospective single-arm HIFU trials found, in 111 who underwent at least 1 postoperative biopsy, an overall positive biopsy rate of 37% with an MRI NPV of between 86% and 97% (depending on definition of clinically significant disease).[56] In a smaller cohort of 26 men Punwani and colleagues[55] demonstrated dynamic contrast-enhanced MRI to have sensitivity and specificity for disease recurrence after focal HIFU as high as 87% and 82%, respectively.

MRI has also been shown to have a high NPV for recurrence after cryotherapy, especially when combined with PSA nadir levels.[57]

Loss of T1-weighted (T1W) contrast enhancement on MRI is suggestive of successful ablation.[26] Conversely, soft tissue enhancement is suggestive of recurrence or failure but might also represent inflammation. A consensus meeting on the role of mpMRI in focal therapy has established that there must be a preoperative mpMRI to compare as baseline. This should ideally occur before biopsy but can take place 8 weeks after biopsy once the biopsy artifact has resolved. A follow-up mpMRI at 6 months to 12 months is recommended to identify failure or recurrence. Some investigators also suggest an mpMRI is performed immediately after ablation (<2 weeks) to predict or identify treatment failure, although this suggestion did not reach consensus and does not seem predictive of subsequent medium-term failure on biopsy.[56] As discussed previously, the radiologist must be experienced, with an arbitrary number of 50 previously supervised reports.[26] This is particularly important after treatment because there are a several changes that can occur to the tissue after treatment, including loss of zonal differentiation, thickening of the prostatic capsule, periprostatic fibrosis, and scarring. This may reflect the different tissue damage mechanisms and immune response profiles that different modalities can induce on the tissue, which then manifest on the mpMRI. After cryotherapy, heterogeneous enhancement intermixed with areas of necrosis and thickening of the prostatic capsule, urethra, and rectal wall are seen on T1W images.[58] After HIFU, ablated areas are nonenhancing hypointense regions on T1W images with 3-mm to 8-mm thick peripheral rims of enhancement that resolve within 3 months to 5 months.[59] PDT induces with areas of enhancement (viable tissue) interposed between nonenhancing low-signal-intensity regions (necrosis) on T1W images.[60] In summary, mpMRI can be used to identify recurrence and guide further diagnosis and treatment.[61]

Biopsy

Biopsies can either be protocol driven or for cause, triggered by rising PSA levels or suspicious MRI findings. There is lack of consensus about whether biopsy should be systematic or targeted. One consensus group comments that systematic biopsies are useful for surveillance of the untreated gland.[46] Conversely, it has been argued that performing biopsies of untreated areas is not assessing treatment success but rather the accuracy of preoperative assessment. In the authors' opinion, if a patient's disease has been accurately classified preoperatively, then follow-up can consist of biopsies targeted to the treated area alone and imaging for both in-field and out-of-field surveillance. Therefore, if protocol biopsies are performed, these should be aimed at determining initial treatment success and thus should be targeted at the treated lesion.[62] There is general consensus that if protocol biopsies are preformed, these should be carried out at 6 months to 12 months post-treatment[46,63,64] because inflammatory and fibrotic changes can resolve sufficiently as soon as 6 months after treatment to make biopsy and grading possible after HIFU.[65]

Special consideration is needed when biopsying the treated area. Muller and colleagues[46] state that the best way to take a biopsy of the treated area is to take 4 to 6 targeted cores from the margins of the ablation zone, including at least 1 sample from within the area of ablated/fibrosed tissue. These 4 to 6 cores from the treated area are essential to account for (1) fibrosis-related gland deformity and (2) the possible slight degree of misregistration even when using a fusion device. In general, MRI-targeted cognitive or fusion biopsies are better than systematic TRUS biopsy at identifying treatment failure due to more accurate sampling of the treated area.

The definition and significance of positive biopsy results also require careful consideration. Study results should be interpreted with caution because there is heterogeneity in the design and reporting of follow-up biopsies.[7] Tumor ablation may be incomplete, which may leave some viable residual disease.[15,19] The clinical significance of this, however, is unknown. There is no difference in disease progression with either whole-gland cryotherapy or radiotherapy.[21] It has also been shown from external beam radiotherapy that biopsies that are technically positive but show good treatment effect do not have significantly different outcomes.[39] There is lack of consensus whether residual low-grade and low-volume cancer is considered treatment failure.[63,64] As with initial diagnosis, however, small and low-grade residual disease is likely to be insignificant, although this presumption needs to be tested. Results from focal ablation series show that 25% of post-treatment biopsies may be positive. Where sufficient data were given to stratify positive biopsies into significant versus nonsignificant, however, only 15% of positive biopsies were deemed significant (Gleason >3, >2 positive).[62] Treatment of patients with positive results includes a period of active surveillance, repeat focal therapy, or whole-gland therapy.[62] Donaldson and colleagues[64] commented that overall retreatment rate should be below 20% because it was argued that retreatment was a positive attribute of the focal therapy strategy.

SUMMARY

Focal ablation of malignancy enables preservation of organ function and minimizes the risk of damage to nearby structures. Recent advances in pathology, imaging, and ablative technology have facilitated a demand for focal ablative technology for prostate cancer. Data suggest fewer significant complications compared with surgery or radiotherapy. Candidates with a clearly identified index lesion are identified with a combination of template, systematic, and/or MRI targeted biopsies. Significant lesions are those greater than 0.5 cm^3 and data suggest that only Gleason pattern 4 and 5 disease has metastatic potential. Treatment should be provided after appropriate training and with robust methods for collection of oncological and functional outcomes or within a defined study, which should ideally be phase II or III. Assessment of outcome is performed using a combination of PSA measurements, MRI, and biopsy.

REFERENCES

1. Gregory A. Prostate cancer breakthrough as new laser treatment destroys tumours with no side effects - mirror online, mirror newsp. 2016. Available at: http://www.mirror.co.uk/science/prostate-cancer-breakthrough-new-laser-8156194. Accessed March 28, 2017.
2. Ahmed HU, El-Shater Bosaily A, Brown LC, et al. Diagnostic accuracy of multi-parametric MRI and TRUS biopsy in prostate cancer (PROMIS): a paired validating confirmatory study. Lancet 2017; 389:815–22.
3. Rud E, Klotz D, Rennesund K, et al. Detection of the index tumour and tumour volume in prostate cancer using T2-weighted and diffusion-weighted magnetic resonance imaging (MRI) alone. BJU Int 2014;114: E32–42.
4. Djavan B, Susani M, Bursa B, et al. Predictability and significance of multifocal prostate cancer in the radical prostatectomy specimen. Tech Urol 1999;5: 139–42. Available at: http://www.ncbi.nlm.nih.gov/pubmed/10527256. Accessed March 20, 2017.
5. Nevoux P, Ouzzane A, Ahmed HU, et al. Quantitative tissue analyses of prostate cancer foci in an unselected cystoprostatectomy series. BJU Int 2012; 110:517–23.
6. Kasivisvanathan V, Emberton M, Ahmed HU. Focal therapy for prostate cancer: rationale and treatment opportunities. Clin Oncol (R Coll Radiol) 2013;25: 461–73.
7. Valerio M, Cerantola Y, Eggener SE, et al. New and established technology in focal ablation of the prostate: a systematic review. Eur Urol 2017; 71:17–34.
8. Azzouzi A-R, Vincendeau S, Barret E, et al. Padeliporfin vascular-targeted photodynamic therapy versus active surveillance in men with low-risk prostate cancer (CLIN1001 PCM301): an open-label, phase 3, randomised controlled trial. Lancet Oncol 2017;18:181–91.
9. Ahmed HU, Arya M, Freeman A, et al. Do low-grade and low-volume prostate cancers bear the hallmarks of malignancy? Lancet Oncol 2012;13:e509–17.
10. Diolombi ML, Epstein JI. Metastatic potential to regional lymph nodes with Gleason score ≤7, including tertiary pattern 5, at radical prostatectomy. BJU Int 2017;119(6):872–8.
11. Eggener SE, Scardino PT, Walsh PC, et al. Predicting 15-year prostate cancer specific mortality after radical prostatectomy. J Urol 2011;185:869–75.
12. Wise AM, Stamey TA, McNeal JE, et al. Morphologic and clinical significance of multifocal prostate cancers in radical prostatectomy specimens. Urology 2002;60:264–9. Available at: http://www.ncbi.nlm.nih.gov/pubmed/12137824. Accessed March 20, 2017.
13. Stamey TA, Freiha FS, McNeal JE, et al. Localized prostate cancer. Relationship of tumor volume to clinical significance for treatment of prostate cancer. Cancer 1993;71:933–8. Available at: http://www.ncbi.nlm.nih.gov/pubmed/7679045. Accessed March 20, 2017.

14. Epstein JI, Walsh PC, Carmichael M, et al. Pathologic and clinical findings to predict tumor extent of non-palpable (stage T1c) prostate cancer. JAMA 1994; 271:368–74. Available at: http://www.ncbi.nlm.nih.gov/pubmed/7506797. Accessed March 20, 2017.

15. Eggener SE, Scardino PT, Carroll PR, et al. Focal therapy for localized prostate cancer: a critical appraisal of rationale and modalities. J Urol 2007; 178:2260–7.

16. Eggener SE, Yousuf A, Watson S, et al. Phase II evaluation of magnetic resonance imaging guided focal laser ablation of prostate cancer. J Urol 2016;196: 1670–5.

17. Choy B, Pearce SM, Anderson BB, et al. Prognostic significance of percentage and architectural types of contemporary Gleason pattern 4 prostate cancer in radical prostatectomy. Am J Surg Pathol 2016;40: 1400–6.

18. Hu Y, Ahmed HU, Carter T, et al. A biopsy simulation study to assess the accuracy of several transrectal ultrasonography (TRUS)-biopsy strategies compared with template prostate mapping biopsies in patients who have undergone radical prostatectomy. BJU Int 2012;110:812–20.

19. Villers A, Puech P, Mouton D, et al. Dynamic contrast enhanced, pelvic phased array magnetic resonance imaging of localized prostate cancer for predicting tumor volume: correlation with radical prostatectomy findings. J Urol 2006;176:2432–7.

20. Nelson AW, Harvey RC, Parker RA, et al. Repeat prostate biopsy strategies after initial negative biopsy: meta-regression comparing cancer detection of transperineal, transrectal saturation and MRI guided biopsy. PLoS One 2013;8:e57480.

21. Moldovan PC, Van den Broeck T, Sylvester R, et al. What is the negative predictive value of multiparametric magnetic resonance imaging in excluding prostate cancer at biopsy? A Systematic review and meta-analysis from the european association of urology prostate cancer guidelines panel. Eur Urol 2017;72(2):250–66.

22. Siddiqui MM, Rais-Bahrami S, Truong H, et al. Magnetic resonance imaging/ultrasound–fusion biopsy significantly upgrades prostate cancer versus systematic 12-core transrectal ultrasound biopsy. Eur Urol 2013;64:713–9.

23. Siddiqui MM, Rais-Bahrami S, Turkbey B, et al. Comparison of MR/ultrasound fusion–guided biopsy with ultrasound-guided biopsy for the diagnosis of prostate cancer. JAMA 2015;313:390.

24. Focal therapy using high-intensity focused ultrasound for localised prostate cancer | Guidance and guidelines | NICE, (n.d.). Available at: https://www.nice.org.uk/guidance/ipg424/chapter/2-The-procedure. Accessed May 13, 2017.

25. Santis D, Henry A, Joniau S, et al. Prostate Cancer EAU -ESTRO -SIOG guidelines on, (n.d.). Available at: https://uroweb.org/wp-content/uploads/EAU-Guidelines-Prostate-Cancer-2016.pdf. Accessed May 13, 2017.

26. Muller BG, Fütterer JJ, Gupta RT, et al. The role of magnetic resonance imaging (MRI) in focal therapy for prostate cancer: recommendations from a consensus panel. BJU Int 2014;113:218–27.

27. Dickinson L, Ahmed HU, Allen C, et al. Magnetic resonance imaging for the detection, localisation, and characterisation of prostate cancer: recommendations from a European consensus meeting. Eur Urol 2011;59:477–94.

28. Onik G, Miessau M, Bostwick DG. Three-dimensional prostate mapping biopsy has a potentially significant impact on prostate cancer management. J Clin Oncol 2009;27:4321–6.

29. van der Kwast TH, Amin MB, Billis A, et al. International Society of Urological Pathology (ISUP) Consensus Conference on Handling and Staging of Radical Prostatectomy Specimens. Working group 2: T2 substaging and prostate cancer volume. Mod Pathol 2011;24:16–25.

30. Nogueira L, Wang L, Fine SW, et al. Focal treatment or observation of prostate cancer: pretreatment accuracy of transrectal ultrasound biopsy and T2-weighted MRI. Urology 2010;75:472–7.

31. Shulman S, Brandt EJ, Yantorno C. Studies in cryo-immunology. II. Tissue and species specificity of the autoantibody response and comparison with iso-immunization. Immunology 1968;14:149–58. Available at: http://www.ncbi.nlm.nih.gov/pubmed/4966655. Accessed March 20, 2017.

32. Simons JW, Sacks N. Granulocyte-macrophage colony-stimulating factor–transduced allogeneic cancer cellular immunotherapy: The GVAX® vaccine for prostate cancer. Urol Oncol 2006;24:419–24.

33. Bastianpillai C, Petrides N, Shah T, et al. Harnessing the immunomodulatory effect of thermal and non-thermal ablative therapies for cancer treatment. Tumour Biol 2015;36:9137–46.

34. Culp SH, Schellhammer PF, Williams MB. Might men diagnosed with metastatic prostate cancer benefit from definitive treatment of the primary tumor? A SEER-based study. Eur Urol 2014;65:1058–66.

35. Kanthabalan A, Shah T, Arya M, et al. The FORECAST study — focal recurrent assessment and salvage treatment for radiorecurrent prostate cancer. Contemp Clin Trials 2015;44:175–86.

36. Agha R, Cooper D, Muir G. The reporting quality of randomised controlled trials in surgery: a systematic review. Int J Surg 2007;5:413–22.

37. Ahmed HU, Berge V, Bottomley D, et al. Can we deliver randomized trials of focal therapy in prostate cancer? Nat Rev Clin Oncol 2014;11:482–91.

38. PART — Surgical Intervention Trials Unit, (n.d.). Available at: https://www.situ.ox.ac.uk/surgical-trials/part. Accessed March 20, 2017.

39. Kurzmitteilung - prostatakrebs: Großstudie PRE-FERE bewertet therapien. Aktuelle Urol 2013;44: 105 [in German].

40. Consort - Welcome to the CONSORT Website, (n.d.). Available at: http://www.consort-statement.org/. Accessed March 20, 2017.

41. Natarajan S, Raman S, Priester AM, et al. Focal laser ablation of prostate cancer: phase I clinical trial. J Urol 2016;196:68–75.

42. Valerio M, Dickinson L, Ali A, et al. A prospective development study investigating focal irreversible electroporation in men with localised prostate cancer: nanoknife electroporation ablation trial (NEAT). Contemp Clin Trials 2014;39:57–65.

43. Shah TT, Arbel U, Foss S, et al. Modeling cryotherapy ice ball dimensions and isotherms in a novel gel-based model to determine optimal cryo-needle configurations and settings for potential use in clinical practice. Urology 2016;91:234–40.

44. Guillaumier S, Hamid S, Charman S, et al. MP18–08 focal Hifu for treatment of localised prostate cancer: a multi-centre registry experience. J Urol 2016;195: e195.

45. Ward JF, Jones JS. Focal cryotherapy for localized prostate cancer: a report from the national Cryo On-Line Database (COLD) Registry. BJU Int 2012; 109:1648–54.

46. Muller BG, van den Bos W, Brausi M, et al. Follow-up modalities in focal therapy for prostate cancer: results from a Delphi consensus project. World J Urol 2015;33:1503–9.

47. Barret E, Harvey-Bryan K-A, Sanchez-Salas R, et al. How to diagnose and treat focal therapy failure and recurrence? Curr Opin Urol 2014;24:241–6.

48. Ray ME, Thames HD, Levy LB, et al. PSA nadir predicts biochemical and distant failures after external beam radiotherapy for prostate cancer: a multi-institutional analysis. Int J Radiat Oncol Biol Phys 2006;64:1140–50.

49. Roach M, Hanks G, Thames H, et al. Defining biochemical failure following radiotherapy with or without hormonal therapy in men with clinically localized prostate cancer: recommendations of the RTOG-ASTRO Phoenix consensus conference. Int J Radiat Oncol Biol Phys 2006;65:965–74.

50. Cox JD, Gallagher MJ, Hammond EH, et al. Consensus Statements on radiation therapy of prostate cancer: guidelines for prostate re-biopsy after radiation and for radiation therapy with rising prostate-specific antigen levels after radical prostatectomy. J Clin Oncol 1999;17:1155.

51. Dhar N, Cher ML, Scionti SM, et al. Focal/partial gland prostate cryoablation: results of 795 patients from multiple centers tracked with the cold registry. J Urol 2009;181:715.

52. Ahmed HU. The index lesion and the origin of prostate cancer. N Engl J Med 2009;361:1704–6.

53. Ganzer R, Robertson CN, Ward JF, et al. Correlation of prostate-specific antigen nadir and biochemical failure after high-intensity focused ultrasound of localized prostate cancer based on the Stuttgart failure criteria - analysis from the @-Registry. BJU Int 2011;108:E196–201.

54. Bahn D, de Castro Abreu AL, Gill IS, et al. Focal cryotherapy for clinically unilateral, low-intermediate risk prostate cancer in 73 men with a median follow-up of 3.7 years. Eur Urol 2012;62: 55–63.

55. Punwani S, Emberton M, Walkden M, et al. Prostatic cancer surveillance following whole-gland high-intensity focused ultrasound: comparison of MRI and prostate-specific antigen for detection of residual or recurrent disease. Br J Radiol 2012; 85:720–8.

56. Dickinson L, Ahmed HU, Hindley RG, et al. Prostate-specific antigen vs. magnetic resonance imaging parameters for assessing oncological outcomes after high intensity-focused ultrasound focal therapy for localized prostate cancer. Urol Oncol 2017;35: 30.e9–15.

57. Hoquetis L, Malavaud B, Game X, et al. MRI evaluation following partial HIFU therapy for localized prostate cancer: a single-center study. Prog Urol 2016;26:517–23.

58. Kalbhen CL, Hricak H, Shinohara K, et al. Prostate carcinoma: MR imaging findings after cryosurgery. Radiology 1996;198:807–11.

59. Rouvière O, Lyonnet D, Raudrant A, et al. MRI appearance of prostate following transrectal HIFU ablation of localized cancer. Eur Urol 2001;40: 265–74.

60. Vargas HA, Wassberg C, Akin O, et al. MR imaging of treated prostate cancer. Radiology 2012; 262:26–42.

61. Moore CM, Robertson NL, Arsanious N, et al. Image-guided prostate biopsy using magnetic resonance imaging-derived targets: a systematic review. Eur Urol 2013;63:125–40.

62. Shah TT, Kasivisvanathan V, Jameson C, et al. Histological outcomes after focal high-intensity focused ultrasound and cryotherapy. World J Urol 2015;33: 955–64.

63. van den Bos W, Muller BG, Ahmed H, et al. Focal therapy in prostate cancer: international multidisciplinary consensus on trial design. Eur Urol 2014; 65:1078–83.

64. Donaldson IA, Alonzi R, Barratt D, et al. Focal therapy: patients, interventions, and outcomes–a report from a consensus meeting. Eur Urol 2015; 67:771–7.

65. Biermann K, Montironi R, Lopez-Beltran A, et al. Histopathological findings after treatment of prostate cancer using high-intensity focused ultrasound (HIFU). Prostate 2010;70:1196–200.

Extent of Lymphadenectomy at Time of Prostatectomy
An Evidence-Based Approach

Annah Vollstedt, MD[a],*, Elias Hyams, MD[b]

KEYWORDS

- Lymphadenectomy • Extended pelvic lymphadenectomy • Prostate cancer
- Radical prostatectomy

KEY POINTS

- Extended pelvic lymph node dissection (PLND) with radical prostatectomy is the most accurate method of prostate cancer staging and includes removing the of external iliac, obturator, and internal iliac lymph nodes.
- Limited or standard PLND templates provide low-yield and inadequate staging.
- Superextended templates include presacral nodes and common iliac nodes to the ureteric crossing, and may detect additional positive lymph nodes; however, these are not routinely performed.
- There is indirect evidence, through retrospective studies, of an oncologic benefit to extended PLND.
- Sentinel lymph node dissection has not been shown to reliably identify at-risk nodes in the surgical management of prostate cancer, and full extended PLND is still required.

INTRODUCTION

Pelvic lymph node dissection (PLND) is a critical staging procedure for men with higher risk prostate cancer, who have nonnegligible risk of lymph node metastasis. Radiographic imaging examinations, including cross-sectional imaging (computed tomography [CT]/MRI) and novel forms of PET/CT (eg, 11C-choline PET), have shown inadequate sensitivity to supplant surgical staging.[1,2] At many centers, PLND has historically been performed with limited templates based on lack of appreciation for anatomic drainage patterns and distribution of nodal disease. Varied anatomic, pathologic and clinical studies have shown that an extended template, including the obturator, external iliac, and internal iliac lymph nodes, is needed for adequate staging. Several studies have shown that removal of presacral and common iliac nodes to the ureteric crossing may find additional positive lymph nodes; however, the clinical impact of these super-extended dissections is unclear. Improved staging is useful for prognostication, but may also valuably inform treatment decisions, given the strong evidence for adjuvant

Disclosures: Neither author has any commercial or financial conflict of interest, or any funding source for this article.

[a] Section of Urology, Dartmouth Hitchcock Medical Center, One Medical Center Drive, Lebanon, NH 03756, USA; [b] Section of Urology, Geisel School of Medicine, Dartmouth College, Dartmouth Hitchcock Medical Center, One Medical Center Drive, Lebanon, NH 03756, USA
* Corresponding author.
E-mail address: Annah.j.vollstedt@hitchcock.org

0094-0143/17/© 2017 Elsevier Inc. All rights reserved.

urologic.theclinics.com

therapy in the setting of pN + disease.[3,4] Unfortunately, however, there is no level 1 evidence for an oncologic benefit of extended PLND (ePLND). Despite limited evidence of therapeutic effect, ePLND to at least the level of internal iliac nodes has become the standard of care for patients at higher risk for lymph node disease.[5–7]

In this article, we review evidence to support an extended template PLND for accurate staging and possible therapeutic benefit in men undergoing radical prostatectomy, and discuss criteria for selecting patients for ePLND.

ANATOMIC LANDMARKS AND NODAL DRAINAGE

Mapping studies have shown that lymphatic drainage from the prostate is variable and complex. Work by Gil-Vernet[8] showed that prostate lymphatics drain into a periprostatic subcapsular network, leading to 3 groups of ducts—ascending ducts from the cranial gland, leading to the external iliac nodes; lateral ducts leading to the hypogastric nodes; and posterior ducts from the caudal prostate leading to the lateral and subaortic sacral nodes. In vivo drainage patterns in patients undergoing PLND with scintographic injections have also been reported. Mattei and colleagues[9] mapped lymphatic spread in 34 patients with organ-confined prostate cancer (who were pN0) through intraprostatic injections of Tc-99m nanocolloid followed by single-photon emission CT fused with CT/MRI, intraoperative gamma probing, and ePLND. These authors found that patients had significant uptake in internal iliac nodes (25%), common iliac nodes (16%), and presacral and pararectal nodes (8%). Sixty-three percent of at-risk nodes were captured with dissection of nodal tissue medial and lateral to internal iliac vessels, versus 38% with the standard template (external iliac and obturator nodes). Seventy-five percent of at-risk nodes were captured with dissection to the ureteric crossing on the common iliac, demonstrating that even higher dissections can theoretically miss nodal metastasis in one-quarter of patients.[9] In a similar study of patients undergoing radical prostatectomy and PLND, Inoue and colleagues[10] injected the prostate with indocyanine green and used fluorescence navigation intraoperatively to map lymphatic drainage, and found that the dominant route of spread was to the internal iliac nodes.

These studies, among others, show that prostate lymphatic drainage extends beyond standard nodal templates (external iliac and obturator nodes) to the level of internal iliac nodes and common iliac nodes.[11–13] Although these mapping studies are useful for understanding drainage patterns, it is important to realize that in the setting of prostate cancer these maps may not be reliable, owing to the lack of congruence between lymphatic drainage and actual cancer dissemination, as well as the fact that lymphatic metastasis itself may alter drainage patterns.[13,14]

RATIONALE FOR EXTENDED PELVIC LYMPHADENECTOMY: IMPROVED STAGING

Studies of the location of positive nodes during PLND provide additional information on the appropriate extent of dissection. Accurate staging is important for varied reasons, including improved prognostication, patient counseling, and enabling prompt adjuvant therapy. Prompt adjuvant therapy is particularly important, given high-level evidence supporting adjuvant therapy for pN + disease.[3,4,15] Accurate staging of pelvic nodes may also influence the details of adjuvant or salvage therapy, for example, the use of concomitant androgen deprivation therapy or higher radiation fields.

It is important to clarify that studies of staging PLND for prostate cancer vary in some important details. One challenge of a cursory read of these studies is that definitions vary; for instance, standard and extended templates do not necessarily have the same anatomic boundaries. In general, ePLND pertains to removal of external iliac, obturator, and internal iliac nodes, although in some studies higher dissection is included. Also, definitions of standard versus limited dissection vary in terms of obturator, external iliac, or both sets of nodes being removed, and the precise landmarks that are used for dissection. It is also important to understand that the populations being evaluated may vary in their underlying risk of lymph node metastasis; indeed, some studies are enriched with low-risk patients for whom any PLND is low yield, and findings may not be representative of what is found in higher risk patients.

Overall, studies of PLND have shown that inclusion of internal iliac nodes in an extended template is necessary for adequate staging. Indeed, Heidenreich and colleagues[16] reported that 25% of positive nodes were found exclusively in the internal iliac packet, and Godoy and colleagues[17] found exclusive metastasis in the hypogastric packet in 31%. For comparison, exclusive nodes were found in the external iliac packet in 11% and obturator packets in 26%.[17] Studies comparing dissections including the internal iliac packet to more limited dissections have shown higher lymph node yields and increased detection of lymph node metastasis with the former.[18,19]

Jung and colleagues[20] found that 25% of positive lymph nodes with ePLND were found in the internal iliac and common iliac packets, and of those with LN+ in internal iliac nodes, three-quarters were found exclusively in that location.

Adding common iliac nodes to the ureteral crossing, as well as presacral nodes, has been shown to decrease risk of incomplete removal of positive nodes from 24% to 3%.[12] As such, some investigators favor adding these packets to the extended dissection.[13,21] Joniau and colleagues[12] found that up to 9% of their cohort had metastases in the presacral region that would have otherwise been missed by more traditional ePLND. In this study, however, staging was similar with ePLND only (32 vs 33 out of 34 patients with accurate staging), whereas removal of all positive nodes (presumably) would have increased from 26 to 30 of 34 patients. Common iliac nodes also may harbor lymph node metastasis, though this has been shown more in mapping studies than in pathologic review of positive nodes.[9,12,22]

Superextended dissection to this level can be performed, but is not generally considered the standard of care based on a shifting risk–benefit ratio with additional dissection. Indeed, although some authors report expeditious and safe superextended dissections, additional manipulation of lymphatic and vascular tissue does increase patient risk.[22] To what extent this risk increases may depend on surgeon experience, and patient anatomy in terms of accessibility of vessels and relevant anatomy. The clinical benefit of improved staging of these nodes remains unclear, although in principle removing as many at-risk nodes within parameters of safety is the goal. One concern with higher dissections in true high-risk patients is that these patients are at risk for microscopic retroperitoneal disease that is not curable.[23,24]

Several studies have attempted to determine whether there are cutoffs for number of resected lymph nodes to ensure adequate staging. Challenges of these studies are that number of lymph nodes may be an unreliable proxy for extent of dissection, because lymph node processing is known to potentially affect the number of detected nodes. In contrast, attempts to identify a numerical threshold may help with quality control in ensuring adequate dissection, and in general the number of removed nodes does reflect the extent of lymphadenectomy. Studies seeking a lymph node threshold, however, have varied in their results. Maccio and colleagues,[25] in a 2016 review of 1690 prostate cancer cases with available histologic and survival data, proposed that a minimum of 10 lymph nodes should be examined for accurate staging. Other studies have suggested a 20 lymph node threshold.[26] Although there is no usable lymph node threshold at present, numerous studies have shown that increased resected lymph nodes is associated with higher yield of detected nodal metastasis.[16]

Templates for PLND are summarized in **Fig. 1.**

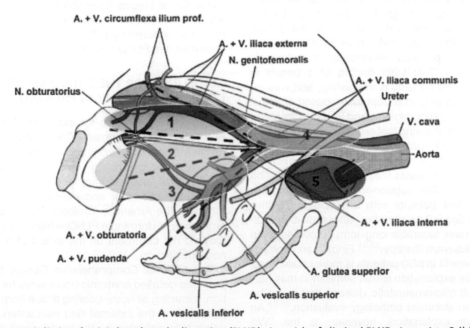

Fig. 1. Anatomic limits of pelvic lymph node dissection (PLND). Area 1 (*red*): limited PLND. Areas 1 to 2 (*blue*): standard PLND. Areas 1 to 3 ± 4 (*green*): extended PLND. Areas 1 to 5 (*purple*): superextended PLND. A, arteria; prof, profunda; N, nervus; V, vena. (Used with permission from Elsevier.) (*From* Spaliviero M, James A. Eastham Hinman's. Pelvic lymph node dissection. In: Atlas of Urologic Surgery. Chapter 78. Elsevier: Philadelphia; 2018. p. 589–602.)

RATIONALE FOR EXTENDED PELVIC LYMPHADENECTOMY: IMPROVED OUTCOMES?

The rationale for extended template PLND also includes a potential oncologic benefit, particularly in patients with low-volume nodal disease. There have been numerous studies showing improvements in biochemical recurrence-free and cancer-specific survival (CSS) with more extensive lymphadenectomy. However, these studies should be interpreted with caution—at times, studied populations vary in their underlying risk of nodal disease or adverse outcomes, the extent of surgical dissection, use of number resected nodes versus anatomic templates as predictors of outcome, and use of adjuvant therapies. Furthermore, these studies are uniformly retrospective and subject to bias; the 1 prospective randomized controlled trial evaluating cancer-specific outcomes of ePLND in intermediate- to high-risk men was retracted owing to data falsification.[27] Nonetheless, it is believed that a subset of patients may have surgical cure in the setting of low-volume N+ disease and this is a commonly cited rationale for extended dissection.[28]

Diverse studies have shown improved oncologic outcomes with more extensive PLND. Abdollah and colleagues[15] reported 315 patients with positive nodes after radical prostatectomy with ePLND, and found that those with a higher number of removed lymph nodes had higher CSS. Schiavina and colleagues[29] reported that more than 10 removed nodes was associated with reduced biochemical recurrence in intermediate- to high-risk patients, regardless of pathologic nodal status. This latter finding of a benefit in node-negative patients is interesting, and was reported separately in a population-based study of Surveillance, Epidemiology, and End Results Medicare patients showing that removal of more than 10 nodes in N0 patients was associated with improved CSS at 10 years.[19] An explanation for benefit in N+ patients may simply be eradication of cancer, further supported by multiple studies showing that patients with low volume positive lymph nodes (<2 or <3 nodes) after radical prostatectomy have favorable long-term outcomes, even without adjuvant therapy.[30,31] Finding an explanation for benefit in pN0 patients is more challenging. A possible explanation is that some men may harbor occult micrometastatic disease that is not be evident on standard pathology evaluation.[32,33] An alternative explanation, however, is the "Will Rogers" effect, in which more accurate staging improves outcomes for both node-positive and node-negative patients (the average prognosis is improved in each group through improved staging). Although these findings are suggestive of oncologic benefit, we are not at a point where we can claim there is a direct benefit from ePLND.

Another useful study in assessing therapeutic effects of ePLND was published by Bivalacqua and colleagues,[18] in which survival outcomes of patients undergoing ePLND versus limited PLND, were compared for 2 surgeons who systematically performed these procedures. Patients undergoing ePLND patients had superior biochemical, metastasis-free, and CSS at median 10.5-year follow-up. Furthermore, patients with a smaller percent involved lymph nodes seem to benefit most (<15% positive). This study further suggests that a subset of patients are achieving oncologic benefit from dissection at least to the level of hypogastric nodes, and patients with low-volume disease are most likely to benefit.

Other studies, interestingly, have shown comparable oncologic outcomes with extended versus limited dissection.[20,34] A large series from the Mayo clinic found that the number of lymph nodes removed was not associated with cancer-specific outcomes among men with node-negative disease; these authors concluded that understaging did not seem to occur.[35] However, this study did include a large proportion of men at lower risk for nodal metastasis (65% had pathologically low-risk disease), which may simply strengthen the argument that these patients did not need PLND in the first place. Other studies have shown that there is not a reduction in biochemical recurrence rates in low-risk men undergoing ePLND,[36] strengthening the argument that PLND is not required in low-risk men.

GUIDELINES FOR THE EXTENT OF PELVIC LYMPHADENECTOMY IN PROSTATE CANCER

Professional guidelines for extent of PLND vary. See **Table 1** for a summary. The National Comprehensive Cancer Network and European Association of Urology (EAU) both recommend an ePLND to at least the internal iliac region in addition to the obturator and external iliac areas.[5,7] Although the American Urologic Association recommends performing a PLND in high-risk patients, they do not comment on the extent of the lymph node dissection.[6]

The National Comprehensive Cancer Network provides detailed anatomic boundaries for dissection, including all node-bearing tissue from an area bounded by the external iliac vein anteriorly, the pelvic side wall laterally, the bladder wall medially, the floor of the pelvis posteriorly, Cooper's ligament distally, and the internal iliac artery proximally.[5] The EAU suggests a similar template.[7]

Table 1
Professional recommendations for PLND in surgical management of prostate cancer

	Criteria for PLND	Anatomic Extent
EAU[7]	Using the Briganti nomogram, Memorial Sloan Kettering Cancer Center, or Roach Formula, a risk of nodal metastases of >5% is an indication to perform an extended PLND	Extended PLND including removal of the nodes overlying the external iliac artery and vein, the nodes within the obturator fossa located cranially and caudally to the obturator nerve and the nodes medial and lateral to the internal iliac artery
AUA[6]	"Generally reserved for patients with higher risk of nodal involvement"	No recommendations
NCCN[5]	Recommends the Memorial Sloan Kettering Cancer Center nomogram (see **Fig. 2**) with using 2% risk of positive nodes as a cutoff for performing a PLND	Extended technique, including removal of all node-bearing tissue from an area bounded by the external iliac vein anteriorly, pelvic side wall laterally, bladder wall medially, floor of pelvis posteriorly, Cooper's ligament distally and internal iliac artery proximally

Abbreviations: AUA, American Urologic Association; EAU, European Association of Urology; NCCN, National Comprehensive Cancer Network; PLND, pelvic lymph node dissection.

These guidelines all emphasize that low-risk patients do not require PLND and that nomograms should be used to stratify patients for risk of lymph node disease. Risk thresholds vary between guidelines, and generally are based on expert opinion. The National Comprehensive Cancer Network Guidelines Panel offers 2% as the cutoff for PLND[5] using the Memorial Sloane Kettering Cancer Center nomogram (**Fig. 2**), whereas the EAU suggests use of a 5% risk threshold using the Briganti nomogram.[7]

Although these nomograms provide objective prediction of risk of lymph node disease, it is important to acknowledge that nomograms themselves vary in their predictive power. Populations on which these nomograms are based may vary in their underlying risk of lymph node disease, as well as the anatomic extent of PLND (eg, standard vs ePLND). For instance, nomograms derived from more limited dissection, such as the Partin tables, may underestimate risk of lymph node disease. Some authors argue for routine use of PLND based on risks of pathologic upgrading and increased post hoc risk,[37] as well as potential benefit of removal of micrometastatic disease that is not evident on traditional pathology evaluation. Generally, however, PLND is reserved for men at increased risk based on cutoffs chosen at the surgeon's discretion.

ROLE OF SENTINEL LYMPH NODE TECHNIQUE

Sentinel lymph node dissection is an approach to lymph node staging and removal that intends to minimize unnecessary surgery by determining if a sentinel node is involved at a critical nexus of drainage. If this node is positive, additional dissection is performed; if not, the patient is spared additional dissection. Sentinel lymph node dissection is used routinely in the treatment of breast cancer and melanoma. However, sentinel lymph node dissection has not proven useful in the surgical management of prostate cancer.

Studies of sentinel lymph node dissection in prostate cancer have generally involved an intraprostatic injection of a radiotracer with intraoperative detection. Studies have shown that sentinel lymph node dissection has low sensitivity for lymph node metastasis,[38] and many sentinel nodes have been found outside of the ePLND template.[39] Investigators have conjectured that the low sensitivity of sentinel lymph node dissection may result from metastasis within lymphatic ducts blocking circulation of the radiotracer[21,40] as well as inaccessibility of important anatomic regions to gamma probing (eg, behind large pelvic blood vessels, presacral nodes). Furthermore, there has not been shown to be a reliable sentinel node or drainage region for the prostate[38]; thus, the complex drainage patterns of the prostate, and multiple primary landing sites in the pelvis, have been obstacles to its adoption.[9,11] Some still argue for sentinel lymph node dissection as an adjunctive procedure to detect aberrant pathways outside standard templates,[38] and EAU guidelines offer sentinel lymph node dissection as an option if the risk of lymph node metastasis is greater than 7%.[41] Nonetheless, this procedure is not currently

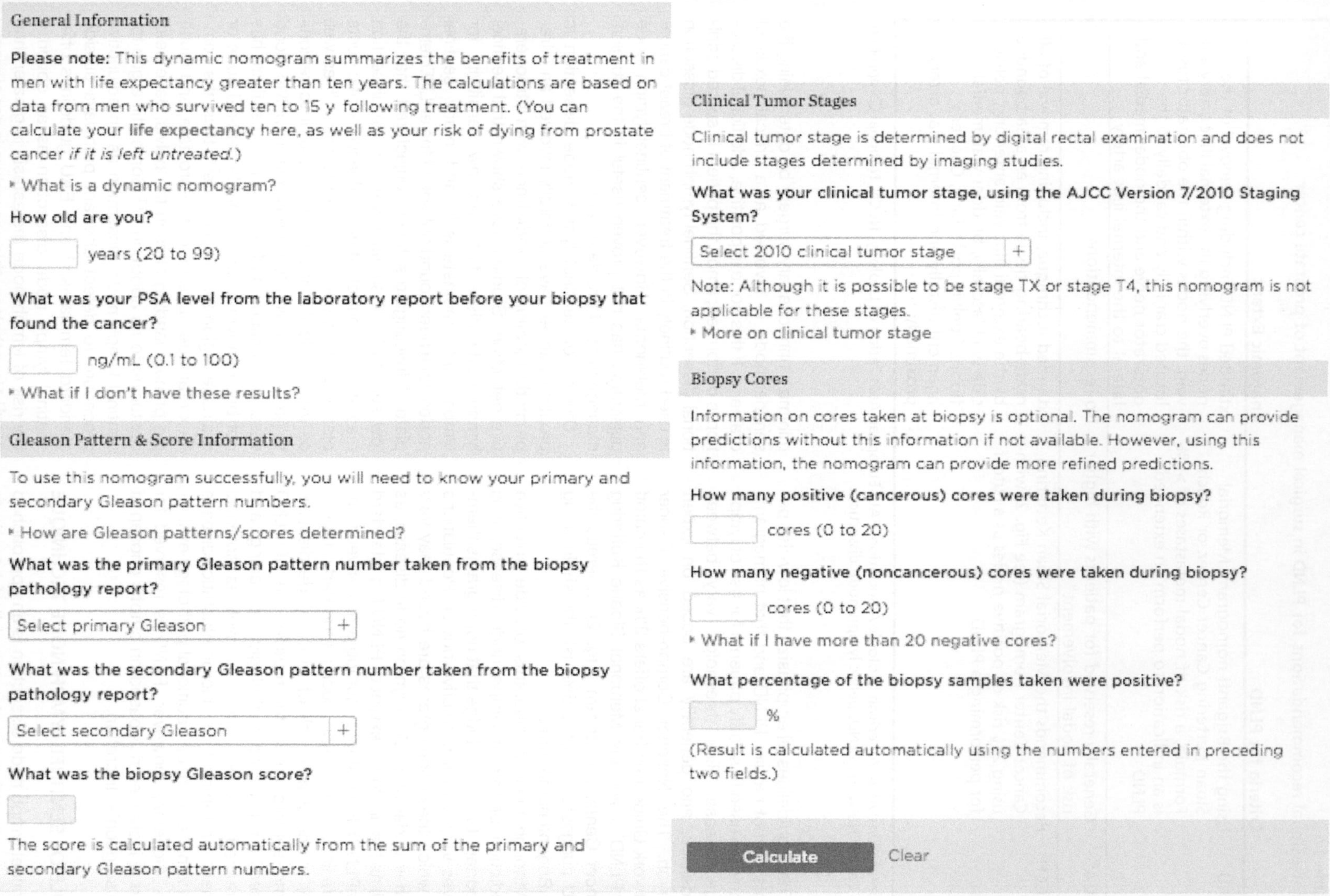

General Information

Please note: This dynamic nomogram summarizes the benefits of treatment in men with life expectancy greater than ten years. The calculations are based on data from men who survived ten to 15 y following treatment. (You can calculate your life expectancy here, as well as your risk of dying from prostate cancer *if it is left untreated*.)

* What is a dynamic nomogram?

How old are you?

[   ] years (20 to 99)

What was your PSA level from the laboratory report before your biopsy that found the cancer?

[   ] ng/mL (0.1 to 100)

* What if I don't have these results?

Gleason Pattern & Score Information

To use this nomogram successfully, you will need to know your primary and secondary Gleason pattern numbers.

* How are Gleason patterns/scores determined?

What was the primary Gleason pattern number taken from the biopsy pathology report?

[Select primary Gleason   +]

What was the secondary Gleason pattern number taken from the biopsy pathology report?

[Select secondary Gleason   +]

What was the biopsy Gleason score?

[   ]

The score is calculated automatically from the sum of the primary and secondary Gleason pattern numbers.

Clinical Tumor Stages

Clinical tumor stage is determined by digital rectal examination and does not include stages determined by imaging studies.

What was your clinical tumor stage, using the AJCC Version 7/2010 Staging System?

[Select 2010 clinical tumor stage   +]

Note: Although it is possible to be stage TX or stage T4, this nomogram is not applicable for these stages.

* More on clinical tumor stage

Biopsy Cores

Information on cores taken at biopsy is optional. The nomogram can provide predictions without this information if not available. However, using this information, the nomogram can provide more refined predictions.

How many positive (cancerous) cores were taken during biopsy?

[   ] cores (0 to 20)

How many negative (noncancerous) cores were taken during biopsy?

[   ] cores (0 to 20)

* What if I have more than 20 negative cores?

What percentage of the biopsy samples taken were positive?

[   ] %

(Result is calculated automatically using the numbers entered in preceding two fields.)

[Calculate]   Clear

Fig. 2. Memorial Sloan Kettering Cancer Center nomogram for predicting the risk of lymph node metastasis. AJCC, American Joint Committee on Cancer; PSA, prostate-specific antigen. (*Data from* https://www.mskcc.org/nomograms/prostate/pre-op. Accessed March 25, 2017.)

standard of care and cannot be reliably used to determine the appropriate extent of PLND.

THE INFLUENCE OF MINIMALLY INVASIVE RADICAL PROSTATECTOMY

The rationale for ePLND holds true for all surgical approaches to radical prostatectomy. Historically, perhaps owing to the learning curve of robotic prostatectomy, there have been lower rates of PLND with robotic compared with open surgery (11%–50% for minimally invasive procedures vs 48%–93% for radical retropubic prostatectomy).[42–45] There has also been discussion about technical limitations of robotic surgery that prohibit dissections within extended templates. Additional experience with robotic prostatectomy and cysto-prostatectomy have revealed that ePLND is safe and feasible with these approaches.[46,47] Because robotic prostatectomy has largely supplanted open surgery, much of the data for the staging and possible therapeutic benefits of ePLND derive from the robotic experience.[48,49]

COMPLICATIONS

In general, ePLND is a safe procedure, although complication rates vary widely in the literature from 2% to 51%.[22,49,50] Although risks are low incidence, they have potential clinical significance, for example, lymphocele, deep venous thrombosis or pulmonary embolism, and injury to blood vessels, nerves, or ureter. Rates of complication in ePLND are uniformly higher than limited PLND in various studies.[51,52] Although meticulous surgical technique has been alleged to reduce risk of lymphocele, a recent randomized trial of titanium clips versus bipolar cautery for control of lymphatic channels found no difference in rates of postoperative lymphocele.[53] Investigators have argued that avoiding dissection lateral to the external iliac artery also decreases risk of lower extremity swelling, or that avoidance of subcutaneous heparin may reduce the risk of lymphocele formation.[37] Technical aspects of PLND vary, but in general the meticulous clipping of lymphatic channels, appropriate selection of patients, and commitment to developing expertise in this procedure are likely the best methods of minimizing morbidity.

Extended PLND can be a challenging and time-consuming procedure that requires commitment by the surgeon. Some authors comment that ePLND can be done expeditiously[54]; however, authors have reported as much as an additional 72 minutes for an extended dissection.[49,50] Indeed, patient habitus and anatomic variation can create technical challenges, and patient comorbid conditions may argue for a more expeditious procedure. Nonetheless, in principle, time constraints should not be a deterrent to performing the appropriate oncologic procedure. Clarifying the therapeutic benefits of PLND will help to convince surgeons to more systematically perform extended dissection.

SUMMARY

Extended PLND, including at minimum obturator, external iliac, and internal iliac nodes, should be performed for patients with higher risk of lymph node metastasis. This procedure in necessary for adequate staging and may have therapeutic benefits in patients with low-volume nodal metastasis. Use of nomograms and criteria for PLND vary, although in general patients with more than a 2% to 5% risk of positive nodes should undergo ePLND. Further research is needed to determine the oncologic benefits of superextended dissection to presacral and common iliac nodes, and to clarify which patient subsets are most likely to benefit. Sentinel lymph node dissection is unfortunately not useful for guiding the extent of PLND owing to various disease-specific and technical issues.

REFERENCES

1. Briganti A, Abdollah F, Nini A, et al. Performance characteristics of computed tomography in detecting lymph node metastases in contemporary patients with prostate cancer treated with extended pelvic lymph node dissection. Eur Urol 2012;61: 1132–8.
2. Budiharto T, Joniau S, Lerut E, et al. Prospective Evaluation of 11-C-choline positron emission tomography/computed tomography and diffusion-weighted magnetic resonance imaging for the nodal staging of prostate cancer with a high risk of lymph node metastases. Eur Urol 2011;60:125–30.
3. Messing EM, Manola J, Yao J, et al. Immediate versus deferred androgen deprivation treatment in patients with node-positive prostate cancer after radical prostatectomy and pelvic lymphadenectomy. Lancet Oncol 2006;7(6):472–9.
4. Jegadeesh N, Liu Y, Zhang C, et al. The role of adjuvant radiotherapy in pathologically lymph node-positive prostate cancer. Cancer 2016; 123(3):512–20.
5. Mohler JL, Antonarakis, ES, Armstrong AJ, et al. NCCN clinical practice guidelines in oncology: prostate cancer Version 2.2017. 2016. Available at: https://www.nccn.org/professionals/physician_gls/pdf/prostate.pdf. Accessed March 25, 2017.

6. Thompson I, Thrasher JB, Aus G, et al. AUA guideline for the management of clinically localized prostate cancer panel: 2007 Update. Available at: https://www.auanet.org/common/pdf/education/clinical-guidance/Prostate-Cancer.pdf. Accessed March 25, 2017.

7. Mottet N, Bellmunt J, Briers E, et al. EUA guidelines on prostate cancer: disease management. 2016. Available at: https://uroweb.org/guideline/prostate-cancer/#6.

8. Gil-Vernet JM. Prostate cancer: anatomical and surgical considerations. Br J Urol 1996;78:161–8. Available at: http://videos-gilvernet.org/articles/Prostate_cancer_anatomical_surgical_considerations.pdf. Accessed on March 17, 2017.

9. Mattei A, Fuechsel FG, Bhatta DN, et al. The template of the primary lymphatic landing sites of the prostate should be revisited: results of a multimodality mapping study. Eur Urol 2008;53(1):118–25.

10. Inoue S, Shiina H, Arichi N, et al. Identification of lymphatic pathway involved in the spreading of prostate cancer by fluorescence navigation approach with intraoperatively injected indocyanine green. Urol Assoc J 2011;5(4):254–9.

11. Nguyen DP, Huber P, Metzger T, et al. A specific mapping study using fluorescence sentinel lymph node detection in patients with intermediate- and high-risk prostate cancer undergoing extended pelvic lymph node dissection. Eur Urol 2016;70:734–7.

12. Joniau S, Van den Bergh L, Lerut E, et al. Mapping of pelvic lymph node metastases in prostate cancer. Eur Urol 2013;63:450–8.

13. Gakis G, Boorjian SA, Briganti A, et al. The role of radical prostatectomy and lymph node dissection in lymph node-positive prostate cancer: a systematic review of the literature. Eur Urol 2014;66:191–9.

14. Janetschek G. Can sentinel pelvic lymph node dissection replace extended pelvic lymph node dissection in patients with prostate cancer? Nat Clin Pract Urol 2007;4:636–7.

15. Abdollah F, Gandaglia G, Suardi N, et al. More extensive pelvis lymph node dissection improves survival in patients with node-positive prostate cancer. Eur Urol 2015;67:212–9.

16. Heidenreich A, Ohlmann CH, Polyakov S. Anatomical extent of pelvic lymphadenectomy in patients undergoing radical prostatectomy. Eur Urol 2007;52:29–37.

17. Godoy G, von Bodman C, Chade DC, et al. Pelvic lymph node dissection for prostate cancer: frequency and distribution of nodal metastases in a contemporary radical prostatectomy series. J Urol 2012;187(6):2082–6.

18. Bivalacqua TJ, Pierorazio PM, Gorin MA, et al. Anatomic extent of pelvic lymph node dissection: impact on long-term cancer-specific outcomes in men with positive lymph nodes at time of radical prostatectomy. Urology 2013;82(3):653–8.

19. Joslyn SA, Konety BR. Impact of extent of lymphadenectomy on survival after radical prostatectomy for prostate cancer. Urology 2006;68(1):121–5.

20. Jung JH, Seo JW, Lim MS, et al. Extended pelvic lymph node dissection including internal iliac packet should be performed during robot-assisted laparoscopic radical prostatectomy for high-risk prostate cancer. J Laparoendosc Adv Surg Tech A 2012;22(8):785–90.

21. Studer UE. Should pelvic lymph node dissection be performed with radical prostatectomy? Yes. J Urol 2010;183:1284–7.

22. Briganti A, Blute ML, Eastham JH, et al. Pelvic lymph node dissection in prostate cancer. Eur Urol 2009;55:1251–65.

23. Briganti A, Suardi N, Capogrosso P, et al. Lymphatic spread of nodal metastases in high-risk prostate cancer: the ascending pathway from the pelvis to the retroperitoneum. Prostate 2012;72(2):186–92.

24. Rigatti P, Suardi N, Briganti A, et al. Pelvic/retroperitoneal salvage lymph node dissection for patients treated with radical prostatectomy with biochemical recurrence and nodal recurrence detected by 11C choline PET/CT. Eur Urol 2011;60:935–43.

25. Maccio L, Barresi V, Domati F, et al. Clinical significance of pelvic lymph node status in prostate cancer: review of 1690 cases. Intern Emerg Med 2016;11:399–404.

26. Weingärtner K, Ramaswamy A, Bittinger A, et al. Anatomical basis for pelvic lymphadenectomy in prostate cancer: results of an autopsy study and implications for the clinic. J Urol 1996;156:1969–71.

27. Ji J, Yuan H, Wang L, et al. Is the impact of the extent of lymphadenectomy in radical prostatectomy related to the disease risk? A single center prospective study. J Surg Res 2012;178(2):779–84.

28. Abdollah F, Karnes RJ, Suardi N, et al. Impact of adjuvant radiotherapy on survival of patients with node-positive prostate cancer. J Clin Oncol 2014;32(35):3939–47.

29. Schiavina R, Manferrari F, Garofalo M, et al. The extent of pelvic lymph node dissection correlates with the biochemical recurrence rate in patients with intermediate- and high-risk prostate cancer. BJU Int 2011;108(8):1262–8.

30. Passoni NM, Abdollah F, Suardi N, et al. Head-to-head comparison of lymph node density and number of positive lymph nodes in stratifying the outcome of patients with lymph node-positive prostate cancer submitted to radical prostatectomy and extended lymph node dissection. Urol Oncol 2014;32(1):29.e21-8.

31. Touijer KA, Mazzola CR, Sjoberg DD, et al. Long-term outcomes of patients with lymph node metastasis treated with radical prostatectomy without adjuvant androgen-deprivation therapy. Eur Urol 2014;65(1):20–5.

32. Pagliarulo V, Hawes D, Brands FH, et al. Detection of occult lymph node metastases in locally advanced node-negative prostate cancer. J Clin Oncol 2006; 24(18):2735–42.

33. Ferrari AC, Stone NN, Kurek R, et al. Molecular load of pathologically occult metastases in pelvic lymph nodes is an independent prognostic marker of biochemical failure after localized prostate cancer treatment. J Clin Oncol 2006;24(19):3081–8.

34. Kim KH, Lim SK, Kim HY, et al. Extended vs standard lymph node dissection in robotassisted radical prostatectomy for intermediate- or high-risk prostate cancer: A propensity score matching analysis. BJU Int 2013;112:216–23.

35. DiMarco DS, Zincke H, Sebo TJ, et al. The extent of lymphadenectomy for pTXNO prostate cancer does not affect prostate cancer outcome in the prostate specific antigen era. J Urol 2005;173(4):1121–5.

36. Rees T, Raison N, Sheikh MI, et al. Is extended pelvic lymph node dissection for prostate cancer the only recommended option? A systematic over-view of the literature. Turk J Urol 2016;42(4):240–6.

37. Bivalacqua TJ, Gorin MA, Walsh PC. Reply: anatomic extent of pelvic lymph node dissection: impact on long-term cancer-specific outcomes in men with positive lymph nodes at time of radical prostatectomy. Urology 2013;82:658–9.

38. Munbauhal G, Seisen T, Gomez FD, et al. Current perspectives of sentinel lymph node dissection at the time of radical surgery for prostate cancer. Cancer Treat Rev 2016;50:228–39.

39. Mottaghy FM, Ameye F, Berkers J, et al. Reliability of sentinel node procedure for lymph node staging in prostate cancer patients at high risk for lymph node involvement. Acta Oncol 2015;54(6):896–902.

40. Weckermann D, Dorn R, Holl G, et al. Limitations of radioguided surgery in high-risk prostate cancer. Eur Urol 2007;51:1549.

41. Heidenreich A, Bellmunt J, Bolla M, et al. EAU guidelines on prostate cancer. Part 1: screening, diagnosis, and treatment of clinically localised disease. Eur Urol 2011;59:61–71.

42. Cooperberg MR, Kane CJ, Cowan JE, et al. Adequacy of lymphadenectomy among men undergoing robot-assisted laparoscopic radical prostatectomy. BJU Int 2010;105:88–92.

43. Feifer AH, Elkin EB, Lowrance WT, et al. Temporal trends and predictors of pelvic lymph node dissection in open or minimally invasive radical prostatectomy. Cancer 2011;117:3933–42.

44. Prasad SM, Keating NL, Wang Q, et al. Variations in surgeon volume and use of pelvic lymph node dissection with open and minimally invasive radical prostatectomy. Urology 2008;72(3):647–52.

45. Briganti A, Bianchi M, Sun M, et al. Impact of the introduction of a robotic training programme on prostate cancer stage migration at a single tertiary referral centre. BJU Int 2013;111:1222–30.

46. Li R, Petros FG, Kukreja JB, et al. Current technique and results for extended pelvic lymph node dissection during robot-assisted radical prostatectomy. Investig Clin Urol 2016;57(Suppl 2):S155–64.

47. Pruthi RS, Wallen EM. Robotic-assisted laparoscopic pelvic lymphadenectomy for bladder cancer: a surgical atlas. J Laparoendosc Adv Surg Tech A 2009;19(1):71–4.

48. Sagalovich D, Calaway A, Srivastava A, et al. Assessment of required nodal yield in a high risk cohort undergoing extended pelvic lymphadenectomy in robotic-assisted radical prostatectomy and its impact on functional outcomes. BJU Int 2013; 111(1):85–94.

49. Katz DJ, Yee DS, Godoy G, et al. Lymph node dissection during robotic-assisted laparoscopic prostatectomy: comparison of lymph node yield and clinical outcomes when including common iliac nodes with standard template dissection. BJU Int 2010;106:391–6.

50. Atug F, Castle E, Srivasta S, et al. Prospective evaluation of concomitant lymphadenectomy in robot-assisted radical prostatectomy: preliminary analysis of outcomes. J Endourol 2006;20(7):514–8.

51. Stone NN, Stock R, Unger P. Laparoscopic pelvic lymph node dissection for prostate cancer: comparison of the extended and modified technique. J Urol 1997;158:1891–4.

52. Briganti A, Chun FK-H, Salonia A, et al. Complications and other surgical outcomes associated with extended pelvic lymphadenectomy in men with localized prostate cancer. Eur Urol 2006;50: 1006–13.

53. Grande P, Di Pierro GB, Mordasini L, et al. Prospective randomized trial comparing titanium clips to bipolar coagulation in sealing lymphatic vessels during pelvis lymph node dissection at the time of robot-assisted radical prostatectomy. Eur Urol 2017;71(2):155–8.

54. Porpiglia F, De Luca S, Bertolo R, et al. Robot-assisted extended pelvic lymph nodes dissection for prostate cancer: personal surgical technique and outcomes. Int Braz J Urol 2015;41(6):1209–19.

Managing Cancer Relapse After Radical Prostatectomy
Adjuvant Versus Salvage Radiation Therapy

Joseph F. Rodriguez, MD[a],*, Stanley L. Liauw, MD[b],
Scott E. Eggener, MD[a]

KEYWORDS

- Prostate • Cancer • Adjuvant • Salvage • Radiotherapy

KEY POINTS

- Disease recurrence following radical prostatectomy is common in men with extraprostatic extension and seminal vesicle invasion with or without positive margins.
- Postoperative adjuvant radiation therapy reduces the risk of risk of biochemical recurrence by approximately half and may improve overall survival.
- Retrospective studies suggest similar efficacy of salvage radiotherapy administered at the time of detectable prostate-specific antigen.
- Patient selection for postoperative radiotherapy is a challenge and current focus of research.

INTRODUCTION

Approximately 1 in 6 men in the United States is diagnosed with prostate cancer.[1] Only 10% to 15% of these men eventually die from their disease, yet more than 25,000 deaths per year are attributed to prostate cancer in the United States.[2] Because of this disparity, identifying those with aggressive disease for early curative therapy while limiting the overtreatment of indolent disease is paramount. Radical prostatectomy (RP) can be curative for men with localized prostate cancer.[3] However, following RP, approximately 30% of men experience biochemical recurrence (BCR), the redetection of prostate-specific antigen (PSA) in the blood, within 10 years.[4–6] The aim of this article was to discuss adjuvant and salvage radiation therapy following RP.

PREDICTING RELAPSE AFTER RADICAL PROSTATECTOMY

Preoperative PSA, pathologic tumor stage (pT), Gleason grade, and margin status have been used to estimate rates of BCR following RP. BCR after RP is most often defined as PSA $\geq$0.2 ng/mL when previously undetectable, although more than 50 definitions have been published.[7] **Table 1** outlines data from more than 10,000 men treated by RP and their associated rates of BCR stratified by risk factors. At 10 years, most men experience BCR with pT3 disease (extraprostatic extension [EPE]; or seminal vesical invasion [SVI]), with or without positive surgical margins (+SMs). For organ-confined cancers, +SMs are associated with a risk of BCR of 30% to 40%, increasing to greater than 50% when associated with

Disclosures: None.
[a] Section of Urology, University of Chicago, The University of Chicago Medicine, 5841 South Maryland Avenue, MC 6038, Chicago, IL 60637, USA; [b] Department of Radiation and Cellular Oncology, University of Chicago, The University of Chicago Medicine, 5758 South Maryland Avenue, MC 9006, Chicago, IL 60637, USA
* Corresponding author.
E-mail address: tony.rodriguez17@gmail.com

Table 1
Percentages of patients with biochemical recurrence at 10 years post-prostatectomy stratified by risk factors

Study	Overview	Risk Factors	%BCR-10 y
8 Centers	1983–2000	+SM	64
Karakiewicz	25 mo med f/u	EPE +SM/−SM	75/54
Urol 2005	39% BCR overall	SVI +SM/−SM	88/80
n = 5831	0% adjuvant	LNI +SM/−SM	92/86
Washington University	1983–2003	Gleason ≥8	68
Roehl	65 mo med f/u	EPE +SM/−SM	47/38
J Urol 2004	32% BCR overall	SVI	74
n = 3478	6% adjuvant	LNI	88
Baylor	1983–1998	+SM	64
Hull	47 mo med f/u	EPE alone	29
J Urol 2002	25% BCR overall	SVI	63
n = 1000	0% adjuvant	LNI	93

Abbreviations: +SM, positive surgical margin; −SM, negative surgical margin; BCR, biochemical recurrence; EPE, extraprostatic extension; f/u, follow-up; LNI, lymph node invasion; med, median; SVI, seminal vesical invasion.

Gleason ≥7 disease.[8] Another strong predictor of BCR, lymph node invasion, has been associated with greater than 85% risk of BCR.[4,6,9]

Nomograms have been developed using these post-RP variables to individualize a patient's risk of disease recurrence. The Stephenson nomogram was modeled from more than 2000 patients treated from 1983 to 2003 at 5 US academic centers.[10] A 10-year progression-free (BCR-free) probability can be predicted from pretreatment PSA, year of RP, SM status, pathologic stage, lymph node status, Gleason score, and time from surgery. An electronic version can be accessed at https://www.mskcc.org/nomograms/prostate/post-op.

The CAPRA-S scoring system was developed from the Cancer of the Prostate Strategic Urologic Research Endeavor (CaPSURE) national disease registry which includes over 3800 patients.[11] It uses many of the same variables as the Stephenson nomogram to assign patients to 1 of 10 risk categories for recurrence at 3 and 5 years following RP (**Table 2**). Both of these tools have been externally validated and can help personalize prognosis and improve decision making.[12,13]

INCREASING UTILIZATION OF RADICAL PROSTATECTOMY FOR LOCALLY ADVANCED DISEASE

Nomograms like Stephenson and CAPRA-S are particularly useful, as the proportion of patients having RP with adverse pathologic features is increasing.[14] Most men choose RP for the initial treatment of localized prostate cancer over other modalities, and that proportion has been increasing since the early 2000s.[15]

Part of this increase in RP may be attributed to decreased utilization of primary hormonal therapy, which at the cost of significant morbidity does not improve overall survival and is not recommended for localized disease.[16] The rise of active surveillance as a management strategy for men with low-risk disease contributes to a higher proportion of men undergoing RP with more advanced disease. Additionally, surgery over radiation for the management of clinically localized, high-risk prostate cancer has been increasing.[17]

Changes in prostate cancer screening may also contribute to the numbers of patients with locally advanced disease undergoing RP. In 2008, the United States Preventative Services Task Force (USPSTF) recommended against PSA screening for patients 75 years and older.[18] This was followed in 2012 by a recommendation discouraging PSA screening for all men.[19] Statistical modeling by Shen and Kumar[20] estimates the "trade-off effect" of PSA screening is 1 less patient with advanced cancer at diagnosis for every 4 patients potentially treated unnecessarily for low-risk disease. Early reports have demonstrated a stage migration following the USPSTF statements toward more advanced disease at diagnosis, thereby increasing the pool of patients with more advanced disease eligible for RP.[21]

PROGNOSIS FOR RELAPSED MEN

BCR can signify cancer in the pelvis (nodal or in the prostatic bed), cancer at a distant site, or the

Table 2
The CAPRA-S scoring system adapted from Cooperberg and colleagues[11]: postsurgical variables are assigned points that are totaled to predict 3-year and 5-year progression-free probability

Variable	Level	Points
PSA	0–6	0
	6.01–10	1
	10.01–20	2
	>20	3
SM	Negative	0
	Positive	2
SVI	No	0
	Yes	2
Gleason	2–6	0
	3+4	1
	4+3	2
	8–10	3
EPE	No	0
	Yes	1
LNI	No	0
	Yes	1

	% Progression-free	
Score	3 y	5 y
0	96.3	94.5
1	95.3	91
2	89.8	83.3
3	80.7	72.8
4	74.9	70.2
5	63.1	42.5
6	49.2	25.9
7	50.9	26.9
8	26.9	12.3
≥9	7.3	0

Abbreviations: EPE, extraprostatic extension; LNI, lymph node invasion; SM, surgical margins; SVI, seminal vesical invasion

presence of residual benign prostatic tissue, with accordingly variable prognoses. In a single-surgeon series with more than 15 years of follow-up, median time to detectable metastasis after BCR was 8 years and to death was an additional 5 years.[22] Although nearly 90% of men with BCR have subsequent PSA progression, a relative minority suffer prostate cancer–specific mortality or even detectable metastasis. Within 15 years of BCR, there is an approximately equal distribution (~33%) of men who have died of prostate cancer, died of other causes, or remain alive.[23,24]

Freedland and colleagues[25] conducted a review of 379 patients with disease recurrence following RP to identify risk factors for prostate cancer–specific mortality. Gleason score, PSA doubling time (PSADT), and time from surgery to BCR were found to be significantly associated. In this series, all patients with BCR more than 3 years after RP and a PSADT ≥15 months were alive at 10 years. Conversely, patients with BCR within 3 years of RP, PSADT less than 3 months, and Gleason 8 to 10 had a median survival of 3 years. A more recent study including more than 2000 patients additionally identified preoperative PSA, pathologic features, and PSA level at BCR as predictors of prostate cancer–specific mortality.[23] Considering all of these variables with an assessment of a patient's life expectancy can help determine whether a patient is likely to die from disease or die with disease.

ADJUVANT RADIATION THERAPY: RECURRENCE AND SURVIVAL

In an effort to decrease BCR and mortality rates following radiation therapy (RT) there have been numerous adjuvant and salvage therapies evaluated, including RT. Although multimodal therapy including RT plays a standard role in other visceral malignancies, such as colon, lung, and breast cancer, postoperative adjuvant RT has not been widely embraced in the treatment of prostate cancer. There are 3 large, randomized controlled trials that study postoperative RT in prostate cancer. Men without known nodal or metastatic disease, but with risk factors for disease recurrence following RP were randomized to either RT within 3 to 4 months after RP or initial observation in each of these trials. An overview is outlined in **Table 3**.

EORTC 22911 (European Organisation for Research and Treatment of Cancer), was originally published in 2005 and updated in 2012.[26] Eligible patients were 75 years or younger, World Health Organization (WHO) performance status ≤1, pathologic stage ≤ T3, and had at least 1 of EPE, SVI, or +SMs, although there was no central review of pathology. Patients were excluded if they had major voiding problems before the receipt of radiation, but this was not clearly defined. A total of 1005 patients were randomized to initial observation versus RT within 16 weeks of surgery and followed until clinical relapse, death, or BCR. Patients were not required to have undetectable PSA before randomization. Median follow-up was 10.6 years, and the primary outcome was BCR-free survival. Biochemical or clinical progression or death within 10 years was observed in 198 (39%) patients in the RT arm versus 311 (62%) in the observation arm

Table 3
Results from the 3 randomized clinical trials of radiation after prostatectomy versus initial observation for men with locally advanced prostate cancer

	EORTC 22911	SWOG 8794	ARO 96-02
	Bolla Lancet 2012	Thompson J Urol 2009	Wiegel Eur Urol 2014
Eligibility	pT2-3N0 EPE, SVI, or +SM	pT2-3N0 EPE, SVI, or +SM	pT3-4N0 EPE, SVI, +/−SM
Patients	n = 1005	n = 425	n = 307
Study period	1992–2001	1988–1997	1997–2004
Age (median)	65 y	64–65 y	64 y
Preoperative PSA (median)	12 ng/mL	~10 ng/mL	9–10 ng/mL
Postoperative PSA	≤0.2 ng/mL in 70%	<0.2 ng/mL in 66%	≤0.2 ng/mL in 100%
Radiation	60 Gy Conventional within 4 mo	60–64 Gy Conventional within 4 mo	60 Gy 3D conformal within 3 mo
Median Follow-up	10.6 y	12.6 y	9.3 y
Endpoints (primary in bold) - Adjuvant vs wait-and-see	**BCR-free survival**: 61.8% vs 39.4% (HR 0.49) NNT = 5 10-y OS: 76.9% vs 80.7% (not significant)	**Metastasis-free survival**: 43% vs 54% (HR 0.71) NNT = 10 OS: 52% vs 41% (HR 0.72) NNT = 10	**BCR-free (10 y)**: 56% vs 35% (HR 0.51) NNT = 5 OS: not powered to detect difference

All 3 trials demonstrate improved biochemical, progression-free (BCR-free) survival. Only the trial with the longest follow-up, SWOG, showed improved overall survival (OS).

Abbreviations: ARO, Arbeitsgemeinschaft Radiologische Onkologie; EORTC, European Organisation for Research and Treatment of Cancer; EPE, extraprostatic extension; HR, hazard ratio; LNI, lymph node invasion; NNT, number needed to treat; PSA, prostate-specific antigen; SM, surgical margins; SVI, seminal vesical invasion; SWOG, Southwest Oncology Group.

(hazard ratio 0.49, *P*<.001). The estimated number of men requiring adjuvant RT to prevent 1 BCR was 5. There was no significant difference in metastases, cancer-specific survival, or overall survival. On subgroup analysis patients ≥70 years showed no significant improvement in BCR-free survival and suffered higher mortality compared with initial observation (43% vs 20%, *P*<.001). The reason for increased mortality in this subset is unclear.

SWOG 8794 (Southwest Oncology Group) was published in 2006 and updated in 2009.[27] Eligible patients had pathologic EPE, SVI, or +SMs. Men were excluded if they had total urinary incontinence or intraoperative pelvic or rectal injury. A total of 425 men were randomized to RT within 16 weeks of surgery or observation. As with the EORTC trial, there was no requirement for undetectable PSA before randomization, and many patients were enrolled in the pre-PSA era. The primary outcome was metastasis-free survival. With the longest median follow-up of the 3 trials at 12.6 years, adjuvant RT was associated with a significantly improved median metastasis-free survival of 14.7 versus 12.9 years (*P* = .016).

Overall survival was also significantly improved with a median overall survival of 15.2 versus 13.3 years (*P* = .023), but there was not improvement in cancer-specific survival. The corresponding estimated number of men requiring adjuvant RT to delay 1 death was 10.[28]

ARO 9602 (Arbeitsgemeinschaft Radiologische Onkologie) is the most recent trial with initial results reported in 2009 followed by an update in 2014.[29] In this multicenter study, patients with up to clinical T3 disease and pathologic T3-4 disease with or without +SM were randomized immediately after surgery to 3-dimensional (3D) conformal RT to occur within 12 weeks of RP versus initial observation. However, if a patient had a detectable PSA before their treatment initiation, they were removed from their assigned arm and placed into a third group. This is a significant difference from SWOG and EORTC, which included nearly a third of patients with detectable PSA in their treatment arms and cannot be considered as "pure" adjuvant trials. This led to 159 patients assigned initial observation and 148 patients who received adjuvant RT out of 388 randomized. The primary outcome of progression-free survival (including BCR, clinical progression, and death) was significantly improved in the adjuvant arm with an overall median follow-up of 9.3 years (56% vs 35%; hazard ratio 0.53, P<.001). As with EORTC, the estimated number needed to treat for BCR-free survival benefit is 5. This study did not show a significant difference in overall survival but was not sufficiently powered for this endpoint.

ADJUVANT RADIATION THERAPY: TOXICITY

The EORTC trial measured morbidity using the WHO and Radiation Therapy Oncology Group (RTOG) toxicity scales, which are organized by organ system. In the RTOG system, 5 grades of toxicity are defined, whereby grade 1 is the mildest (eg, no medicines necessary) and grade 5 indicates death from toxicity. For example, grade 2 late bladder toxicity indicates moderate frequency or intermittent gross hematuria, whereas grade 4 indicates severe hemorrhagic cystitis that is life-threatening and requires blood transfusion. There was no grade 4 toxicity reported in the EORTC trial, but there was more grade 3 toxicity in the adjuvant arm, primarily within the first 3 years after treatment (5.3% vs 2.5%). Grade ≥ 2 or genitourinary toxicity was increased (21% vs 13%), but there was no significant difference for gastrointestinal toxicities. There were more late adverse events of any kind in the treatment group (71% vs 60%), but the vast majority were grade 1 or grade 2. The EORTC trial did not directly evaluate erectile function or continence.

The SWOG trial did not include graded assessment of complications. Patients who received adjuvant radiotherapy had more bowel tenderness and urgency for 2 years after treatment and worse urinary frequency until 5 years after treatment. Erectile function was not affected by radiation; however, the reported rate of erectile dysfunction for each group was 94%. There were higher rates of urethral strictures (17.8% vs 9.5%), total urinary incontinence (6.5% vs 2.8%), and rectal complications (3.3% vs 0%) for men assigned initial RT.

A subset of 217 of the SWOG patients participated in a health-related quality of life study.[30] Overall, patients who received adjuvant radiation therapy had worse quality of life for approximately 2 years, after which the trend reversed and patients had significantly better quality of life at 5 years. This was presumably related to less prevalent patient-reported radiation toxicity with time and more men in the observation group eventually requiring salvage treatment with systemic therapy.

The ARO trial reported adverse events in a similar fashion to the EORTC trial. Three-dimensional conformal RT was used, which is likely to decrease toxicity compared with the conventional RT used in the other 2 adjuvant trials. There was no assessment of continence or erectile dysfunction. There was no grade 4 toxicity. There were 3 grade 3 genitourinary events in the radiation therapy arm (2%) versus none in the others. One urethral stricture occurred in the observation arm and 2 in the treatment arm. Including any grade toxicity, the adverse event rate was 21.9% for treatment versus 3.7% for initial observation.

In all 3 trials, severe urinary incontinence was a contraindication to radiation, and none were designed to determine the effect of RT on continence beyond the gross description of total urinary incontinence reported in SWOG. Suardi and colleagues[31] used a detailed multivariable analysis to identify predictors of continence following RP and found a strong association between adjuvant RT and incontinence. Of note, the median radiation dose in this experience was 70 Gy, which is substantially higher than the dose used in the randomized trials. Conversely, a subset of 100 patients from EORTC were prospectively evaluated using a validated system to measure incontinence, and there was no discernable difference in continence between those that received RT and those that did not; notably there was minimal nerve-sparing or bladder neck preservation in this cohort.[32] A recent retrospective analysis showed decreased recovery of erectile function as well as urinary continence in patients receiving RT following RP, especially if RT was received within the first year of RP.[33] It is possible that RT may limit a patient's level of continence recovery. Further work is necessary in this area to better evaluate the effects of dose and timing of radiation on the potential to either limit postoperative recovery or contribute toxicity. A recent comparative study suggests that a delay of 7 months between surgery and radiation may help to limit the development of urinary morbidity.[34]

It is important to note the delivery of radiation therapy has evolved since the adjuvant trials were conducted. Using modern techniques, such as intensity-modulated radiation therapy (IMRT), there may be minimal bladder and bowel toxicity.[35,36] Even at doses of 70 Gy, IMRT has been associated with less toxicity compared with 3D conformal RT, demonstrating a wider therapeutic window.[37] Acute and late toxicities with pelvic IMRT including the nodal beds have also been shown to be decreased relative to SWOG and EORTC data, particularly for gastrointestinal side effects.[38] Patient-reported quality of life in the genitourinary, gastrointestinal, and sexual domains has been reported to be unchanged at 4 years after postoperative radiation.[35]

Despite improvements in the delivery of RT and the evidence the 3 randomized trials provide to support the use of adjuvant RT, there has not been any appreciable increased utilization. Surveillance, Epidemiology, and End Results data from 2000 to 2007 shows a steady 10% to 15% utilization of adjuvant RT for patients with at least 1 risk factor.[39] In the National Cancer Database from 2004 to 2011, the utilization of adjuvant RT remained approximately 10% for eligible patients.[40]

Many physicians may remain concerned about overtreatment, and point out at least 2 major issues with the clinical applicability of the randomized controlled trials. For one, although all 3 trials showed an improvement in BCR-free survival, only the SWOG trial demonstrated an improvement in the more clinically relevant endpoints of metastasis-free and overall survival. The significance of overall survival has been questioned in a secondary analysis of this study revealing imbalances between the treatment and observation groups in their baseline risks for competing causes of mortality. When comorbidity was accounted for, including a difference of mean ages between the group of 1.7 years, an overall survival benefit with adjuvant radiation was no longer apparent.[41]

Second, no trial compared adjuvant (undetectable PSA) with early salvage (detectable PSA) therapy. Many believe an early salvage approach can spare men who were never destined to recur from side effects and cost, while still providing oncologic benefit. Nearly a third of patients in SWOG and EORTC had detectable PSA before treatment assignment so these studies actually included salvage patients. Additionally, RT was not delivered in the initial observation groups until PSA was more than 1 ng/mL in up to half of cases, and was often administered at suboptimal doses by today's standards. There are multiple studies ongoing to address these limitations, which are discussed later in this article.

SALVAGE RADIATION THERAPY

There are a multitude of retrospective studies suggesting the effectiveness of salvage RT over observation. Stephenson and colleagues[42] analyzed a retrospective cohort of 501 patients treated with salvage RT at 5 tertiary care centers between 1987 and 2002. Radiation delivery was nonstandardized, and median pretreatment PSA was 0.7 ng/mL. Over a median follow-up of 45 months, 50% of men achieved and maintained an undetectable PSA and 10% developed metastases, 4% died of

prostate cancer, and 4% died of other causes. Trock and colleagues[43] reviewed a cohort of patients with BCR who went on to have salvage RT versus no salvage treatment. Prostate cancer–specific survival was significantly improved on a multivariate model with a median follow-up of 6 years (hazard ratio [HR] 0.32; 95% confidence interval 0.19–0.54, $P<.01$). Similar findings have been demonstrated in other cohorts.[44,45]

There are no completed randomized trials of adjuvant versus early salvage RT, and retrospective studies have shown mixed results. Trabulsi and colleagues[46] compared 96 patients who received adjuvant RT with 96 patients who received salvage RT after matching according to preoperative PSA, Gleason score, SVI, margin status, and follow-up from surgery. The 5-year BCR-free rate for the adjuvant RT was better at 75% versus 66% for salvage RT (HR 1.6, $P = .49$). A study by Budiharto and colleagues[47] comparing patients who received adjuvant versus salvage RT placed patients into groups based on the presence of lymphovascular invasion (LVI). Patients who received salvage RT had worse BCR-free survival in all combinations of LVI and margin status except for $-SM/+LVI$. Superiority of adjuvant RT was most apparent in the $-SM/-LVI$ cohort in which 5-year BCR-free survival was 90% versus 60% ($P<.001$). However, a major limitation to these studies is the exclusion of patients who elected initial observation and did not recur in the salvage RT arms. Thus, all patients in the salvage RT groups had already recurred, reflecting a more aggressive cancer phenotype compared with an adjuvant group in which only approximately 50% are expected to recur based on data from the randomized trials.

A large analysis accounting for this bias was conducted by Briganti and colleagues[48] on 890 pT3N0 patients treated between 1991 and 2007 who elected either adjuvant RT or initial observation followed by salvage RT at the time of disease recurrence. All patients had pelvic lymph node dissection and an "early" PSA recurrence of ≤ 0.5 ng/mL (median, 0.2 ng/mL) at the time of salvage RT. Approximately half (n = 390) of the patients who underwent initial observation required salvage RT and were matched to patients who underwent adjuvant RT (n = 390). There were no differences in 2-year and 5-year BCR-free survival rates with a median follow-up of 47 months. More recently, Fossati and colleagues[49] reported a matched analysis with a median 93 months of follow-up, and observed there was no difference in metastasis-free or overall survival between adjuvant and salvage RT. Subanalysis in the 2 prior studies showed no difference in BCR-free survival, metastasis, or death even when patients were stratified according to pathologic stage, margin status, and pretreatment PSA.

For salvage RT to have similar effectiveness to adjuvant RT, it must routinely be administered at a low PSA. Nearly 50% of men will have a durable response if they are treated when PSA ≤0.5 ng/mL versus only 18% if PSA greater than 1.5 ng/mL.[50] King[51] used Poisson statistics to estimate 5-year BCR-free survival rates based on PSA at the time of RT. He found the expected control rate for those with PSA less than 0.01 ng/mL is approximately 75%, and drops approximately 2.6% for each additional 0.1 ng/mL increase in PSA.[51] King's[51] hypothesis is supported by results of a recent retrospective study that found an increased rate of distant metastasis in patients receiving salvage RT at a PSA between 0.2 and 0.5 ng/mL versus those who were treated between 0.01 and 0.2 ng/mL.[52] However, men treated at very low PSA may have a greater proportion of benign prostate or relatively indolent cancers causing detectable PSA. Aggressive cancers, including those with micrometastases, may be more likely to recur at a higher first detectable PSA, potentially biasing comparisons in retrospective studies. It is possible that a salvage approach in some high-risk patients may miss a window of curative potential compared with adjuvant treatment.

Risk-adapted treatment strategies have been proposed in which patients most likely to recur are encouraged to undergo adjuvant therapy, whereas lower-risk patients may be more confidently managed with observation and an early salvage approach, if necessary.

Prognostic tools, such as CAPRA-S or nomograms predicting response to salvage radiation are available to guide decisions.[53] Alternatively, a genomic classifier (GC) score has been developed based on the expression levels of 22 genes in the prostate cancer.[54] In a cohort of patients who did not receive adjuvant or salvage RT, low, intermediate, and high-risk GC scores were associated with a 12%, 31%, and 47% risk of metastasis within 10 years, respectively.[55] In a separate study among men with high GC score, the 5-year metastasis rate was 6% for men treated with adjuvant RT (defined as PSA ≤0.2 ng/mL) versus 23% for those treated with salvage RT (defined as PSA >0.2 ng/mL).[56] One model suggested this risk-adjusted strategy of adjuvant versus salvage RT based on GC score could ultimately generate cost savings compared with treating all eligible patients with adjuvant RT.[57] Although GC score has been shown to add precision to risk stratification based on clinically available information, the gain is relatively modest and available data comes only from retrospective studies.[58]

RESTAGING IN SALVAGE RT

PSA can be detected in the blood following RP as the result of any combination of benign tissue in the prostate bed, residual cancer in the pelvis, or extrapelvic disease, most commonly in the bones and/or retroperitoneum. Adjuvant or salvage RT offers a potential benefit only to those patients with residual cancer within the pelvis. Selecting these patients is a challenge and remains an area of active research.

Treatment failure following post-RP RT is mostly attributed to cancer beyond the radiation field. Several clinical factors have been associated with failure of salvage radiation, and by inference may suggest whether a patient harbors occult metastatic disease. A review of more than 1500 patients who received salvage RT determined a PSADT less than 10 months was the most significant predictor of failure.[53] A high pre-radiotherapy PSA was also a poor sign, and frequently led to treatment failure. These factors as well as Gleason score, pathologic stage, margin status, lymph node status, use of neoadjuvant androgen deprivation, and RT dose were incorporated into a nomogram predicting 6-year, BCR-free survival. The test's ability to discriminate patient risks is modest. The clinical applicability of nomograms to "rule-out" distant disease and positive salvage RT response is limited considering, often, treatment should be administered before the ability to calculate a PSADT. Additionally, many high-risk patients did achieve a durable response from salvage RT especially if they were treated at a lower PSA. Of note, as patients with a short PSADT may in fact be the subset most likely to experience a reduction in cancer mortality with salvage radiation, doubling time per se may not be a useful tool for patient selection.[43]

Unfortunately, most conventionally available imaging modalities do not provide much additional help in identifying patients with metastatic disease. At a PSA ≤0.5 ng/mL, transrectal ultrasound can detect disease in the prostate fossa in 14% of patients. Endorectal coil MRI may perform slightly better, with a yield of approximately 25% at a PSA ≤0.3 ng/mL; most of these recurrences will be at or near the vesicourethral anastomosis.[59,60] Positive findings can be useful for radiation treatment planning, but the subsequent impact on clinical outcome remains undefined. Furthermore, because distant disease is not ruled out, local imaging may not aid in patient selection for salvage therapy.[61]

Computerized tomography (CT) and skeletal scintigraphy (bone scan) are important components of initial prostate cancer staging, but are rarely positive in the setting of an early BCR. CT detected disease in fewer than 15% of men who had a mean PSA of 12.4 ng/mL.[62,63] Bone scans similarly reveal metastases in fewer than 5% of patients with BCR and PSA less than 10 ng/mL.[62] Given these characteristics, CT and/or bone scan need not be offered routinely to all patients at the time of BCR.[61] Restaging bone scans can be considered, however, in patients with symptoms, PSA greater than 10 ng/mL, PSADT of less than 6 months, or PSA velocity greater than 0.5 ng/mL per month, due to a much higher rate of detectable metastasis in this cohort.[64]

Various PET tracers have been investigated in conjunction with CT or MRI to improve the ability to localize disease recurrence. Traditional PET with ^{18}F-fluorodeoxyglucose performs poorly in detecting prostate cancer due to the low metabolic activity of prostate cancer cells and obfuscation around the bladder and urethra due to tracer excretion.[65] Choline PET tracers were introduced in the late 1990s to try to overcome these limitations. Radiolabeled choline is preferentially absorbed by cancer cells requiring substrate for cell wall synthesis, and exhibits minimal excretion in the urine.[66] Multiple retrospective studies have shown good performance of ^{18}F-Choline PET/CT when PSA is >2 ng/mL with both sensitivity and specificity greater than 70%.[67–69] With an estimated positive predictive value of approximately 90%, this test can be used to exclude patients from salvage local therapy when distant disease is found. At lower PSA values, the range when salvage RT success rates are most favorable, the sensitivity drops significantly, thereby limiting its use in the routine selection of patients for salvage RT. Similar test characteristics have been reported for an amino acid analog radiotracer, ^{18}F-Fluciclovine.[70]

An alternative radiotracer target under investigation is prostate-specific membrane antigen (PSMA). PSMA is a membrane protein overexpressed in prostate cancer cells.[71] Radiolabeled ^{68}Ga-PSMA PET/CT is both more sensitive and specific than ^{18}F-Choline PET, especially when PSA is less than 0.5 ng/mL.[72] In a study of 319 patients with BCR, ^{68}Ga-PSMA PET was positive in more than 80% of all patients and in approximately 50% of patients with PSA less than 0.5 ng/mL.[73] Among the 42 patients who subsequently had biopsy or surgery, cancer was identified in all 42. Although these patients may have been selected for surgery or biopsy based on having more obviously positive imaging, the results are impressive and imaging with this and other PSMA-specific radiotracers merit further investigation.

FUTURE DIRECTIONS

In the past decade, the role for postoperative radiation after RP has become more established. However, there remain several areas of need for future research. Perhaps the most significant area of need is to improve patient selection, for either adjuvant or salvage radiation. Although some patients with high-risk pathology after prostatectomy may fail locally and will benefit from further treatment, there is also a subset of men who will have distant disease either at the time of, or very early after prostatectomy who will not derive benefit from additional local therapy. Clinical or pathologic factors, such as PSA level, stage, or margin status, are likely to be inadequate to select patients for further therapy, in part due to heterogeneity within particular subgroups at risk. As an example, recent studies showing a benefit for radiation for men with lymph node–positive disease have challenged the traditional conceptual framework that nodal metastases are a surrogate for distant failure. It is plausible to think that a favorable subset of men with lymph node involvement may still derive a reduction in cancer mortality from radiation.[74] Genomic classifiers[56] and novel imaging[73] hold promise to improve patient selection, but neither is likely to accurately identify all men who will benefit from further local therapy. The optimal timing of postoperative radiation is another area of investigation, which when answered may either improve the efficacy of therapy, or limit overtreatment with adjuvant therapy. There are multiple ongoing clinical trials that seek to compare adjuvant and salvage RT.[75–77] **Table 4** shows an overview of current clinical trials. Finally, for men who do undergo postoperative radiation, therapy should be tailored to balance benefit and risk. Several methods of intensifying treatment exist, including increasing radiation dose, expanding volume of coverage (eg, pelvic lymph nodes), and prescribing concurrent hormonal therapy. Clinical trials regarding dose[78] and volume (RTOG 0534) will soon be reported. Meanwhile, 2 trials have recently been published[79,80] demonstrating improved disease outcomes with hormonal therapy. The optimal duration of hormonal therapy remains an open question, as does the potential role of integrating other systemic agents including novel hormonal agents or chemotherapy.

AMERICAN UROLOGIC ASSOCIATION/ AMERICAN SOCIETY FOR RADIATION ONCOLOGY GUIDELINES

In 2013 the American Urologic Association (AUA) and the American Society for Radiation Oncology

Table 4
Current clinical trials comparing adjuvant and salvage radiation therapy

	RADICALS	RAVES	GETUG
Title	Radiotherapy and Androgen Deprivation In Combination After Local Surgery	Adjuvant vs Early Salvage. A Phase III Multi-centre Randomised Trial Comparing Adjuvant Radiotherapy (RT) with Early Salvage RT in Patients with Positive Margins or Extraprostatic Disease Following Radical Prostatectomy	[a]Randomized, Multicenter Study Comparing Immediate Adjuvant RT with Hormonal Therapy vs RT Until Biochemical Relapse with Hormonal Therapy in Patients With Prostate Cancer pT3R1N0 or pNx at Intermediate Risk
Study start date	October 2007	March 2009	December 2007
Estimated enrollment	4236 - Canada, UK, Denmark, Ireland	333 - Australia, New Zealand	718 - France (multicenter)
Randomization	Immediate vs early salvage RT and: no hormone therapy, short hormone therapy, long-term hormone therapy	Immediate vs early salvage RT (within 4 mo following first PSA ≥0.2 ng/mL)	Immediate radiohormonal therapy vs early salvage radiohormonal therapy
Primary outcome	Disease-specific survival	Biochemical recurrence	Biochemical Recurrence at 5 y
Status	Closed Accrual 12/2016	Closed accrual 12/2015 and Estimated completion 12/2026	Actively recruiting

Abbreviations: GETUG, Groupe d' Étude des Tumeurs Uro-Génitales; PSA, prostate-specific antigen; RAVES, Radiotherapy–Adjuvant Versus Early Salvage.
[a] Abbreviated title.

(ASTRO) issued a joint set of 9 guidelines regarding adjuvant and salvage therapy after RP.[81] The guidelines are built on a framework of shared patient-physician decision making, and recognize the current lack of data to inform these decisions. They dictate as clinical principle that patients should be informed before RP about the potential benefits of additional therapy when adverse pathologic features are identified. Additionally, when patients have adverse RP pathology they should be offered adjuvant RT after a discussion of the risks and benefits; notably, this is the only recommendation supported by grade A evidence, and therefore considered a standard of care by AUA/ASTRO. A similar discussion should occur with regard to salvage RT at the time of PSA recurrence if patients did not elect adjuvant treatment. In this setting, a restaging evaluation can be considered, and patients should be informed that RT effectiveness is greatest at lower levels of PSA. The full guidelines can be found through the AUA Web site (https://www.auanet.org/education/guidelines/radiation-after-prostatectomy.cfm).

SUMMARY

An increasing proportion of patients are undergoing RP for locally advanced disease. There are clinical, pathologic, and genomic factors that can be used to personalize risk assessment of disease recurrence following RP and estimate the likelihood of responding favorably to radiation. For those with high-risk features, adjuvant RT has been proven to reduce biochemical recurrence, and may improve overall survival. A reasonable alternative is observation followed by consideration of salvage RT at the time of detectable PSA. Current trials will further elucidate the risks and benefits of post-RP therapy, including the timing of radiation and methods to improve treatment.

REFERENCES

1. Siegel RL, Miller KD, Jemal A. Cancer statistics, 2015: cancer statistics, 2015. CA Cancer J Clin 2015;65(1):5–29.
2. Cancer statistics review, 1975-2013-SEER statistics. Available at: https://seer.cancer.gov/csr/1975_2013/. Accessed March 7, 2017.

3. Bill-Axelson A, Holmberg L, Garmo H, et al. Radical prostatectomy or watchful waiting in early prostate cancer. N Engl J Med 2014;370(10): 932–42.

4. Roehl KA, Han M, Ramos CG, et al. Cancer progression and survival rates following anatomical radical retropubic prostatectomy in 3,478 consecutive patients: long-term results. J Urol 2004;172(3):910–4.

5. Han M, Partin AW, Zahurak M, et al. Biochemical (prostate specific antigen) recurrence probability following radical prostatectomy for clinically localized prostate cancer. J Urol 2003;169(2):517–23.

6. Hull GW, Rabbani F, Abbas F, et al. Cancer control with radical prostatectomy alone in 1,000 consecutive patients. J Urol 2002;167(2 Pt 1):528–34.

7. Cookson MS, Aus G, Burnett AL, et al. Variation in the definition of biochemical recurrence in patients treated for localized prostate cancer: the American Urological Association Prostate Guidelines for localized prostate cancer update panel report and recommendations for a standard in the reporting of surgical outcomes. J Urol 2007;177(2):540–5.

8. Karakiewicz PI, Eastham JA, Graefen M, et al. Prognostic impact of positive surgical margins in surgically treated prostate cancer: multi-institutional assessment of 5831 patients. Urology 2005;66(6): 1245–50.

9. Messing EM, Manola J, Yao J, et al. Immediate versus deferred androgen deprivation treatment in patients with node-positive prostate cancer after radical prostatectomy and pelvic lymphadenectomy. Lancet Oncol 2006;7(6):472–9.

10. Stephenson AJ, Scardino PT, Eastham JA, et al. Postoperative nomogram predicting the 10-year probability of prostate cancer recurrence after radical prostatectomy. J Clin Oncol 2005;23(28): 7005–12.

11. Cooperberg MR, Hilton JF, Carroll PR. The CAPRA-S score. Cancer 2011;117(22):5039–46.

12. Tilki D, Mandel P, Schlomm T, et al. External validation of the CAPRA-S score to predict biochemical recurrence, metastasis and mortality after radical prostatectomy in a European Cohort. J Urol 2015; 193(6):1970–5.

13. Punnen S, Freedland SJ, Presti JC Jr, et al. Multi-institutional validation of the CAPRA-S score to predict disease recurrence and mortality after radical prostatectomy. Eur Urol 2014;65(6):1171–7.

14. Lowrance WT, Elkin EB, Yee DS, et al. Locally advanced prostate cancer: a population-based study of treatment patterns. BJU Int 2012;109(9): 1309–14.

15. Martin JM, Handorf EA, Kutikov A, et al. The rise and fall of prostate brachytherapy: use of brachytherapy for the treatment of localized prostate cancer in the national cancer data base. Cancer 2014;120(14): 2114–21.

16. Lu-Yao GL, Albertsen PC, Moore DF, et al. Survival following primary androgen deprivation therapy among men with localized prostate cancer. JAMA 2008;300(2):173–81.

17. Cooperberg MR, Carroll PR. Trends in management for patients with localized prostate cancer, 1990-2013. JAMA 2015;314(1):80–2.

18. U.S. Preventive Services Task Force. Screening for prostate cancer: U.S. Preventive Services Task Force recommendation statement. Ann Intern Med 2008;149(3):185–91.

19. Moyer VA. Screening for prostate cancer: U.S. Preventive Services Task Force recommendation statement. Ann Intern Med 2012;157(2):120–34.

20. Shen X, Kumar P. Trade-off between treatment of early prostate cancer and incidence of advanced prostate cancer in the prostate screening era. J Urol 2016;195(5):1397–402.

21. Reese AC, Wessel SR, Fisher SG, et al. Evidence of prostate cancer "reverse stage migration" toward more advanced disease at diagnosis: data from the Pennsylvania Cancer Registry. Urol Oncol 2016;34(8):335.e21-8.

22. Pound CR, Partin AW, Eisenberger MA, et al. Natural history of progression after PSA elevation following radical prostatectomy. JAMA 1999;281(17):1591–7.

23. Brockman JA, Alanee S, Vickers AJ, et al. Nomogram predicting prostate cancer–specific mortality for men with biochemical recurrence after radical prostatectomy. Eur Urol 2015;67(6):1160.

24. Bianco FJ Jr, Scardino PT, Eastham JA. Radical prostatectomy: long-term cancer control and recovery of sexual and urinary function ("trifecta"). Urology 2005;66(5 Suppl):83–94.

25. Freedland SJ, Humphreys EB, Mangold LA, et al. Risk of prostate cancer–specific mortality following biochemical recurrence after radical prostatectomy. JAMA 2005;294(4):433–9.

26. Bollá M, van Poppel H, Tombal B, et al. Postoperative radiotherapy after radical prostatectomy for high-risk prostate cancer: long-term results of a randomised controlled trial (EORTC trial 22911). Lancet 2012;380(9858):2018–27.

27. Thompson IM, Tangen CM, Paradelo J, et al. Adjuvant radiotherapy for pathological T3N0M0 prostate cancer significantly reduces risk of metastases and improves survival: long-term followup of a randomized clinical trial. J Urol 2009; 181(3):956–62.

28. Daly T, Hickey BE, Lehman M, et al. Adjuvant radiotherapy following radical prostatectomy for prostate cancer. Cochrane Database Syst Rev 2011;12: CD007234.

29. Wiegel T, Bartkowiak D, Bottke D, et al. Adjuvant radiotherapy versus wait-and-see after radical prostatectomy: 10-year follow-up of the ARO 96–02/AUO AP 09/95 trial. Eur Urol 2014;66(2):243–50.

30. Moinpour CM, Hayden KA, Unger JM, et al. Health-related quality of life results in pathologic stage C prostate cancer from a southwest oncology group trial comparing radical prostatectomy alone with radical prostatectomy plus radiation therapy. J Clin Oncol 2008;26(1):112–20.

31. Suardi N, Gallina A, Lista G, et al. Impact of adjuvant radiation therapy on urinary continence recovery after radical prostatectomy. Eur Urol 2014;65(3): 546–51.

32. Van Cangh PJ, Richard F, Lorge F, et al. Adjuvant radiation therapy does not cause urinary incontinence after radical prostatectomy: results of a prospective randomized study. J Urol 1998;159(1):164–6.

33. Zaffuto E, Gandaglia G, Fossati N, et al. Early postoperative radiotherapy is associated with worse functional outcomes in patients with prostate cancer. J Urol 2017;197(3 Pt 1):669–75.

34. van Stam M-A, Aaronson NK, Pos FJ, et al. The effect of salvage radiotherapy and its timing on the health-related quality of life of prostate cancer patients. Eur Urol 2016;70(5):751–7.

35. Corbin KS, Kunnavakkam R, Eggener SE, et al. Intensity modulated radiation therapy after radical prostatectomy: early results show no decline in urinary continence, gastrointestinal, or sexual quality of life. Pract Radiat Oncol 2013;3(2):138–44.

36. Melotek JM, Liao C, Liauw SL. Quality of life after post-prostatectomy intensity modulated radiation therapy: pelvic nodal irradiation is not associated with worse bladder, bowel, or sexual outcomes. PLoS One 2015;10(10):e0141639.

37. Goenka A, Magsanoc JM, Pei X, et al. Improved toxicity profile following high-dose postprostatectomy salvage radiation therapy with intensity-modulated radiation therapy. Eur Urol 2011;60(6): 1142–8.

38. Alongi F, Fiorino C, Cozzarini C, et al. IMRT significantly reduces acute toxicity of whole-pelvis irradiation in patients treated with post-operative adjuvant or salvage radiotherapy after radical prostatectomy. Radiother Oncol 2009;93(2):207–12.

39. Hoffman KE, Nguyen PL, Chen M-H, et al. Recommendations for post-prostatectomy radiation therapy in the United States before and after the presentation of randomized trials. J Urol 2011; 185(1):116–20.

40. Kalbasi A, Swisher-McClure S, Mitra N, et al. Low rates of adjuvant radiation in patients with nonmetastatic prostate cancer with high-risk pathologic features. Cancer 2014;120(19):3089–96.

41. Zakeri K, Rose BS, Gulaya S, et al. Competing event risk stratification may improve the design and efficiency of clinical trials: secondary analysis of SWOG 8794. Contemp Clin Trials 2013;34(1):74–9.

42. Stephenson AJ, Shariat SF, Zelefsky MJ, et al. Salvage radiotherapy for recurrent prostate cancer after radical prostatectomy. JAMA 2004;291(11): 1325–32.

43. Trock BJ, Han M, Freedland SJ, et al. Prostate cancer-specific survival following salvage radiotherapy vs observation in men with biochemical recurrence after radical prostatectomy. JAMA 2008;299(23): 2760–9.

44. Loeb S, Roehl KA, Viprakasit DP, et al. Long-term rates of undetectable PSA with Initial observation and delayed salvage radiotherapy after radical prostatectomy. Eur Urol 2008;54(1):88–96.

45. Tsien C, Griffith KA, Sandler HM, et al. Long-term results of three-dimensional conformal adjuvant and salvage radiotherapy after radical prostatectomy. Urology 2003;62(1):93–8.

46. Trabulsi EJ, Valicenti RK, Hanlon AL, et al. A multi-institutional matched-control analysis of adjuvant and salvage postoperative radiation therapy for pT3-4N0 prostate cancer. Urology 2008;72(6): 1298–302.

47. Budiharto T, Perneel C, Haustermans K, et al. A multi-institutional analysis comparing adjuvant and salvage radiation therapy for high-risk prostate cancer patients with undetectable PSA after prostatectomy. Radiother Oncol 2010;97(3): 474–9.

48. Briganti A, Wiegel T, Joniau S, et al. Early salvage radiation therapy does not compromise cancer control in patients with pT3N0 prostate cancer after radical prostatectomy: results of a match-controlled multi-institutional analysis. Eur Urol 2012;62(3):472–87.

49. Fossati N, Karnes RJ, Boorjian SA, et al. Long-term impact of adjuvant versus early salvage radiation therapy in pT3N0 prostate cancer patients treated with radical prostatectomy: results from a multi-institutional series. Eur Urol 2017;71(6): 886–93.

50. King CR. The timing of salvage radiotherapy after radical prostatectomy: a systematic review. Int J Radiat Oncol Biol Phys 2012;84(1):104–11.

51. King CR. Adjuvant radiotherapy after prostatectomy: does waiting for a detectable prostate-specific antigen level make sense? Int J Radiat Oncol Biol Phys 2011;80(1):1–3.

52. Abugharib A, Jackson WC, Tumati V, et al. Very early salvage radiotherapy improves distant metastasis-free survival. J Urol 2017;197(3 Pt 1):662–8.

53. Stephenson AJ, Scardino PT, Kattan MW, et al. Predicting the outcome of salvage radiation therapy for recurrent prostate cancer after radical prostatectomy. J Clin Oncol 2007;25(15): 2035–41.

54. Karnes RJ, Bergstralh EJ, Davicioni E, et al. Validation of a genomic classifier that predicts metastasis following radical prostatectomy in an at risk patient population. J Urol 2013;190(6):2047–53.

55. Ross AE, Johnson MH, Yousefi K, et al. Tissue-based genomics augments post-prostatectomy risk stratification in a natural history cohort of inter-mediate- and high-risk men. Eur Urol 2016;69(1): 157–65.

56. Den RB, Yousefi K, Trabulsi EJ, et al. Genomic classifier identifies men with adverse pathology af-ter radical prostatectomy who benefit from adju-vant radiation therapy. J Clin Oncol 2015;33(8): 944–51.

57. Lobo JM, Trifiletti DM, Sturz VN, et al. Cost-effective-ness of the decipher genomic classifier to guide individualized decisions for early radiation therapy after prostatectomy for prostate cancer. Clin Genito-urin Cancer 2017;15(3):e299–309.

58. Cooperberg MR, Davicioni E, Crisan A, et al. Com-bined value of validated clinical and genomic risk stratification tools for predicting prostate cancer mortality in a high-risk prostatectomy cohort. Eur Urol 2015;67(2):326–33.

59. Leventis AK, Shariat SF, Slawin KM. Local recur-rence after radical prostatectomy: correlation of US features with prostatic fossa biopsy findings. Radi-ology 2001;219(2):432–9.

60. Liauw SL, Pitroda SP, Eggener SE, et al. Evaluation of the prostate bed for local recurrence after radical prostatectomy using endorectal magnetic reso-nance imaging. Int J Radiat Oncol 2013;85(2): 378–84.

61. Beresford MJ, Gillatt D, Benson RJ, et al. A systematic review of the role of imaging before salvage radiotherapy for post-prostatectomy biochemical recurrence. Clin Oncol 2010;22(1): 46–55.

62. Kane CJ, Amling CL, Johnstone PAS, et al. Limited value of bone scintigraphy and computed tomography in assessing biochemical failure after radical prostatectomy. Urology 2003;61(3): 607–11.

63. Johnstone PA, Tarman GJ, Riffenburgh R, et al. Yield of imaging and scintigraphy assessing biochemical failure in prostate cancer patients. Urol Oncol 1997; 3(4):108–12.

64. Gomez P, Manoharan M, Kim SS, et al. Radionuclide bone scintigraphy in patients with biochemical recurrence after radical prostatectomy: when is it indicated? BJU Int 2004;94(3):299–302.

65. Hofer C, Laubenbacher C, Block T, et al. Fluorine-18-fluorodeoxyglucose positron emission tomogra-phy is useless for the detection of local recurrence after radical prostatectomy. Eur Urol 1999;36(1): 31–5.

66. Hara T, Kosaka N, Kishi H. PET imaging of prostate cancer using carbon-11-choline. J Nucl Med 1998; 39(6):990–5.

67. Krause BJ, Souvatzoglou M, Tuncel M, et al. The detection rate of [11C]Choline-PET/CT depends on the serum PSA-value in patients with biochemical recurrence of prostate cancer. Eur J Nucl Med Mol Imaging 2008;35(1):18–23.

68. Giovacchini G, Picchio M, Coradeschi E, et al. Predictive factors of [11C]choline PET/CT in pa-tients with biochemical failure after radical prosta-tectomy. Eur J Nucl Med Mol Imaging 2010;37(2): 301–9.

69. Vees H, Buchegger F, Albrecht S, et al. 18F-choline and/or 11C-acetate positron emission tomography: detection of residual or progressive subclinical dis-ease at very low prostate-specific antigen values (<1 ng/mL) after radical prostatectomy. BJU Int 2007;99(6):1415–20.

70. Schuster DM, Nanni C, Fanti S. PET tracers beyond FDG in prostate cancer. Semin Nucl Med 2016; 46(6):507–21.

71. Sweat SD, Pacelli A, Murphy GP, et al. Prostate-spe-cific membrane antigen expression is greatest in prostate adenocarcinoma and lymph node metasta-ses. Urology 1998;52(4):637–40.

72. Morigi JJ, Stricker PD, van Leeuwen PJ, et al. Pro-spective comparison of 18F-fluoromethylcholine versus 68Ga-PSMA PET/CT in prostate cancer pa-tients who have rising PSA after curative treatment and are being considered for targeted therapy. J Nucl Med 2015;56(8):1185–90.

73. Afshar-Oromieh A, Avtzi E, Giesel FL, et al. The diag-nostic value of PET/CT imaging with the 68Ga-labelled PSMA ligand HBED-CC in the diagnosis of recurrent prostate cancer. Eur J Nucl Med Mol Imag-ing 2015;42(2):197–209.

74. Abdollah F, Karnes RJ, Suardi N, et al. Impact of adjuvant radiotherapy on survival of patients with node-positive prostate cancer. J Clin Oncol 2014; 32(35):3939–47.

75. Pearse M, Fraser-Browne C, Davis ID, et al. A Phase III trial to investigate the timing of radiotherapy for prostate cancer with high-risk features: background and rationale of the radiotherapy – Adjuvant Versus Early Salvage (RAVES) trial. BJU Int 2014; 113(Suppl 2):7–12.

76. Parker C, Sydes MR, Catton C, et al. Radiotherapy and androgen deprivation in combination after local surgery (RADICALS): a new Medical Research Council/National Cancer Institute of Canada phase III trial of adjuvant treatment after radical prostatec-tomy. BJU Int 2007;99(6):1376–9.

77. Triptorelin and radiation therapy in treating patients who have undergone surgery for intermediate-risk stage III or stage IV prostate cancer - Full text view - ClinicalTrials.gov. Available at: https://clinicaltrials.gov/ct2/show/NCT00667069. Accessed March 29, 2017.

78. Ghadjar P, Hayoz S, Bernhard J, et al. Acute toxicity and quality of life after dose-intensified salvage radi-ation therapy for biochemically recurrent prostate

cancer after prostatectomy: first results of the randomized trial SAKK 09/10. J Clin Oncol 2015; 33(35):4158–66.

79. Shipley WU, Seiferheld W, Lukka HR, et al. Radiation with or without antiandrogen therapy in recurrent prostate cancer. N Engl J Med 2017;376(5):417–28.

80. Carrie C, Hasbini A, de Laroche G, et al. Salvage radiotherapy with or without short-term hormone therapy for rising prostate-specific antigen concentration after radical prostatectomy (GETUG-AFU 16): a randomised, multicentre, open-label phase 3 trial. Lancet Oncol 2016;17(6):747–56.

81. Thompson IM, Valicenti RK, Albertsen P, et al. Adjuvant and salvage radiotherapy after prostatectomy: AUA/ASTRO guideline. J Urol 2013;190(2): 441–9.

Newly Diagnosed Metastatic Prostate Cancer: Has the Paradigm Changed?

Shivashankar Damodaran, MBBS, MCh[a],
Christos E. Kyriakopoulos, MD[b], David F. Jarrard, MD[c],*

KEYWORDS

- Prostate cancer (PCa) • Hormone-sensitive prostate cancer (HSPC)
- Androgen deprivation therapy (ADT) • Docetaxel • Androgen axis inhibitors

KEY POINTS

- Median overall survival is almost 4 times the failure-free survival and metastatic castration-resistant prostate cancer (CRPC) makes up most of the survival time in patients with metastatic prostate cancer. Three major phase III studies combining ADT with docetaxel in patients with newly diagnosed metastatic prostate cancer have been recently reported.
- The GETUG-AFU 15 trial failed to show a survival advantage for chemohormonal therapy over ADT alone, although progression-free survival (clinical and biochemical) and prostate-specific antigen control were improved.
- The role of surgery and newer androgen receptor pathway inhibitors in metastatic hormone-sensitive prostate cancer is currently being studied.
- Early chemohormonal therapy for hormone-sensitive metastatic prostate cancer leads to improved overall survival and should be used for good performance patients with moderate and high-volume metastatic disease.

INTRODUCTION

Metastatic prostate cancer (mPCa) carries a dismal 5-year survival rate of 29.3%.[1] This is in stark contrast to the nearly 100% 5-year survival for low-volume organ-confined disease. The conventional treatment of PCa has been androgen deprivation therapy (ADT) ever since the landmark discovery of androgen ablation for metastatic PCa by Charles Huggins and Clarence Hodges in 1941.[2] In a retrospective review from the National Cancer Center, the median time for progression to metastatic castration-resistant PCa (mCRPC) was found to be 13.1 months and 19.3 months in patients with and without radiologic evidence of metastasis at initiation of ADT, respectively.[3] A systematic review of 12 studies including 71,179 patients found that 10% to 20% of patients with

Disclosure statement: The authors have no disclosures, nor any commercial or financial conflicts of interest nor funding sources.
[a] Urologic Oncology, Department of Urology, University of Wisconsin School of Medicine and Public Health, 1111 Highland Avenue, Madison, WI 53705-2281, USA; [b] Department of Medicine, University of Wisconsin School of Medicine and Public Health, 600 Highland Avenue, Madison, WI 53792-0001, USA; [c] Department of Urology, University of Wisconsin School of Medicine and Public Health, Uiniversity of Wisconsin Carbone Cancer Center, 600 Highland Avenue, Madison, WI 53705, USA
* Corresponding author.
E-mail address: jarrard@urology.wisc.edu

Urol Clin N Am 44 (2017) 611–621
http://dx.doi.org/10.1016/j.ucl.2017.07.008
0094-0143/17/© 2017 Elsevier Inc. All rights reserved.

urologic.theclinics.com

mPCa develop mCRPC within 5 years of follow-up.[4]

The survival of PCa in metastatic patients is being more clearly defined and has changed in the modern era. James and colleagues,[5] reported a median failure-free survival (FFS) of 11 months (2-year FFS of 29%) for patients with newly diagnosed metastatic PCa enrolled in the recent Systemic Therapy in Advancing or Metastatic PCa: Evaluation of Drug Efficacy (STAMPEDE) trial. The median overall survival (OS) was 42 months (2-year OS was 72%) in this same cohort. The finding that median OS is almost 4 times the median FFS demonstrates that the mCRPC now makes up most of the survival time rather than being a short terminal phase with limited treatment options. Furthermore, in the same study, it was observed that the median time to the next therapy was 20 months for the control arm and 15.4 months for the experimental arm, emphasizing that important time is lost in waiting for CRPC transition. Median OS times in the Southwest Oncology Group (SWOG) trials cited by Tangen and colleagues[6] ranged from 32 months in the oldest trial to 49 months in the more recent one, demonstrating improved survival in more modern studies similar to the results reported in STAMPEDE.[7]

Metastatic hormone-sensitive PCa (mHSPC) is a heterogeneous disease that consists of both androgen receptor (AR)-positive and AR-negative cells. ADT eventually selects a clonal population that is capable of surviving without AR-mediated signaling.[8] The mechanisms of overcoming androgen loss during CRPC transition include autocrine androgen production, amplification of AR protein and mechanisms that bypass the AR, such as coactivators and trans activators. Some of the most important of these biologically heterogeneous mechanisms involve cancer stem cells, receptor tyrosine kinases, and neuroendocrine differentiation (NE). Cells that have a "stemlike" phenotype are potentially resistant to ADT and can differentiate into androgen-independent cells.[9,10] The activation of the PI3/Akt tyrosine kinase signaling by deletion, mutation, and methylation silencing of PTEN tumor suppressor gene function is thought to be caused by selective pressure caused by ADT.[11–13] NE differentiation also occurs in an adenocarcinoma prostate-specific antigen (PSA)-secreting environment under the selection pressure of ADT. These cells effectively progress to CRPC through the production of neurosecretory peptides in potentially up to 25% of advanced cancers.[11,12] AR gene amplification is another important mechanism by which PCa cells acquire resistance to conventional ADT and these cells are a target for second-line hormonal therapy[14,15] Thus, CRPC is now known to be the consequence of selective pressure exerted by ADT on mHSPC, which induces clonal selection and the growth of androgen-independent clones.[16–21]

Docetaxel was initially approved for the treatment of metastatic CRPC in 2004 based on 2 separate studies that for the first time confirmed a survival benefit in that setting.[22,23] Despite the small increase in OS (2.4 months in TAX 327 and 1.9 months in SWOG 99–16, respectively), it was approved for the treatment and paved the way to subsequent studies that saw an increasing number of newer agents for CRPC management.[24] Subsequently, combining docetaxel with ADT in the hormone-sensitive setting emerged as an appealing strategy to delay development of CRPC and prolong survival. The rationale behind this approach was some degree of resistance to ADT is already present at the time of diagnosis, a phenomenon that is thought to be proportional to the tumor burden. Early chemotherapy could potentially eradicate the hormone-resistant subpopulation, thus prolonging the time to CRPC transition. In support of this hypothesis, simultaneous castration and treatment with paclitaxel in mouse models was found to be superior to sequential administration.[25] Engrafted mice receiving chemohormonal therapy showed delayed median time to progression compared with those treated with sequential castration and chemotherapy. The explanation for the synergistic activity of taxanes and ADT was provided by Zhu and colleagues in 2010,[26] when they showed that taxanes blocked the microtubule-mediated AR nuclear localization by androgens, thus effectively blocking AR-signaling pathways. In addition to the potential synergistic effect of taxanes to ADT, a proportion of patients might be too frail at the time of development of CRPC and thus might miss the opportunity to receive treatment with a potent chemotherapeutic agent.[27]

Discussion

To date, 3 large-scale phase III studies have examined the role of docetaxel in HSPC:

- *GETUG-AFU 15* (Groupe d'Etude des Tumeurs Uro-Genital and Association Française d'Urologie)
- *CHAARTED* (Chemo-Hormonal therapy vs Androgen Ablation Randomized Trial for Extensive Disease in PCa)
- *STAMPEDE* (Systemic Therapy in Advancing or Metastatic PCa: Evaluation of Drug Efficacy)

These studies have driven the recent change in paradigm regarding the early treatment with docetaxel and ADT in metastatic HSPC.

Groupe d'Etude des Tumeurs Uro-Genital and Association Française d'Urologie

The GETUG-AFU 15 was the first phase III study published that compared ADT alone versus ADT plus docetaxel.[28] A total of 385 men with mHSPC were enrolled in 29 centers in France and 1 in Belgium. Eligible patients were required to have biopsy-proven PCa with radiologic evidence of metastasis, Karnofsky score above 70, minimum life expectancy of 3 months, and adequate hepatic and renal function.

Treatment plan Patients were 1:1 randomized to ADT versus ADT in combination with docetaxel. Treatment with ADT included orchiectomy or luteinizing hormone releasing hormone (LHRH) agonists, alone or in combination with steroidal antiandrogens. In addition, patients in the chemohormonal therapy arm received docetaxel 75 mg/m^2 every 3 weeks for a maximum of 9 cycles. The primary end point of the study was OS, with clinical progression-free survival (PFS) and biochemical PFS being secondary endpoints. Patients who had started ADT within 2 months of the study enrollment were included and efficacy analysis.

Evaluation The initial assessment included clinical history, physical examination, weight, and Karnofsky performance status. Imaging (computed tomography [CT] scan and bone scan as indicated), electrocardiography, and blood investigation, including serum PSA, were done within 30 days of treatment initiation. Patients in the chemohormonal arm underwent clinical and laboratory evaluation every 3 weeks while receiving chemotherapy and every 3 months thereafter, whereas patients in the ADT-alone arm were evaluated every 3 months. Imaging studies were repeated every 3 months. For patients remaining on study for more than 42 months, clinical, laboratory, and radiographic evaluations were spaced out to every 6 months. Biochemical PFS was defined as PSA decrease of at least 50% and an increase of at least 50% above the nadir, with an absolute increase of 5 ng/mL. For patients without PSA nadir less than 50%, progression was defined as a PSA increase of at least 25% above the nadir and 5 ng/mL, both confirmed by a confirmatory testing. Clinical progression was defined as progression of preexisting lesions with Response Evaluation Criteria in Solid Tumors (RECIST) or appearance of new bone lesions, whichever occurred first.

Results Between October 2004 and December 2008, 192 patients were randomly assigned to receive ADT plus docetaxel and 193 to receive ADT alone. A total of 71% of the patients who participated had metastatic disease at diagnosis. The median number of cycles of treatment with docetaxel was 8, with fewer than half of all patients receiving all 9 cycles. Median follow-up was 50 months (interquartile range 39–63). Median OS was not significantly different between the 2 arms (58.9 months for the chemohormonal arm vs 54.2 months for the ADT-alone arm [hazard ratio (HR) 1.01, 95% confidence interval (CI) 0.75–1.36]). However, a significantly longer biochemical PFS (22.9 vs 12.9 months; HR 0.72; 95% CI 0.57–0.91; $P = .005$) and clinical PFS (23.5 vs 15.4 months; HR 0.75; 95% CI 0.59–0.94; $P = .015$), respectively, was observed in the patients receiving chemohormonal therapy.

In a subsequent report of GETUG-AFU 15 with a longer median follow-up of 83.9 months, there was a numerically improved OS for the chemohormonal therapy group, but this did not reach statistical significance (62.1 months vs 48.6 months; HR 0.88; 95% CI 0.68–1.14; $P = .3$). Of note, the initial design of that study did not include tumor volume as a stratification factor. A subsequent retrospective analysis based on tumor volume was conducted and again failed to reach statistical significance for OS for high-volume patients on docetaxel + ADT compared with patients with high-volume disease on ADT alone (39.8 months vs 35.1 months; HR 0.78; 95% CI 0.56–1.09; $P = .14$). The investigators concluded that the addition of chemotherapy to ADT does not improve OS compared with ADT alone, although PFS (clinical and biochemical) and PSA control were improved.

E3805 the Chemo-Hormonal therapy vs Androgen Ablation Randomized Trial for Extensive Disease in Prostate Cancer Trial

This landmark trial was the first one to show that the addition of 6 cycles of docetaxel 75 mg/m^2 every 3 weeks to standard ADT significantly improved outcomes in men with metastatic HSPC.[29] The study was designed in 2005 by the Eastern Cooperative Oncology Group (now ECOG-ACRIN) and enrolled patients through ECOG, SWOG, the Alliance for Clinical Trials in Oncology, and NRG Oncology (a merged group that includes the National Surgical Adjuvant Breast and Bowel Project, the Radiation Therapy Oncology Group, and the Gynecologic Oncology Group), and the Clinical Trials Support Unit. The primary objective of the study was to determine whether the addition of docetaxel to ADT could improve the OS in patients with newly diagnosed mHSPC. Eligible patients were required to have either a pathologic diagnosis of metastatic PCa or an elevated serum PSA with clinical features consistent with metastatic disease and an ECOG performance status between 0 and 2. Furthermore, patients who had received ADT in the adjuvant setting were allowed to enroll as long as the duration of treatment was less than 24 months and it had stopped at least 12 months before the development of metastatic disease. Patients who had already started ADT had a window period of 120 days before randomization.

Treatment plan Patients were randomly assigned to 2 arms: ADT alone versus ADT plus docetaxel. Docetaxel dose was 75 mg per square meter of body-surface area given every 3 weeks for up to 6 cycles. Patients developing significant toxicities from docetaxel were allowed 2 dose reductions to 65 mg and 55 mg per square meter respectively, as clinically indicated. Patient stratification was done according to age (<70 years vs ≥70 years), ECOG performance status (0 or 1 vs 2), planned use of combined androgen blockade for more than 30 days, prior usage of agents approved for prevention of skeletal-related events in castration-resistant disease (zoledronic acid or denosumab), duration of prior ADT (<12 months vs ≥12 months) and tumor volume (high vs low). High-volume disease was defined as the presence of visceral metastases or ≥4 bone lesions with at least 1 lesion beyond the vertebral bodies and pelvis. This study design was unique among the contemporary trials in stratifying patients based on tumor volume.

Evaluation Patients in the ADT-alone arm were followed every 3 months, whereas patients in the ADT plus docetaxel arm were followed every 3 weeks for the duration of chemotherapy and every 3 months thereafter. PSA levels were measured at each scheduled visit. Imaging in the form of CT of the abdomen and pelvis, technetium-99m bone scan and radiography or CT of the chest, as clinically indicated were performed at baseline, as clinically indicated as well as at the time of development of CRPC. Disease progression on imaging was determined according to the RECIST. A complete PSA control was defined as a PSA level of less than 0.2 ng per milliliter on 2 consecutive measurements at least 4 weeks apart. Serologic progression was defined as an increase in the PSA level of more than 50% above the nadir reached after the initiation of ADT, with 2 consecutive increases at least 2 weeks apart. The date of a first recorded increase of more than 50% above the nadir was deemed the date of progression.

Results From July 2006 through 2012, a total of 790 patients were enrolled and underwent randomization.[30] The mean follow-up duration was 28.9 months, with 136 deaths in the ADT-alone group and 101 deaths in the combination group. The mean age was 64 years in the combination group and 63 in ADT-alone group. In both groups, approximately 85% of the patients were white, approximately 70% had an ECOG performance status score of 0, and approximately 65% had high-volume disease. A total of 60% had a Gleason score of 8 or higher. The median OS was 57.6 months in the chemohormonal arm versus 44 months in the ADT-alone arm, thus conferring an improvement of 13.6 months in OS (HR 0.61; 95% CI 0.47–0.80; P<.001). The improvement in OS was more pronounced in the high-volume disease subgroup (49.2 months vs 32.2 months; HR 0.60; 95% CI 0.45–0.81; P<.001). In contrast, there was no statistically significant difference in the OS with the addition of docetaxel for the low-volume group (64 months vs not reached, HR 1.04; 95% CI 0.70–1.55; P = .11). In addition to OS, the median time to CRPC was also prolonged in the chemohormonal arm compared with ADT-alone arm (20.2 months vs 11.7 months; HR 0.61; 95% CI 0.51–0.72; P<.001), as well as the median time for clinical progression (33 months vs 19.8 months; HR 0.61; 95% CI 0.50–0.75; P<.001).

In a more recent report of the CHAARTED trial with a longer follow-up of 53.7 months, the initial results were confirmed (OS of 57.6 months for ADT plus docetaxel vs 47.2 months for ADT alone; HR 0.73 [0.59–0.89]; P = .0018). However, even though patients with high-volume disease were clearly found to benefit from the addition of docetaxel (OS 51.2 months vs 34.4 months; HR 0.63 [0.50–0.79]; P<.0001), for low-volume patients, the addition of docetaxel was not found to confer a survival benefit (OS 63.5 months vs NR (not reported) for ADT alone; HR 1.04 [0.70–1.55]; P = .86).[30] Another subgroup analysis in patients with de novo disease showed a median OS of 48 months in high-volume disease treated with chemohormonal therapy compared with high-volume disease treated with ADT alone (48.0 vs 34.1 months; HR 0.63 [0.49–0.81]; P<.001).

The investigators concluded that the addition of 6 cycles of docetaxel to ADT during the initiation of treatment for high-volume metastatic HSPC was associated with a significant improvement in OS, longer time to development of CRPC, better PSA control at 1 year of follow-up, higher cancer-specific survival, and a substantially longer OS.

Systemic Therapy in Advancing or Metastatic Prostate Cancer: Evaluation of Drug Efficacy

This innovative multiarm, multistage trial incorporated a phase II/III approach to assess the impact of hormonal therapy at the time of initiation of long-term hormonal therapy. This trial added much needed evidence to the findings of CHAARTED trial. It showed a definitive survival benefit from early chemohormonal therapy with docetaxel in patients with HSPC.[31] Newly diagnosed metastatic, node-positive, or high-risk locally advanced (with at least 2 features from T3/4, Gleason score of 8–10, and PSA $\geq$40 ng/mL); or previously treated with radical surgery, radiotherapy, or both and relapsing with high-risk features were used as inclusion criteria.

Treatment plan A total of 2962 previously untreated patients with both metastatic and nonmetastatic PCa were randomly assigned in a 2:1:1:1 ratio to the following arms.

- ADT (n = 1184)
- ADT plus zoledronic acid (n = 593)
- ADT plus docetaxel (n = 592)
- ADT plus zoledronic acid and docetaxel (n = 593)

Patients in the ADT arm received LHRH agonist, antagonist, or antiandrogen, with orchiectomy allowed as an alternative for drug therapy. Six 3-weekly cycles of zoledronic acid (4 mg) was followed by once-a-month dosing up to 2 years. Docetaxel (75 mg/m^2) was given along with prednisolone for six 3-weekly cycles and trial therapy was discontinued after intolerable side effects or disease progression.

Evaluation Patients were followed-up every 6 weeks for 6 months, every 12 weeks for 2 years, and every 6 months for 5 years. PSA was measured at every follow-up visit and other tests were done at the clinician's discretion. The lowest value of PSA within 24 weeks of starting treatment was considered as the nadir value. The primary endpoints were OS and FFS. FFS was defined as time from randomization to onset of biochemical failure, local or systemic progression, or death from prostate cancer. Biochemical failure was defined as PSA increase of 50% above nadir and absolute increase by 4 ng/mL and confirmed by retesting.

Results After a median follow-up of 43 months, the primary endpoint of OS was significantly improved for patients who received docetaxel in combination with ADT versus patients who received ADT alone (81 months for the combination arm vs

71 months for the ADT-alone arm; HR 0.78; 95% CI 0.66–0.93; P = .006), as well as for the patients who received both docetaxel and zoledronic acid versus the patients who received neither docetaxel nor zoledronic acid (76 months vs 71 months; HR 0.82; 95% CI 0.69–0.97; P = .022). Maximal benefit was seen in the subset of patients with metastasis, with a 15-month improvement in OS (60 months vs 45 months; HR 0.76; 95% CI 0.62–0.92; P = .005). Median FFS and 5-year FFS were better in the chemohormonal arm compared with the ADT arm (37 months and 38% vs 20 months and 28%).

This study again confirmed that the addition of docetaxel to standard ADT alone was associated with an improvement in median OS, with an HR of 0.78 and a difference in median survival of 10 months. There was statistically significant improvement in the secondary endpoints of PCa-specific survival and FFS. The time for the onset of first skeletal-related event was also significantly prolonged in the chemohormonal therapy group.

VARIATIONS BETWEEN OUTCOMES IN THESE STUDIES

Even though all 3 aforementioned trials used a similar treatment design, there were significant differences in the patient populations that could explain the differences in outcomes (**Table 1**). One possible explanation is regarding the patient population. In the GETUG trial, the control arm that received ADT alone had an overall better survival compared with the patients in the control arms of the CHAARTED and STAMPEDE trials (54 months in GETUG versus 44 months in CHAARTED and 45 months in STAMPEDE [metastatic subgroup]). In addition, the 9 cycles of chemotherapy were poorly tolerated by patients in the GETUG trial and consequently, only 48% of the patients completed chemotherapy compared with 74% and 77% in CHAARTED and STAMPEDE, respectively (**Table 2**).

The timing of chemotherapy could also have played a role in the improved survival seen in CHAARTED and STAMPEDE trials. Patients were enrolled within a window of 120 days before randomization in the CHAARTED and 12 weeks in the STAMPEDE, respectively. In contrast, in the GETUG-AFU15, patients were enrolled within 2 months of starting ADT and 47% actually enrolled within 15 days of starting ADT. There is a transient period of increased hepatic clearance of docetaxel after castration. However, the duration of this altered clearance is not known and could offer an explanation for the observed differences between the trials.[32] Another reason for

Table 1
Phase III chemohormonal trials: outcome analyses

Phase III Study	GETUG-AFU15		CHAARTED		STAMPEDE	
	ADT + Doc	ADT	ADT + Doc	ADT	ADT + Doc	ADT
Median age, y	63	64	64	63	65	65
Percentage of metastatic disease	67	75	72.8	72.8	N/A	N/A
Median OS (mOS), mo	62.1	48.6	57.6	44	60[a]	45[a]
Median biochemical progression-free survival (bPFS)	22.9	12.9	20.2	11.7	N/A	N/A
HR (95% CI) for mOS	0.88 (0.68–1.14)		0.61 (0.47–0.80)		0.76 (0.62–0.9)	
HR (95% CI) for bPFS	0.72 (0.57–0.91)		0.61 (0.51–0.72)		0.61 (0.53–0.71)	

Abbreviations: ADT, androgen deprivation therapy; CHAARTED, Chemo-Hormonal therapy vs Androgen Ablation Randomized Trial for Extensive Disease in Prostate Cancer; CI, confidence interval; Doc, docetaxel; GETUG-AFY15, Groupe d'Etude des Tumeurs Uro-Genital and Association Française d'Urologie; HR, hazard ratio; NA, not available; STAMPEDE, Systemic Therapy in Advancing or Metastatic Prostate Cancer: Evaluation of Drug Efficacy.
[a] mOS in the STAMPEDE trial is for the metastatic hormone-sensitive prostate cancer cohort.

increased survival in CHAARTED and STAMPEDE could be due to treatment with newer antiandrogens. The GETUG-AFU 15 was the first of these trials and most participants developed CRPC at a time that neither abiraterone nor enzalutamide were widely available.

Among the 3 phase III trials, only the CHAARTED trial used stratification based on tumor volume and reported a statistically significant improvement in OS for patients with high-volume disease, as well as a numerically but nonstatistically significant improvement in OS for the low-volume group. One of the reasons for the difference in the GETUG trial could be because more than half of the patients (52%) had low-volume disease. No comparisons based on tumor volume have been done so far in the STAMPEDE trial, however 61% of patients had metastatic disease at the time of enrollment. Newer imaging techniques in development, such as sodium fluoride–PET/CT (NaF-PET/CT),[33,34] have emerged as very useful clinical tools in detecting bone

Table 2
Phase III chemohormonal trials: design and toxicities

Phase III Trial	GETUG-AFU15	CHAARTED	STAMPEDE
Disease category	M1	M1	High-risk N0M0, N1M0, M1
Performance status	KPS ≥70	ECOG 0–2	WHO 0–2
Median follow-up, mo	50	28.9	43
No. of chemotherapy cycles	9	6	6
Adverse events, n (%)	72 (38)	114 (29)	288 (52)
Adverse events type, n (%)	Neutropenia 40 (21) Febrile neutropenia 6 (3) Abnormal LFT 3 (2)	Neutropenia 47 (12.1) Febrile neutropenia 24 (6.1) Fatigue 16 (4.1)	Febrile neutropenia 84 (15) Neutropenia 66 (12) GI symptoms 45 (8)
Treatment-related deaths, n (%)	4 (2)	1 (0.2)	2 (0.3)

The 3 most common Grade 3 and above adverse events are compared between the trials.
Abbreviations: CHAARTED, Chemo-Hormonal therapy vs Androgen Ablation Randomized Trial for Extensive Disease in Prostate Cancer; ECOG, Eastern Cooperative Oncology Group performance status; GETUG-AFY15, Groupe d'Etude des Tumeurs Uro-Genital and Association Française d'Urologie; GI, gastrointestinal; KPS, Karnofsky Performance Status; LFT, liver function test; STAMPEDE, Systemic Therapy in Advancing or Metastatic Prostate Cancer: Evaluation of Drug Efficacy; WHO, World Health Organization Performance Status.

metastasis and defining functional tumor burden, which could prove valuable in selecting patients with high tumor burden for chemohormonal therapy in the future.

THE APPLICATION OF OTHER ANDROGEN AXIS AGENTS IN METASTATIC HORMONE-SENSITIVE PROSTATE CANCER

The development of several newer oral agents to disrupt the androgen axis has resulted in their routine use in CRPC. These include enzalutamide, an androgen axis inhibitor with multiple sequential actions in the AR pathway, including competitive inhibition of androgen binding to receptors and inhibition of AR nuclear translocation and DNA interaction.[35] Abiraterone is another androgen axis inhibitor, which blocks androgen biosynthesis by inhibiting steroidal enzyme 17 α-hydroxylase/C17, 20-lyase (CYP17). This causes suppression of androgen synthesis in testicular, adrenal, and prostatic tumor tissues.[36] Apalutamide is structurally and pharmacologically similar to enzalutamide, acting as a selective competitive antagonist of the AR, but has greater potency and reduced central nervous system permeation with improved adverse events profile.[37,38] Orteronel is functionally similar to abiraterone as a steroidal biosynthesis inhibitor, but it is selective for 17,20-lyase relative to 17α-hydroxylase, which reduces need for concomitant corticosteroids unlike abiraterone.[39]

Enzalutamide

Enzalutamide has shown significant survival benefits in patients with mCRPC, both before and after treatment with docetaxel. In a randomized placebo-controlled phase III trial (AFFIRM) involving 1199 patients with chemotherapy-progressed mCRPC, enzalutamide-treated patients had an improved median OS (18.4 months vs 13.6 months; HR 0.63; P<.001).[35] In another phase III trial involving 1717 chemotherapy-naïve mCRPC (PREVAIL), enzalutamide-treated patients had a 65% radiographic PFS (rPFS) at 12 months, as compared with 14% among patients receiving placebo (81% risk reduction; HR 0.19; CI 0.15–0.23; P<.001). There was also a 29% risk reduction of death, which was the coprimary endpoint studied (HR 0.71; 95% CI 0.60–0.84; P<.001).[40]

A phase II single-arm study of enzalutamide as monotherapy in mHSPC showed PSA declines to a similar degree as GnRH agonists.[41] A Phase III study comparing enzalutamide with conventional antiandrogen + LHRH agonists or surgical castration as first-line treatment for mHSPC (ENZAMET, NCT02446405) is currently recruiting participants.

The primary endpoint is OS and secondary endpoints are PFS (Clinical and PSA), adverse events, and health-related quality of life, and cost effectiveness. Another study comparing enzalutamide + ADT versus placebo + ADT (NCT02677896) is currently recruiting and primary endpoints of this trial include rPFS, with multiple secondary endpoints including OS, time to CRPC and time to first skeletal-related event. Both are expected to be completed by 2020.

Abiraterone

Abiraterone as a CYP 17 inhibitor has shown survival benefit in the mCRPC setting, both before and after treatment with docetaxel. In a phase III randomized placebo-controlled trial (COU-AA-301) involving 1195 patients with mCRPC who had progressed on docetaxel, OS was longer in the abiraterone acetate–prednisone group than in the placebo-prednisone group (14.8 vs 10.9 months; HR 0.65; 0.54–0.77; P<.001). All secondary endpoints, including PFS, time to PSA progression, and PSA response rate were significantly better in the abiraterone group.[36] In another randomized phase III trial (NCT00887198) to assess coprimary endpoints of radiographic PFS and OS in chemotherapy-naïve patients, abiraterone showed an improved radiographic PFS of 16.5 compared with 8.3 months with prednisone alone (HR 0.53; 0.45–0.62; P<.001) and an improved OS (median not reached, vs 27.2 months; HR 0.75; 95% CI 0.61–0.93; P = .01).[42]

A phase III trial examining OS as a primary endpoint in mHSPC treated with abiraterone acetate with low-dose prednisone plus ADT compared with ADT alone (NCT01715285) is ongoing. Coprimary endpoints are OS and radiographic PFS and the results are expected by 2018. Similarly, a multicenter phase III study (PEACE1, NCT01957436) is comparing PFS and OS in patients with mHSPC with 4 treatment arms: (1) ADT; (2) ADT with abiraterone acetate; (3) ADT with local radiotherapy; and (4) ADT with abiraterone acetate and local radiotherapy. The coprimary end points are OS and PFS, and results are expected in 2018.

Apalutamide

This potent antiandrogen demonstrated durable PSA response and safety in a phase II trial in mHSPC; 89% of patients had ≥50% PSA decline at 12 weeks, which was the primary endpoint and median time to PSA progression was 24.0 months.[43] A phase III trial comparing Apalutamide + ADT to ADT (TITAN; NCT02489318) in the setting of mHSPC is under way. It is estimated to enroll 1000 patients and the coprimary end points are radiographic PFS and OS, with results expected by 2020.

Orteronel

This selective adrenal androgen synthesis inhibitor (17 20 lyase inhibitor) demonstrated marked and durable PSA declines in phase II trials in mHSPC. In this study involving 39 patients with nonmetastatic PCa with rising PSA, 35 patients had a PSA decrease of greater than 30% and 6 (16%) achieved PSA $\leq$0.2 ng/mL at 3 months.[39] In a phase III randomized placebo-controlled multi-institutional trial (ELM-PC 4), 2353 patients were randomized to receive Orteronel + prednisolone or placebo + prednisolone, with primary end points of rPFS and OS, determined in the intention-to-treat population. Both radiographic and PFS were superior in the Orteronel arm; median rPFS was 13.8 months versus 8.7 months (HR 0.71; 95% CI 0.63–0.80; P<.0001) and median OS was 31.4 months versus 29.5 months (HR 0.92; 95% CI 0.79–1.08; P = 0.31).[44] A phase III trial comparing Orteronel + ADT with Bicalutamide + ADT (S1216; NCT01809691) is currently recruiting an estimated 1300 participants. The primary endpoint is OS and the results are expected by 2022.

The results of the previously mentioned phase III trials are expected to elucidate the role of newer antiandrogens in the setting of mHSPC. However, at present their role in the early management of mHSPC is considered exploratory.

Future Directions

Given data that docetaxel has demonstrated efficacy in mHSPC in randomized phase III trials and the proven efficacy of Cabazitaxel in advanced PCa, addition of Cabazitaxel with ADT for chemohormonal therapy is being examined in clinical trials. A randomized phase III trial comparing Cabazitaxel and ADT with ADT alone in mHSPC for high-risk disease is currently recruiting participants (SensiCab; NCT01978873). The primary endpoint is OS, with PFS and PSA control as secondary endpoints. Results are expected in 2018. Other validated chemotherapy agents active in the CRPC will likely be applied to earlier disease in the future based on the findings of the CHAARTED and other trials.

An issue that has arisen is control of the primary tumor in the face of metastatic disease, an approach that is being used successfully for other diseases, including renal cancer.[45] In a feasibility study to look at effect of radical prostatectomy (RP) after ADT, patients treated with ADT + RP combination showed a delayed time to CRPC transition and had a significantly better PFS and CSS.[46] Two recent population-based database analyses from the United States and Europe have suggested a beneficial role of surgery/radiation in mPCa.[47,48] With lengthening time of survival in patients with CRPC this is likely to demonstrate improvements for a subset of patients. Several phase II trials examining these issues are ongoing (NCT01751438 and NCT02716974) with results expected in 2018.

SUMMARY

Metastatic HSPC is a heterogeneous disease and recent studies have shown that patients with metastatic disease spend most of their remaining life in the castration-resistant state. There has been

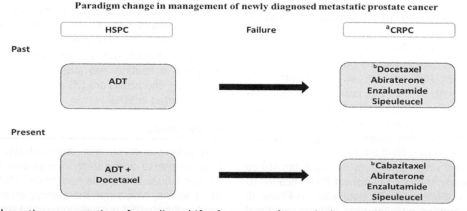

Fig. 1. Schematic representation of paradigm shift of treatment for newly diagnosed metastatic HSPC. Randomized mature trials suggest the addition of docetaxel chemotherapy at the initiation of ADT results in a cancer-specific improvement in survival. After failure of ADT, other options are available for metastatic CRPC. [a] First line treatment options for mCRPC. [b] Docetaxel and Cabazitaxel preferred for symptomatic CRPC.

a paradigm change in the therapeutic approach to mHSPC with recently published phase III studies confirming a survival advantage with chemohormonal therapy (**Fig. 1**). A recent abstract on the analysis of use indicates that chemohormonal therapy is being used for 65% of high-volume and 35% of low-volume mHSPC. The updated National Comprehensive Cancer Network (NCCN) guidelines recommend chemohormonal therapy for all adequately fit men with newly diagnosed mHSPC, regardless of the disease burden.[49]

ADDENDUM

At the time of publication, results from the recent LATITUDE trial using abiraterone and ADT have been reported[50] further supporting a role for the application of other agents at the time of initiating ADT. The median overall survival was significantly longer in the abiraterone group than in the placebo group (not reached vs 34.7 months) (hazard ratio for death, 0.62, 95% confidence interval [CI], 0.51–.76; P<.001).

REFERENCES

1. National Cancer Institute. Stat Facts: Prostate Cancer. Available at: https://seer.cancer.gov/statfacts/html/prost.html. Accessed March 15, 2017.

2. Denmeade SR, Isaacs JT. A history of prostate cancer treatment. Nat Rev Cancer 2002;2(5):389–96.

3. Sharifi N, Dahut WL, Steinberg SM, et al. A retrospective study of the time to clinical endpoints for advanced prostate cancer. BJU Int 2005; 96(7):985–9.

4. Kirby M, Hirst C, Crawford ED. Characterizing the castration-resistant prostate cancer population: a systematic review. Int J Clin Pract 2011;65(11): 1180–92.

5. James ND, Spears MR, Clarke NW, et al. Survival with newly diagnosed metastatic prostate cancer in the "docetaxel era": data from 917 patients in the control arm of the STAMPEDE Trial (MRC PR08, CRUK/06/019). Eur Urol 2015;67(6): 1028–38.

6. Tangen CM, Hussain MH, Higano CS, et al. Improved overall survival trends of men with newly diagnosed M1 prostate cancer: a SWOG phase III trial experience (S8494, S8894 and S9346). J Urol 2012;188:1164–9.

7. Ahmed M, Li LC. Adaptation and clonal selection models of castration-resistant prostate cancer: current perspective. Int J Urol 2013;20:362–71.

8. Attar RM, Takimoto CH, Gottardis MM. Castration-resistant prostate cancer: locking up the molecular escape routes. Clin Cancer Res 2009;15:3251–5.

Available at: https://www.ncbi.nlm.nih.gov/pubmed/19447877.

9. Collins AT, Berry PA, Hyde C, et al. Prospective identification of tumorigenic prostate cancer stem cells. Cancer Res 2005;65:10946–51.

10. Shah RB, Mehra R, Chinnaiyan AM, et al. Androgen-independent prostate cancer is a heterogeneous group of diseases: lessons from a rapid autopsy program. Cancer Res 2004;64:9209–16.

11. Craft N, Chhor C, Tran C, et al. Evidence for clonal outgrowth of androgen-independent prostate cancer cells from androgen-dependent tumors through a two-step process. Cancer Res 1999;59:5030–6.

12. Zhu ML, Kyprianou N. Androgen receptor and growth factor signaling cross-talk in prostate cancer cells. Endocr Relat Cancer 2008;15:841–9.

13. Whang YE, Wu X, Suzuki H, et al. Inactivation of the tumor suppressor PTEN/MMAC1 in advanced human prostate cancer through loss of expression. Proc Natl Acad Sci U S A 1998;95:5246–50.

14. Koivisto P, Kononen J, Palmberg C, et al. Androgen receptor gene amplification: a possible molecular mechanism for androgen deprivation therapy failure in prostate cancer. Cancer Res 1997;57:314–9.

15. Palmberg C, Koivisto P, Kakkola L, et al. Androgen receptor gene amplification at primary progression predicts response to combined androgen blockade as second line therapy for advanced prostate cancer. J Urol 2000;164:1992–5.

16. Scher HI, Sawyers CK. Biology of progressive, castration-resistant prostate cancer: directed therapies targeting the androgen-receptor signaling axis. J Clin Oncol 2005;23:8253–61.

17. Nelson PS. Molecular states underlying androgen receptor activation: a framework for therapeutics targeting androgen signalling in prostate cancer. J Clin Oncol 2012;30:644–6.

18. Mostaghel EA, Marck BT, Plymate SR, et al. Resistance to CYP17A1 inhibition with abiraterone in castration-resistant prostate cancer: induction of steroidogenesis and androgen receptor splice variants. Clin Cancer Res 2011;17:5913–25.

19. Fenton MA, Shuster TD, Feting Am, et al. Functional characterization of mutant androgen receptors from androgen-independent prostate cancer. Clin Cancer Res 1997;3:1383–8.

20. Antonarakis ES, Lu C, Wang H, et al. AR-V7 and resistance to enzalutamide and abiraterone in prostate cancer. N Engl J Med 2014;371:1028–38.

21. Stanbrough M, Bubley GJ, Ross K, et al. Increased expression of genes converting adrenal androgens to testosterone in androgen-independent prostate cancer. Cancer Res 2006;66:2815–25.

22. Tannock IF, de Wit R, Berry WR, et al. Docetaxel plus prednisone or mitoxantrone plus prednisone for advanced prostate cancer. N Engl J Med 2004; 351:1502–12.

23. Petrylak DP, Tangen CM, Hussain MH, et al. Docetaxel and estramustine compared with mitoxantrone and prednisone for advanced refractory prostate cancer. N Engl J Med 2004;351:1513–20.

24. Suzman DL, Antonarakis ES. Castration-resistant prostate cancer: latest evidence and therapeutic implications. Ther Adv Med Oncol 2014;6:167–79.

25. Eigl BJ, Eggener SE, Baybik J, et al. Timing is everything: preclinical evidence supporting simultaneous rather than sequential chemo hormonal therapy for prostate cancer. Clin Cancer Res 2005;11:4905–11.

26. Zhu ML, Horbinski CM, Garzotto M, et al. Tubulin-targeting chemotherapy impairs androgen receptor activity in prostate cancer. Cancer Res 2010;70:7992–8002.

27. Kyriakopoulos CE, Liu G. Chemohormonal therapy for hormone-sensitive prostate cancer: a review. Cancer J 2016;22(5):322–5.

28. Gravis G, Fizazi K, Joly F, et al. Androgen-deprivation therapy alone or with Docetaxel in noncastrate metastatic prostate cancer (GETUG-AFU 15): a randomised, open-label, phase 3 trial. Lancet Oncol 2013;14:149–58.

29. Sweeney CJ, Chen YH, Carducci M, et al. Chemo hormonal therapy in metastatic hormone-sensitive prostate cancer. N Engl J Med 2015;373:737–46.

30. Caffo O, Biasco E, Facchini G, et al. Long term efficacy and QOL data of chemohormonal therapy (C-HT) in low and high volume hormone naïve metastatic prostate cancer (PrCa). Switzerland: European Society of Medical Oncology; 2016. Available at: http://oncologypro.esmo.org/Meeting-Resources/ESMO-2016/Long-term-efficacy-and-QOL-data-of-chemohormonal-therapy-C-HT-in-low-and-high-volume-hormone-naive-metastatic-prostate-cancer-PrCa-E3805-CHAARTED-trial. Accessed March 15, 2017.

31. James ND, Sydes MR, Clarke NW, et al. Addition of Docetaxel, Zoledronic acid, or both to first-line long-term hormone therapy in prostate cancer (STAMPEDE): survival results from an adaptive, multiarm, multistage, platform randomised controlled trial. Lancet 2016;387:1163–77.

32. Franke RM, Carducci MA, Rudek MA, et al. Castration-dependent pharmacokinetics of Docetaxel in patients with prostate cancer. J Clin Oncol 2010;28(30):4562–7.

33. Apolo AB, Lindenberg L, Shih JH, et al. Prospective study evaluating Na18F-positron emission tomography/computed tomography (NaF-PET/CT) in predicting clinical outcomes and survival in advanced prostate cancer. J Nucl Med 2016;57:886–92.

34. Liu G, Perlman S, Perk T, et al. Quantitative total bone imaging (QTBI) in patients with metastatic castration-resistant prostate cancer (CRPC) using NaF PET/CT. J Clin Oncol 2015;33(suppl 7) [abstract: 180].

35. Scher HI, Fizazi K, Saad F, et al. Increased survival with enzalutamide in prostate cancer after chemotherapy. N Engl J Med 2012;367(13):1187–97.

36. de Bono JS, Logothetis CJ, Molina A, et al. Abiraterone and increased survival in metastatic prostate cancer. N Engl J Med 2011;364:1995–2005.

37. Ya-Xiong T. Pharmacology and therapeutics of constitutively active receptors. Elsevier Science; 2014. p. 351. ISBN: 978-0-12-417206-7.

38. Clegg NJ, Wongvipat J, Joseph JD, et al. ARN-509: a novel antiandrogen for prostate cancer treatment. Cancer Research 2012;72(6):1494–503.

39. Hussain M, Corn PG, Michaelson MD, et al. Prostate Cancer Clinical Trials Consortium, a program of the Department of Defense Prostate Cancer Research Program and the Prostate Cancer Foundation. Phase II study of single-agent orteronel (TAK-700) in patients with nonmetastatic castration-resistant prostate cancer and rising prostate-specific antigen. Clin Cancer Res 2014;20(16):4218–27.

40. Beer TM, Armstrong AJ, Rathkopf DE, et al. Enzalutamide in metastatic prostate cancer before chemotherapy. N Engl J Med 2014;371(5):424–33.

41. Tombal B, Borre M, Rathenborg P, et al. Enzalutamide monotherapy in hormone-naive prostate cancer: primary analysis of an open-label, single-arm, phase 2 study. Lancet Oncol 2014;15(6):592–600.

42. Ryan CJ, Smith MR, de Bono JS, et al. Abiraterone in metastatic prostate cancer without previous chemotherapy. N Engl J Med 2013;368:138–48.

43. Smith MR, Antonarakis ES, Ryan CJ, et al. Phase 2 study of the safety and antitumor activity of apalutamide (ARN-509), a potent androgen receptor antagonist, in the high-risk nonmetastatic castration-resistant prostate cancer cohort. Eur Urol 2016;70(6):963–70.

44. Saad F, Fizazi K, Jinga V, et al. Orteronel plus prednisone in patients with chemotherapy-naive metastatic castration-resistant prostate cancer (ELM-PC4): a double-blind, multicentre, phase 3, randomised, placebo-controlled trial. Lancet Oncol 2015;16(3):338–48.

45. Bamias A, Tzannis K, Papatsoris A, et al. Prognostic significance of cytoreductive nephrectomy in patients with synchronous metastases from renal cell carcinoma treated with first-line sunitinib: a European multiinstitutional study. Clin Genitourin Cancer 2014;12(5):373–83.

46. Heidenreich A, Pfister D, Porres D. Cytoreductive radical prostatectomy in patients with prostate cancer and low volume skeletal metastases: results of a feasibility and case-control study. J Urol 2015;193(3):832–8.

47. Culp SH, Schellhammer PF, Williams MB. Might men diagnosed with metastatic prostate cancer benefit from definitive treatment of the primary tumor? A SEER-Based Study. Eur Urol 2014;65(6):1058–66, ISSN: 0302-2838.

48. Gratzke C, Engel J, Stief CG. Role of radical prostatectomy in metastatic prostate cancer: data from the Munich Cancer Registry. Eur Urol 2014;66(3): 602–3.

49. National Comprehensive Cancer Network. Clinical practice guidelines in oncology version 2.2016: prostate cancer. Available at: http://www.nccn.org/professionals/physician_gls/pdf/prostate.pdf. Accessed March 11, 2016.

50. Fizazi K, Tran N, Fein L, et al. Abiraterone plus prednisone in metastatic, castration-sensitive prostate cancer. N Engl J Med 2017;377:352–60.

The Role of Local Therapy for Oligometastatic Prostate Cancer
Should We Expect a Cure?

Rajesh Nair, FRCS (Urol), FEBU, MSc[a],
Benjamin W. Lamb, FRCS (Urol), PhD[a],
Nicolas Geurts, MD, FEBU[a], Omar Alghazo, MBBS[a],
Wayne Lam, FRCS (Urol), MSc[b],
Nathan Lawrentschuk, MBBS, PhD[a,c],
Declan G. Murphy, MB BCh, FRACS, FRCS (Urol)[a,d],*

KEYWORDS

- Prostate cancer • Oligometastatic disease • Radical prostatectomy • Radical radiotherapy
- PSMA-PET

KEY POINTS

- There are data to suggest that an oligometastatic state may confer a better outcome than higher-volume metastases.
- Such patients may be considered for aggressive approaches, including radical treatment of the primary cancer.
- The definition of oligometastatic state remains contentious, and superior imaging is challenging the traditional paradigm based on conventional imaging.
- Nonrandomized data suggest a survival benefit for patients who undergo treatment of the primary despite metastatic disease at diagnosis.
- Prospective trials are underway to assess this hypothesis, otherwise treatment of the primary in men with oligometastatic disease should be considered experimental.

INTRODUCTION

The so-called oligometastatic state is defined as limited metastatic burden amenable to aggressive local therapy in an attempt to achieve long-term survival. First described by Hellman and Weichselbaum in 1995,[1] these investigators postulated a theory that tumors, when in a state of oligometastasis, are at a transition point between localized disease and widespread metastases.[2,3] However, it remains contentious whether a truly oligometastatic state can be reliably identified, and therefore whether aggressive approaches directed toward such patients are warranted or reasonable.

Disclosures: None.
[a] Division of Cancer Surgery, Peter MacCallum Cancer Centre, 305 Grattan Street, Melbourne, Victoria 3000, Australia; [b] Department of Urology, The University of Hong Kong, 9/F, Knowles Building Pok Fu Lam Road, Pok Fu Lam, Hong Kong SAR, China; [c] Department of Surgery, Austin Health, University of Melbourne, Parkville, 145 Studley Rd, Heidelberg Victoria 3084, Australia; [d] Sir Peter MacCallum Cancer centre, Department of Oncology, University of Melbourne, 305 Grattan Street, Melbourne VIC 3000, Australia
* Corresponding author. Department of Genitourinary Oncology, The Peter MacCallum Cancer Centre, 305 Grattan Street, Melbourne, Victoria 3000, Australia.
E-mail address: declan.murphy@petermac.org

Urol Clin N Am 44 (2017) 623–633
http://dx.doi.org/10.1016/j.ucl.2017.07.013
0094-0143/17/© 2017 Elsevier Inc. All rights reserved.

It is not known whether metastatic lesions in the oligometastatic state directly disseminate to other, distant sites of disease in the metastatic state, or whether the oligometastases facilitate disease progression by the primary tumor through the release of circulating growth factors.[4,5] Nevertheless, the treatment of the primary cancer in the oligometastatic state does seem to delay or interrupt the development of further metastatic disease in some, but not all, situations. This phenomenon has been observed in several cancer types, including renal cell carcinoma and colorectal, ovarian, and breast cancer.[6–8] In prostate cancer specifically, it is accepted that widespread metastatic disease accounts for more than 90% of prostate cancer–specific mortality,[9] and accordingly there is a conceptual argument that, by delaying this end stage of disease, perhaps at a point when the metastatic burden is low, clinicians can improve survival for men with prostate cancer. It was shown several years ago that there was a significant difference in overall survival in patients with prostate cancer who had fewer than 5 metastases at the time of diagnosis,[10] although the stratification of the number of metastases that should be considered oligo remains contentious.

The current standard of treatment of men with localized prostate cancer, with an otherwise expected longevity of more than 10 years, is curative therapy, achieved through radical prostatectomy or radiotherapy.[11] In contrast, when evidence of metastatic disease is present, albeit minimal metastatic disease (pelvic lymph node disease), the traditional treatment paradigm says that cure is no longer possible. Consequently, these patients have been commenced on systemic androgen deprivation therapy (ADT).[11–13] However, as alluded to earlier, there is emerging evidence that treatment of the primary tumor, and even metastatic deposits, in the context of metastatic and lymph node–positive prostate cancer may confer a survival benefit.[14–17]

However, not all men with metastatic prostate cancer benefit from potentially toxic local therapy, and as such the ability to accurately distinguish patients in the oligometastatic state, who may respond more favorably, is crucial before embarking on aggressive treatment.[18] With greater understanding of prostate cancer genomics, advances in imaging techniques, such as [11C] choline or prostate-specific membrane antigen (PSMA) PET, used in the diagnostic and surveillance setting,[19,20] and an increase in the number of clinical trials recruiting patients with prostate cancer, the detection of oligometastatic disease has increased. With this increase in detection has come an enthusiasm for treatment.

The foundation for successful treatment probably requires more than aggressive local control alone. It is likely that a multimodal approach to therapy is required, encompassing local consolidative therapy to the prostate, metastasis-directed therapy (including surgery or radiation), and systemic chemohormonal therapy.[21]

Current literature regarding both the diagnosis and treatment of oligometastatic disease remains limited. The definition of oligometastatic disease varies between studies and thus extrapolation of data in existing systematic reviews carries its own statistical prejudice. It is widely acknowledged that the data on treatment are drawn largely from nonrandomized trials, retrospective cohorts, and post-hoc analyses of prospective studies, all of which carry inherent bias, significantly limiting the findings. This article evaluates the available evidence in order to establish whether local treatment of oligometastatic prostate cancer is a feasible, safe, and beneficial strategy in an enlarging cohort of patients for whom traditional treatment paradigms are in a state of flux.

DEFINING OLIGOMETASTATIC PROSTATE CANCER

Most studies and trials have defined oligometastasis in prostate cancer according to the number of metastatic lesions. Most vary between 3 and 5 metastases,[2–9,11] although 1 study included patients with 10 or fewer lesions.[12] Other studies have defined the oligometastatic state according to site of lesions, with lymph node, bone, and extrapelvic metastases commonly used as site-specific criteria.[21] In addition, 1 previous study used the size of the metastases as part of their inclusion criteria, and defined oligometastasis in prostate cancer if there was only bone involvement, with each lesion less than half the size of the vertebral body.[22]

There is some validity to using either the number or site of metastases as the definition of oligometastasis in prostate cancer. A recent study by Sridharan and colleagues[23] showed that bone metastases contribute more than those of other sites to the development of widespread metastases, and that having more than 3 bone metastases had a major impact on prostate cancer–specific mortality.

However, the Achilles heel of all such strategies to define oligometastatic disease is that such a definition is a function of imaging sensitivity.[21,24] In prostate cancer, conventional imaging, typically using computed tomography (CT) scanning, or bone scintigraphy with technetium-99m, has very poor accuracy for identifying metastatic disease.

However, novel functional imaging techniques, such as 11C-choline and 18Ga-PSMA–PET/CT, has recently shown increased sensitivity to prostate cancer metastases.[20] As such, there seems to be a migration in the staging of patients with prostate cancer, and it is likely that the definition of the oligometastatic state will change according to the results of studies evaluating this technology. However, at present, a widely accepted definition of oligometastatic disease is the presence of 3 or fewer metastases based on conventional imaging, and this is the definition agreed at the St Gallen Consensus on Advanced Prostate Cancer.[25]

Furthermore, in some cases, oligometastatic disease progresses rapidly to widespread metastatic disease, whereas in others it takes a more gradual course. An imaging modality only ever captures a snapshot in time: is the bone scan with 3 lesions truly a stable state, or is it just a snapshot of a rapidly disseminating cascade? Early genomic studies suggest that there are potentially underlying molecular phenotypic variabilities that could account for this phenomenon.[18] This biological component should therefore also be integrated into the evolving definition of oligometastatic prostate cancer so that it better reflects the prognosis of the disease for each case.

RATIONALE FOR LOCAL TREATMENT OF THE PRIMARY IN OLIGOMETASTATIC PROSTATE CANCER
Surgical Treatment of Oligometastatic Prostate Cancer

It is important to remember that there is no level 1 evidence with respect to treatment of the primary in metastatic prostate cancer, and guidelines uniformly recommend systemic treatment as the standard of care. Data on treatment are drawn largely from nonrandomized trials, retrospective cohorts, and post-hoc analyses of prospective studies, all of which carry inherent bias, and should be interpreted with caution.

Nevertheless, there are some data that support the role of cytoreductive prostatectomy in metastatic disease, and these data are considered here. Frohmuller and colleagues found that radical prostatectomy combined with ADT in patients with T1-2, pN1-2 prostate cancer was associated with improved survival and quality of life outcomes compared with patients treated with ADT alone.[26] In addition, in a study evaluating patients who developed M1 disease, those patients who had previously undergone a radical prostatectomy had longer prostate cancer–specific survival than men who had undergone radiotherapy. Further data have emerged from post-hoc secondary analysis of data from the SWOG (Southwest Oncology Group) 8894 study, in which patients with metastatic disease were randomized to orchidectomy and placebo or flutamide. Patients who had previously undergone radical prostatectomy had a survival benefit compared with those who had not. **Table 1** presents data from several retrospective reviews on radical prostatectomy in patients with metastatic prostate cancer. Although these publications suggest some benefit from so-called cytoreductive surgery, studies have been limited either by lack of a control group, retrospective nature, or post-hoc analysis, as well as limited long-term survival beyond 5 years. It is well known that men who are likely to undergo surgery in this cohort are fitter, have less burden of metastatic disease, and are more likely to respond to systemic treatment, thereby introducing likely selection bias. Accordingly, a criticism of such data is that it is possible that patients would have responded well regardless of surgery or radiotherapy.

Apart from any potential survival benefit, the effect on radical prostatectomy in the prevention of local symptoms of prostate cancer has been used

Table 1
Outcomes of radical prostatectomy in metastatic (M1) prostate cancer

Study Reference	Number of Patients	No Local Treatment	No Local Resection	RP	RP or Brachytherapy	5-y OS	5-y CSS
Heidenreich et al,[28] 2015	61	38 (on ADT)	NA	23 (after ADT)	NA	91.3% RP vs 78.9% (NLT) P = .048	95.6% (RP) vs 84.2% (NLT) P = .043
Gratzke et al,[43] 2014	1538	NA	7811	74	NA	55% RP vs 21% NLR P<.01	NA
Culp et al,[42] 2014	8185	7811	NA	NA	245	67.4% RP vs 52.6% NLT P<.001	75.8% RP vs 61.3% NLT P<.001

Abbreviations: CSS, cancer-specific survival; NA, not applicable; NLR, no local resection; NLT, no local treatment; OS, overall survival; RP, radical prostatectomy.

as a driver to justify the use of surgery in the oligometastatic setting. Local complications of advanced prostate cancer include urinary retention, catheterization with subsequent requirement for transurethral resection of the prostate, ureteric obstruction, bleeding, requirement for palliative radiotherapy (RT), urinary diversion, or even pelvic exenteration. Frazier and colleagues[27] found that, of the patients undergoing exploratory pelvic lymph node dissection with frozen section, 24.6% of those with node-positive disease who did not have surgery, and were treated with ADT alone, had symptomatic local progression of the disease, compared with 9.5% who underwent radical prostatectomy and ADT. It has also been found that, among patients who developed castration-resistant disease, treatment with radical prostatectomy or radiation reduced complications compared with no local therapy (54.6% vs 32.6%). In addition, outcomes favored radical prostatectomy more than radiation treatment.[27]

The question of safety is paramount when applying radical prostatectomy to locally advanced tumors in the metastatic setting. The benefit from multimodality treatment must outweigh the morbidity and mortality associated with aggressive local control. Heidenreich and colleagues[28] performed radical prostatectomy in 23 patients in the setting of metastatic disease (3 or fewer bone metastases and prostate-specific antigen [PSA] level <1.0 ng/mL following ADT) and recorded complications to a similar degree as is found in the high-risk localized setting (Clavien-Dindo grade 1 = 17.4%, grade 2 = 8.7%, grade 3 = 13%, and no grade 4 or 5 complications).[28] The investigators also highlighted that none of the operated patients in the study went on to develop symptoms of local progression, compared with 28.9% of the 38 patients who did not have surgery.

In theory, if surgically feasible, metastasectomy is potentially beneficial by reducing tumor burden and improving survival in patients with low-volume metastatic disease. However, evidence of surgical monotherapy in the treatment of oligometastatic prostate cancer has been limited to case reports. In total, 13 case reports were available. All reported patients had low-volume metastatic disease, with location of solitary metastases suitable for surgical resection. The commonest site of oligometastatic prostate cancer treated by surgery were testis (n = 4) and lung (n = 4). At present, with very limited evidence, metastasis-directed surgical resection in prostate cancer aiming for cure cannot be recommended as a routine procedure but could be considered in individual patients following multidisciplinary review, or as part of a clinical trial.

Multimodal Treatment of Oligometastatic Prostate Cancer

O'Shaughnessy and colleagues recently investigated the use of multimodal treatment in patients with castration-naive metastatic prostate cancers. Twenty patients with M1a/M1b oligometastatic prostate cancer were included.[29] All identifiable and radiologically visible disease was treated sequentially with androgen deprivation, radical prostatectomy with pelvic and retroperitoneal lymphadenectomy, and stereotactic body radiotherapy to sites of bone metastasis or the primary site. Ninety-five percent of patients achieved an undetectable PSA, and in 20% PSA remained undetectable following testosterone recovery for up to 46 months. This study showed that, in carefully selected patients with oligometastatic disease at presentation, it is feasible to eliminate all detectable disease with multimodal treatment, with short-term to medium-term biochemical response.

Despite the limitations of the evidence to date, it is reasonable to conclude that the effective management of oligometastatic prostate cancer requires a 3-fold approach: First, management of local disease by radical treatment; second, targeted treatment of metastases by surgery if located at operable sites, or stereotactic body radiotherapy; third, systematic treatment with ADT or chemotherapy for occult disease.

LIMITATIONS OF THE EVIDENCE FOR TREATING THE PRIMARY IN OLIGOMETASTATIC DISEASE

Although, at face value, the evidence for treatment of the primary in oligometastatic prostate cancer may be convincing, it must be interpreted with caution. There is currently no level 1 evidence from randomized trials suggesting that local treatment of the primary tumor in metastatic prostate cancer improves survival. Many of the studies are epidemiologic or are nonrandomized and therefore have significant methodological limitations (selection bias in particular), which limits the scope of their findings.

Defining the oligometastatic state in prostate cancer is controversial and has varied across published studies and trials currently in progress. Review of published reports and active clinical trials confirms wide variability in how oligometastatic prostate cancer has been defined: 6 studies (38%) imposed a limit of 3 metastases[30] (https://clinicaltrials.gov/ct2/show/NCT02680587). Three studies (19%) include up to 4 metastases[31] (https://clinicaltrials.gov/ct2/show/NCT02489357), 5 metastases,[32] 1 (6%) up to 10 metastases, another (https://clinicaltrials.gov/ct2/show/NCT02020070), and 1 (6%) does not strictly define an upper limit of lesions (https://clinicaltrials.gov/ct2/show/NCT01859221). Eight of the 16 reports specified sites of metastasis that were considered in defining oligometastatic disease. Some investigators argue that the concept of an oligometastatic state is a misnomer, and that oligometastasis represents a snapshot of a continuum between localized and metastatic disease.[33]

Many studies have examined local therapy for the primary tumor in nodal disease and showed improved outcomes when radical prostatectomy (RP) or RT to the primary tumor was used. However, these studies have significant limitations, the most serious being the inevitable selection bias of treating surgeons in the decision of whether or not to proceed with treatment. Furthermore, other factors likely to have an impact on the study outcomes, such as characteristics of the disease (lymph node burden) and neoadjuvant and adjuvant treatments, varied between studies, and were not consistently reported.[34–38]

Post-hoc analyses of subgroup data from randomized controlled trials have generated conflicting data. Thompson and colleagues[39] compared patients who received either RP or RT before enrollment into the SWOG 8894 trial with men who did not receive any prior local therapy. Prior RP was associated with a statistically significant decrease in the risk of death relative to those who did not undergo RP. This study was limited by its post-hoc nature but also by a lack of data on the stage of prostate cancer in each group, which is a potential bias the investigators cannot account for in the data. Furthermore, a potential confounder is the significantly increased time from diagnosis to study entry, representing possible lead-time bias. Similarly, Halabi and colleagues,[40] who analyzed pooled data from 9 clinical trials investigating men with progressive prostate cancer while on ADT, had the same confounder in their retrospective analysis, although the investigators found no association between improved survival and previous RP. Both studies have significant limitations in methodology and, as such, should be viewed as hypothesis generating, not definitive.[41]

The effect of prior local treatment on metastatic prostate cancer has been investigated from population level databases in the United States and Europe with consistent findings of improved outcomes in men with prior local treatment. Such population data have strengths, including large sample size. However, such studies also have significant flaws. Because of the retrospective analysis, the investigators were unable to account for known clinical and pathologic predictors of survival, such as comorbidities, other treatments, and metastatic burden, that may have significant effects on survival beyond the variable of interest, which was prior local treatment.[42–44]

IMAGING TECHNIQUES IN REDEFINING METASTATIC DISEASE

Traditional curative treatment of localized prostate cancer has only been advocated in the nonmetastatic setting.[11] At present, the standard for staging prostate cancer, in order to determine eligibility for potentially curative treatment, is cross-sectional imaging (CT or MRI and technetium-99m [99mTc] bone scan or single-photon emission CT [SPECT]). However, over the past few years, significant advancements in imaging techniques have been made, specifically in PET imaging.[45–47] Emerging evidence is beginning to redefine the understanding of prostate cancer, with the result that the concepts and definitions of organ-confined, oligometastatic and polymetastatic disease may also change.

18F-Sodium Fluoride PET

18F-sodium fluoride (Na18F) is a bone-specific tracer that was introduced to clinical practice more than 50 years ago. Na18F-PET imaging enables detection of osteoblastic metastases by targeting areas of bone remodeling in a similar fashion to 99mTc–methylene diphosphonate. It has recently been used in PET imaging of metastatic prostate cancer, showing higher sensitivity and specificity than 99mTc–methylene diphosphate planar and SPECT imaging.[48] The main limitation is a reliance on additional CT or MRI imaging to evaluate the potential for soft tissue metastases.[21] Moreover, Na18F activity is frequently seen to overlap in both benign and metastatic disease, and there remains no standardized method to quantify Na18F PET/CT findings.[48]

2-[18F]-Fluoro-2-deoxy-D-glucose PET

2-[18F]-fluoro-2-deoxy-D-glucose (FDG) is a commonly used tracer for assessing solid malignancies, acting as a surrogate-radiolabeled marker for glucose metabolism. Its use in metastatic prostate cancer is limited by its low sensitivity for detecting bone metastases,[49] which is a reflection of poor glucose metabolism in bone. In addition, FDG avidity varies depending on the natural history of the disease, being low in untreated prostate cancer, and increasing as patients develop castration-resistant prostate cancer and docetaxel-refractory prostate cancer.[50]

18F-Choline and 11C-Choline PET

18F-choline and 11C-choline show similar diagnostic accuracies in metastatic prostate cancer.

Uptake is shown in both osteoblastic and osteolytic lesions. Choline PET/CT has been shown in most studies to have a higher diagnostic accuracy for staging compared with conventional bone scan, and has the advantage of detecting both bone and soft tissue metastases.[49] The main concern with choline PET imaging is its sensitivity and specificity at lower PSA levels, limiting its use in the assessment of biochemical failure.[51]

Prostate-Specific Membrane Antigen

Recently, PSMA tracers for use in SPECT and PET imaging have shown encouraging results. The most studied imaging modality so far is 68Ga-PSMA–PET/CT, which has shown promise because of its high sensitivity for detecting early recurrence after local treatment of organ-confined prostate cancer.[47] Although PSMA is not exclusively expressed in the prostate, it does show significant overexpression compared with the surrounding tissue, rendering it of value as a biological tracer.[47] It is expressed in a large proportion of prostate cancers, and the degree of PSMA expression has been found to correlate with several predictors of tumor aggressiveness, such as hormone sensitivity and higher tumor grade, as well as increased risk of progression.[52,53] The results of several studies have recently been published, highlighting the merits of PSMA-PET/CT rather than conventional imaging in the assessment of biochemical recurrence, and although most trials are small, the current trend in evidence shows 68Ga-PSMA–PET/CT to be more effective in early detection of recurrent prostate cancer compared with conventional imaging techniques.[20,45,47] The role of PSMA in primary staging of prostate cancer is unclear, but a recent study including 130 patients undergoing a pelvic lymphadenectomy has identified sensitivity (65.9%) and specificity rates (98.9%) for pelvic lymph nodes identified by PSMA-PET[54] **(Fig. 1)**.

Several molecular imaging modalities that are now available in clinical practice may shed new light on the understanding of the biology of prostate cancer. The challenge remains to define the role of PSMA and newer imaging modalities in the diagnosis and management of prostate cancer, and there is a need for future randomized trials evaluating outcomes of localized treatment of oligometastatic prostate cancer.

END POINTS IN OLIGOMETASTATIC PROSTATE CANCER: IS A CURE REALLY EXPECTED?

Patients presenting with advanced prostate cancer account for approximately one-third of prostate cancer deaths in the United States, with an average

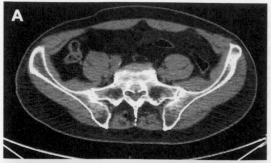

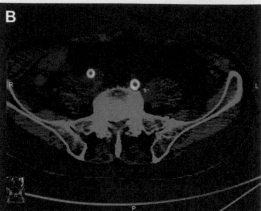

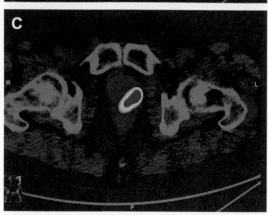

Fig. 1. (A) Axial image from CT scan of a patient with prostate cancer showing no evidence of lymphadenopathy under CT criteria. (B) Axial image from 68Ga-PSMA–PET/CT scan at same location as in panel (A), showing uptake of tracer at iliac lymph nodes on left and right side. (C) Axial image from 68Ga-PSMA–PET/CT scan showing uptake of tracer in primary prostate tumor.

age of 73 years and a median survival of approximately 3 years.[55] However, most patients who die from prostate cancer are those who recur after radical treatment. Men with oligometastatic disease belong to both groups and accordingly, discussion of a cure may not adequately represent the complexity of the disease. It may be more appropriate to discuss disease control. Studies of adjuvant prostate cancer treatment assessing overall survival show a median time from enrollment to the end of recruitment of 11.5 years,[56] showing a lengthy, and often variable, time from localized disease to death from prostate cancer. Furthermore, the risk of death from prostate cancer is affected by the patient's age and comorbidities.[57]

It is clear from the literature on the treatment of men with oligometastatic prostate cancer that there is no agreement on what might be considered success in assessing outcomes.[33] Several different outcome measures could be used, including a decrease in PSA, improvement in radiographic appearance, and prolonged castration-free survival, which is likely the most common end point in current use. However, this end point is problematic because there is little agreement about when ADT should be initiated in these patient populations. Clearly, the best way to prolong castration-free survival is to not write the prescription. Without clearly defined and validated outcome measures, it may be tempting just to target lesions increasingly seen on PSMA-PET/CT with treatments such as stereotactic ablative radiotherapy[58] or salvage robotic lymphadenectomy,[59] both of which are feasible treatments, but questionable in their utility.[33,60]

It is therefore necessary for investigators to use validated outcomes as surrogates for overall survival in order to monitor the effect of treatment and expedite the findings of clinical studies.[61] Such surrogates, or intermediate clinical end points (ICEs), have previously been defined in the Intermediate Clinical Endpoints in Cancer of the Prostate (ICECaP) project[56] and are set out in **Table 2**. Given the variation in the natural history of oligometastatic prostate cancer, the heterogeneity of patients in age and comorbidity, and the numerous different treatment regimens used, identifying ICEs will be challenging. Moreover, end points may be confounded by the treatments given; for example, some men may have depressed testosterone levels following neoadjuvant or adjuvant ADT, which affect PSA levels.

Moreover, ADT may affect overall survival by increasing non–prostate cancer death through cardiovascular morbidity, thereby confusing the association of PSA with overall survival. Sweeney and colleagues[56] therefore suggested identifying subgroups with the highest risk of prostate cancer death within trials to minimize the impact of non–prostate cancer death on prostate cancer–related end points.

FUTURE DIRECTIONS OF RESEARCH
Imaging in Oligometastatic Prostate Cancer

PSMA-targeted imaging is gaining interest, with data showing high sensitivity to small-volume sites of prostate cancer that are not detectable on conventional imaging.[62] The ongoing proPSMA (Prospective Evaluation of 68Ga-PSMA–PET/CT for Recurrence Detection of Prostate Cancer and Its Impact on Patient Management) study, a single-arm, phase III imaging trial, is designed to prospectively evaluate the impact of 68Ga-PSMA–PET/CT on the therapeutic management of patients with biological recurrent prostate cancer and negative, equivocal, or oligometastatic disease after routine imaging diagnostic work-up (http://findanexpert.unimelb.edu.au/display/grant101823#Awards). Such data will not only provide information on the utility of PSMA-targeted imaging but are predicted to shift the objective with regard to the diagnosis of oligometastatic prostate cancer. It may be that the 20% to 30% of men who progress following radical therapy for localized disease will, with more sensitive imaging, be recategorized as men with metastatic disease, which will fundamentally change the way clinicians think about treating such patients.

Local Treatment in Oligometastatic Prostate Cancer

Randomized trials of local therapy for oligometastatic prostate cancer are currently underway, and it is hoped that they will resolve some of the criticism that has been leveled at the existing evidence for the benefit of treatment in this field.

Radiotherapy to the primary tumor
The Systemic Therapy in Advancing or Metastatic Prostate Cancer (STAMPEDE) trial was established to further evaluate multimodal therapy in the treatment of metastatic prostate cancer (http://www.stampedetrial.org/). With 10 arms in the STAMPEDE trial, this unique multiarm, multistage study has already changed the standard of care for men with prostate cancer and continues to assess the effects of additional agents, including abiraterone, enzalutamide, and most recently metformin. Arm H is assessing the added effect of radiotherapy to the prostate for men diagnosed with M1 prostate cancer versus standard of care with 1200 patients, 600 of whom will be allocated to RT. A similar prospective multicenter study from Holland A randomised study about the effect on survival of hormonal therapy versus hormonal therapy plus local external radiation therapy in patients with primary diagnosed metastasised (M+) prostate cancer (HORRAD) randomizing patients with metastatic prostate cancer to hormonal therapy or hormonal therapy and RT has finished recruitment (http://www.controlled-trials.com/ISRCTN06890529).

Table 2
End points in use to measure outcomes in men with oligometastatic disease

Intermediate Clinical End Point	Measure	Author	Trial/Notes
Time to biochemical failure	<1.5 y, <2 y, <2.5 y	Denham	TROG 96.01
PSA doubling time	<12m, <15m, ≤3 mo	Denham, D'Amico	TROG 96.01, CAPSURE and CPDR
PSA nadir	PSA nadir >0.5 ng/mL	Denham, D'Amico	TROG 96.01 and a DFCI
End-of-treatment PSA		D'Amico	TROG 96.01 and a DFCI
DFS	PSA of 25 ng/mL or greater, initiation of treatment, and disease-free survival	Ray	RTOG92-02
MFS	MFS at 3 y, not 5 y		
DFS	First evidence of recorded clinical recurrence (local/regional progression and/or distant metastases confirmed by imaging or histologic evidence) or death from any cause	Sweeney et al	Can be applied to radiation and prostatectomy trials; may be affected by use of ADT; eg, prognosis different at DFS for MCPc with ADT vs de-novo mCSPC without ADT
MFS	Documented metastatic disease or death from any cause	Sweeney et al	Excludes local progression events
EFS	Any documented disease event (same as DFS plus biochemical failure) or death from any cause	Sweeney et al	
Time to biochemical failure defined according to local therapy	Prostatectomy: PSA level >0.2 ng/mL Postradiation increase of >2 ng/mL above nadir PSA level	Cookson Roach	Confounded by recovery of testosterone after adjuvant ADT; ADT for increasing PSA level after local therapy; salvage therapy; long lead time with death from other causes

Abbreviations: DFS, disease-free survival; EFS, event-free survival; MFS, metastasis-free survival.

Surgery or radiotherapy to the primary tumor

Chapin and colleagues in North America are carrying out a multicenter, randomized, phase 2 study to evaluate whether treatment with systemic therapy in combination with local therapy in distant metastatic disease (M1) is more effective than systemic therapy alone (https://clinicaltrials.gov/ct2/show/NCT01751438).

The safety of this treatment combination will also be studied. Patients who progress within 6 months will not be randomized to the treatment arms but will be evaluated as a separate group in order to gather data on this group of patients with a poor prognosis. Crucially, the study is open to men with all volumes of metastatic disease so long as they show no evidence of progression at 6 months. This feature of eligibility is interesting because it may accommodate

potential problems with eligibility that may be found in studies limited to oligometastatic disease, especially with advances in imaging techniques that are emerging. Furthermore, this study allows the treating physicians to initiate therapy, including surgery, or radiotherapy as they see fit, with randomization helping to correct for any selection bias for or against systemic therapy alone. In the United Kingdom a feasibility study, Testing radical prostatectomy in men with oligometastatic prostate cancer that has spread to the bone (TRoMbone), is recruiting patients with oligometastatic disease (defined by conventional imaging), who will be randomized to RP plus standard treatment, versus standard treatment alone (http://trendsinmenshealth.com/news/trombone-calls-recruits/). Both studies, as well as providing important data from randomized allocation, will have the advantage that they have not defined what standard therapy should be, thereby protecting the trial design against changes to standard therapy as other studies mature.

Metastasis-directed therapy

Although there are many studies investigating metastasis-directed therapy in oligometastatic disease, OLigometastatic Prostate CancEr Trial (ORIOLE) and Surveillance or metastasis-directed Therapy for OligoMetastatic Prostate cancer recurrence (STOMP) will provide evidence from randomized patients. The ORIOLE study is designed to randomize men with oligometastatic prostate cancer who have failed primary treatment to observation versus Stereotactic Body Radiation Therapy (SBRT) in order to determine whether it is possible to delay the use of hormonal therapy and/or prevent other bone metastases from developing elsewhere in the body (https://clinicaltrials.gov/ct2/show/NCT02680587). In addition, the study will use an investigational radioactive drug called 18F-DCFPyL to further assess the spread of metastatic disease. Similarly, the Belgian STOMP study will be randomizing men with oligometastatic prostate cancer to surveillance or metastasis-directed therapy in the form of surgery or SBRT.[63]

Multimodal therapy

Several studies are underway to assess the benefits and safety of multimodal therapy and, although they are not randomized, it is hoped they will yield important information to inform future randomized trials. A study from Memorial Sloan Kettering Cancer Center is assessing the benefits of multimodal therapy by assessing the effect on prostate cancer of ipilimumab with degarelix before RP, followed by more degarelix and ipilimumab after the surgery (https://clinicaltrials.gov/ct2/show/NCT02020070). Similarly, Johns Hopkins is undertaking a study assessing the safety of consolidative therapy to metastases with SBRT after systemic therapy and definitive prostatectomy or radiotherapy to the prostate. It is hoped that both studies will generate interesting data that can go on to inform future randomized comparative studies to inform future best practice (https://clinicaltrials.gov/ct2/show/NCT02716974?term=NCT02716974&rank=1).

SUMMARY

The widespread use of local and ablative treatment of oligometastatic prostate cancer outside the setting of clinical trials remains uncertain. Although there is a promising and growing bank of evidence, current standard of care has not been sufficiently challenged. There remain insufficient conclusions regarding cancer-specific and overall survival and the outcomes of the prospective trials are eagerly awaited.

Standardization in the definition of oligometastasis must extend beyond the number of metastases to include the genetic and biological basis of the disease as it is further characterized. Individualized therapeutic strategies are likely to be based on these divisions. A combination of local therapy, which has been shown to be safe, may negate the need for palliative treatment to the prostate in the future. In addition, the combination of metastasis-directed therapy and systemic chemohormonal treatment might prolong metastasis-free intervals with limited systemic toxicity.

At present, to expect a cure of oligometastatic prostate cancer remains a goal and not a certainty. However, the pace at which clinical, molecular, and genetic research is being driven may make this goal a reality sooner rather than later.

REFERENCES

1. Hellman S, Weichselbaum RR. Oligometastases. J Clin Oncol 1995;13:8–10.
2. Vogelstein B, Kinzler KW. The multistep nature of cancer. Trends Genet 1993;9:138–41.
3. Rinker-Schaeffer CW, Partin AW, Isaacs WB, et al. Molecular and cellular changes associated with the acquisition of metastatic ability by prostatic cancer cells. Prostate 1994;25:249–65.
4. Gupta GP, Massague J. Cancer metastasis: building a framework. Cell 2006;127:679–95.
5. Norton L, Massague J. Is cancer a disease of self-seeding? Nat Med 2006;12:875–8.
6. Dabestani S, Marconi L, Bex A. Metastasis therapies for renal cancer. Curr Opin Urol 2016;26:566–72.
7. Mesko S, Sandler K, Cohen J, et al. Clinical outcomes for stereotactic ablative radiotherapy in oligometastatic and oligoprogressive gynecological malignancies. Int J Gynecol Cancer 2017;27:403–8.
8. Kucharczyk MJ, Parpia S, Walker-Dilks C, et al. Ablative therapies in metastatic breast cancer: a systematic review. Breast Cancer Res Treat 2017;164(1):13–25.
9. Man YG, Gardner WA. Bad seeds produce bad crops: a single stage-process of prostate tumor invasion. Int J Biol Sci 2008;4:246–58.
10. Singh D, Yi WS, Brasacchio RA, et al. Is there a favorable subset of patients with prostate cancer who develop oligometastases? Int J Radiat Oncol Biol Phys 2004;58:3–10.
11. Heidenreich A, Bastian PJ, Bellmunt J, et al. EAU guidelines on prostate cancer. part 1: screening, diagnosis, and local treatment with curative intent–update 2013. Eur Urol 2014;65:124–37.

12. Sharifi N, Gulley JL, Dahut WL. Androgen depriva- tion therapy for prostate cancer. JAMA 2005;294: 238–44.

13. Perlmutter MA, Lepor H. Androgen deprivation ther- apy in the treatment of advanced prostate cancer. Rev Urol 2007;9(Suppl 1):S3–8.

14. James ND, Spears MR, Clarke NW, et al. Failure-free survival and radiotherapy in patients with newly diagnosed nonmetastatic prostate cancer: data from patients in the control arm of the STAMPEDE trial. JAMA Oncol 2016;2(3):348–57.

15. Lin CC, Gray PJ, Jemal A, et al. Androgen depriva- tion with or without radiation therapy for clinically node-positive prostate cancer. J Natl Cancer Inst 2015;107 [pii:djv119].

16. Rusthoven CG, Carlson JA, Waxweiler TV, et al. The impact of definitive local therapy for lymph node- positive prostate cancer: a population-based study. Int J Radiat Oncol Biol Phys 2014;88:1064–73.

17. Aoun F, Peltier A, van Velthoven R. A comprehensive review of contemporary role of local treatment of the primary tumor and/or the metastases in metastatic prostate cancer. Biomed Res Int 2014;2014:501213.

18. Rubin P, Brasacchio R, Katz A. Solitary metastasis: illusion versus reality. Semin Radiat Oncol 2006;16: 120–30.

19. Lee ST, Lawrentschuk N, Scott AM. PET in prostate and bladder tumors. Semin Nucl Med 2012;42:231–46.

20. Perera M, Papa N, Christidis D, et al. Sensitivity, specificity, and predictors of positive 68Ga-pros- tate-specific membrane antigen positron emission tomography in advanced prostate cancer: a system- atic review and meta-analysis. Eur Urol 2016;70: 926–37.

21. Tosoian JJ, Gorin MA, Ross AE, et al. Oligometa- static prostate cancer: definitions, clinical outcomes, and treatment considerations. Nat Rev Urol 2017; 14(1):15–25.

22. Tabata K, Niibe Y, Satoh T, et al. Radiotherapy for oli- gometastases and oligo-recurrence of bone in pros- tate cancer. Pulm Med 2012;2012:541656.

23. Sridharan S, Steigler A, Spry NA, et al. Oligometa- static bone disease in prostate cancer patients treated on the TROG 03.04 RADAR trial. Radiother Oncol 2016;121:98–102.

24. Reeves F, Murphy D, Evans C, et al. Targeted local therapy in oligometastatic prostate cancer: a promising potential opportunity after failed primary treatment. BJU Int 2015;116:170–2.

25. Gillessen S, Omlin A, Attard G, et al. Management of patients with advanced prostate cancer: recommen- dations of the St Gallen Advanced Prostate Cancer Consensus Conference (APCCC) 2015. Ann Oncol 2015;26(8):1589–604.

26. Frohmüller HG, Theiss M. Radical prostatectomy in the management of localized prostate cancer. Eur J Surg Oncol 1995;21(4):336–40.

27. Frazier II HA, Robertson JE, Paulson DF. Does radical prostatectomy in presence of positive pelvic lymph no- des enhace survival?, world jurol 1994;2(6):308–12.

28. Heidenreich A, Pfister D, Porres D. Cytoreductive radical prostatectomy in patients with prostate can- cer and low volume skeletal metastases: results of a feasibility and case-control study. J Urol 2015; 193:832–8.

29. O'Shaughnessy MJ, McBride SM, Vargas HA, et al. A Pilot Study of a Multimodal Treatment Paradigm to Accelerate Drug Evaluations in Early-stage Metastatic Prostate Cancer Urology 2017;102:164–72. http://dx. doi.org/10.1016/j.urology.2016.10.044. Epub 2016 Nov 22.

30. Berkovic P, De Meerleer G, Delrue L, et al. Salvage stereotactic body radiotherapy for patients with limited prostate cancer metastases: deferring androgen deprivation therapy. Clin Genitourin Can- cer 2013;11:27–32.

31. Schick U, Jorcano S, Nouet P, et al. Androgen depri- vation and high-dose radiotherapy for oligometa- static prostate cancer patients with less than five regional and/or distant metastases. Acta Oncol 2013;52:1622–8.

32. Ahmed KA, Barney BM, Davis BJ, et al. Stereotactic body radiation therapy in the treatment of oligometa- static prostate cancer. Front Oncol 2012;2:215.

33. Murphy DG, Sweeney CJ, Tombal B. "Gotta catch 'em all", or do we? Pokemet approach to metastatic prostate cancer. Eur Urol 2017;72:1–3.

34. Bhindi B, Rangel LJ, Mason RJ, et al. Impact of radical prostatectomy on long-term oncologic out- comes in a matched cohort of men with pathological node positive prostate cancer managed by castra- tion. J Urol 2017;198(1):86–91.

35. Zagars GK, Pollack A, von Eschenbach AC. Addi- tion of radiation therapy to androgen ablation im- proves outcome for subclinically node-positive prostate cancer. Urology 2001;58:233–9.

36. Steuber T, Budaus L, Walz J, et al. Radical prostatec- tomy improves progression-free and cancer-specific survival in men with lymph node positive prostate cancer in the prostate-specific antigen era: a confir- matory study. BJU Int 2011;107(11):1755–61.

37. Boorjian SA, Thompson RH, Siddiqui S, et al. Long- term outcome after radical prostatectomy for pa- tients with lymph node positive prostate cancer in the prostate specific antigen era. J Urol 2007;178: 864–71.

38. Briganti A, Karnes JR, Da Pozzo LF, et al. Two pos- itive nodes represent a significant cut-off value for cancer specific survival in patients with node posi- tive prostate cancer. A new proposal based on a two-institution experience on 703 consecutive N+ patients treated with radical prostatectomy, extended pelvic lymph node dissection and adju- vant therapy. Eur Urol 2009;55:261–70.

39. Thompson IM, Tangen C, Basler J, et al. Impact of previous local treatment for prostate cancer on subsequent metastatic disease. J Urol 2002;168: 1008–12.

40. Halabi S, Vogelzang NJ, Ou SS, et al. The impact of prior radical prostatectomy in men with metastatic castration recurrent prostate cancer: a pooled analysis of 9 cancer and leukemia group B trials. J Urol 2007;177:531–4.

41. Bayne CE, Williams SB, Cooperberg MR, et al. Treatment of the primary tumor in metastatic prostate cancer: current concepts and future perspectives. Eur Urol 2016;69(5):775–87.

42. Culp SH, Schellhammer PF, Williams MB. Might men diagnosed with metastatic prostate cancer benefit from definitive treatment of the primary tumor? A SEER-based study. Eur Urol 2014;65: 1058–66.

43. Gratzke C, Engel J, Stief CG. Role of radical prostatectomy in metastatic prostate cancer: data from the Munich Cancer Registry. Eur Urol 2014;66(3):602–3.

44. Sooriakumaran P, Karnes J, Stief C, et al. A multi-institutional analysis of perioperative outcomes in 106 men who underwent radical prostatectomy for distant metastatic prostate cancer at presentation. Eur Urol 2016;69(5):788–94.

45. Morigi JJ, Fanti S, Murphy D, et al. Rapidly changing landscape of PET/CT imaging in prostate cancer. Curr Opin Urol 2016;26:493–500.

46. Murphy DG, Hofman M, Lawrentschuk N, et al. Bringing clarity or confusion? The role of prostate-specific membrane antigen positron-emission/computed tomography for primary staging in prostate cancer. BJU Int 2017;119:194–5.

47. Maurer T, Eiber M, Schwaiger M, et al. Current use of PSMA-PET in prostate cancer management. Nat Rev Urol 2016;13:226–35.

48. Oldan JD, Hawkins AS, Chin BB. (18)F sodium fluoride PET/CT in patients with prostate cancer: quantification of normal tissues, benign degenerative lesions, and malignant lesions. World J Nucl Med 2016;15:102–8.

49. Cook GJ, Azad G, Padhani AR. Bone imaging in prostate cancer: the evolving roles of nuclear medicine and radiology. Clin Transl Imaging 2016; 4:439–47.

50. Simoncic U, Perlman S, Liu G, et al. Comparison of NaF and FDG PET/CT for assessment of treatment response in castration-resistant prostate cancers with osseous metastases. Clin Genitourin Cancer 2015;13:e7–17.

51. Leiblich A, Stevens D, Sooriakumaran P. The utility of molecular imaging in prostate cancer. Curr Urol Rep 2016;17:26.

52. Sathianathen NJ, Lamb A, Nair R, et al. Updates of prostate cancer staging: prostate-specific membrane antigen. Investig Clin Urol 2016;57:S147–54.

53. Rowe SP, Gorin MA, Allaf ME, et al. PET imaging of prostate-specific membrane antigen in prostate cancer: current state of the art and future challenges. Prostate Cancer Prostatic Dis 2016;19(3):223–30.

54. Maurer T, Gschwend JE, Rauscher I, et al. Diagnostic efficacy of gallium-PSMA positron emission tomography compared to conventional imaging in lymph node staging of 130 consecutive patients with intermediate to high risk prostate cancer. J Urol 2016;195:1436–43.

55. Wu JN, Fish KM, Evans CP, et al. No improvement noted in overall or cause-specific survival for men presenting with metastatic prostate cancer over a 20-year period. Cancer 2014;120:818–23.

56. Sweeney C, Nakabayashi M, Regan M, et al. The development of intermediate clinical endpoints in cancer of the prostate (ICECaP). J Natl Cancer Inst 2015;107. djv261.

57. Briganti A, Spahn M, Joniau S, et al. Impact of age and comorbidities on long-term survival of patients with high-risk prostate cancer treated with radical prostatectomy: a multi-institutional competing-risks analysis. Eur Urol 2013;63:693–701.

58. Decaestecker K, De Meerleer G, Lambert B, et al. Repeated stereotactic body radiotherapy for oligometastatic prostate cancer recurrence. Radiat Oncol 2014;9:135.

59. Montorsi F, Gandaglia G, Fossati N, et al. Robot-assisted salvage lymph node dissection for clinically recurrent prostate cancer. Eur Urol 2016;72(3): 432–8.

60. Maurer T, Murphy DG, Hofman MS, et al. PSMA-PET for lymph node detection in recurrent prostate cancer: how do we use the magic bullet? Theranostics 2017;7:2046–7.

61. Prentice RL. Surrogate and mediating endpoints: current status and future directions. J Natl Cancer Inst 2009;101:216–7.

62. van Leeuwen PJ, Emmett L, Ho B, et al. Prospective evaluation of 68Gallium-prostate-specific membrane antigen positron emission tomography/computed tomography for preoperative lymph node staging in prostate cancer. BJU Int 2017; 119:209–15.

63. Decaestecker K, De Meerleer G, Ameye F, et al. Surveillance or metastasis-directed therapy for oligometastatic prostate cancer recurrence (STOMP): study protocol for a randomized phase II trial. BMC Cancer 2014;14:671.

Approach to the Patient with High-Risk Prostate Cancer

Matthew Mossanen, MD[a], Ross E. Krasnow, MD[a],
Paul L. Nguyen, MD[b,c], Quoc D. Trinh, MD[a,c],
Mark Preston, MD, MPH[a,c], Adam S. Kibel, MD[a,c,*]

KEYWORDS

- Prostate cancer • High risk • Management

KEY POINTS

- There are multiple definitions of high risk prostate cancer and each definition is associated with a different prognosis.
- Men classified as having high-risk disease warrant treatment because durable outcomes can be achieved.
- Radical prostatectomy, radiation therapy, and androgen deprivation therapy play pivotal roles in the management of men with high-risk disease, and potentially in men with metastatic disease.
- The optimal combinations of therapeutic regimens are an evolving area of study and future work looking into therapies for men with high-risk disease will remain critical.

INTRODUCTION

Prostate cancer (PC) is the second most common cancer in men, accounting for 1 in 5 new cancer diagnoses in the United States.[1] In 2016, more than 180,000 new cases were diagnosed and more than 26,000 men died of disease.[1] Although the majority of men are diagnosed with low- or intermediate-risk disease, upwards of 15% of men are diagnosed with high-risk disease.[2–4] Importantly, the incidence of high-risk and metastatic PC seems to be increasing.[5] Although this has been attributed in part to the 2012 recommendation by the US Preventive Services Task Force against screening for PC, the true long-term impact of these recommendations on advanced disease and mortality remains to be determined.[6]

In the face of these changes in disease presentation, the management of high-risk disease is evolving. Recent examinations in patterns of care suggest continued undertreatment of high-risk disease and overtreatment of low-risk disease.[7] Men with high-risk disease have a higher relative risk of PC-specific mortality than men with intermediate-risk disease.[8] Moreover, because they represent a substantial proportion of PC patients at legitimate risk of metastatic disease and death, our treatment must evolve to improve cure rates in this population.[9] In this review, we discuss the approach to management of men with high-risk PC, including diagnosis and treatment strategies.

DEFINITION OF HIGH-RISK DISEASE

Multiple schemas exist to define high-risk PC. However, there is a lack of consensus on which is the optimal definition. The 3 components that comprise

Disclosure Statement: No disclosures.
[a] Division of Urology, Brigham and Women's Hospital, Harvard Medical School, 45 Francis Street, Boston, MA 02115, USA; [b] Department of Radiation Oncology, Brigham and Women's Hospital, Harvard Medical School, 45 Francis Street, Boston, MA 02115, USA; [c] Dana-Farber Cancer Institute, Harvard Medical School, Boston, MA, USA
* Corresponding author.
E-mail address: akibel@bwh.harvard.edu

Urol Clin N Am 44 (2017) 635–645
http://dx.doi.org/10.1016/j.ucl.2017.07.009

the definition of PC typically include Gleason grade, prostate-specific antigen (PSA), and rectal examination findings.[10] **Table 1** provides commonly used definitions incorporating these parameters. Other definitions use additional readily available clinical data to provide a more precise risk of failure. For example, the Cancer of the Prostate Risk Assessment (CAPRA) score uses age, PSA, clinical stage, Gleason score, and positive biopsy cores to predict risk of recurrence for localized disease.[11] The Kattan nomograms do not categorize patients into risk groups, but instead give a probability of 5-year treatment failure after radical prostatectomy or radiation by using multiple clinical variables including PSA, Gleason score, and clinical stage.[12]

A clear benefit to standard risk stratification is clear communication with the patients as to their disease state. However, the risk of recurrence varies greatly depending on the definition used for the same patient. An evaluation of 4708 patients treated with radical prostatectomy at Memorial Sloan-Kettering Cancer Center examined 8 different definitions of high-risk disease and found that, depending on the definition used, the proportion of patients defined as high risk ranged from 3% to 38% and 5-year relapse-free probability varied between 49% and 80%.[13] Revision of risk stratifications has been an active area of research and will likely continue to evolve in the future.[14] Consistent schemas are critical because, with standard definitions, providers may better determine ideal treatment strategies for patients, compare outcomes across clinical studies, and share expectations for clinical outcomes with patients.[15]

SCREENING

The impact of US Preventive Services Task Force recommendations on primary care and urologist practice patterns differs and optimal PSA screening strategy is in evolution, but does not clearly apply to men at high risk for PC, particularly aggressive disease.[21] Screening of men at risk for aggressive disease should consider additional factors. A family history of high-grade, high stage, or lethal PC is particularly important because cancer-specific survival in parents predicts survival from PC in their children.[22] The survival of a son correlates linearly with the survival of his father.[23] In addition, ethnic background is important because African American men may have up to a 60% higher risk of developing PC than Caucasians and have a worse prognosis[24] with an approximately 2-fold increased risk of diagnosis and death owing to PC.[25] Unfortunately, the rates of PSA screening are lower in African Americans when compared with non-Hispanic whites throughout multiple geographic regions in the United States.[26] As a result of the increased risk of death owing to PC in African American men, more frequent PSA testing and aggressive treatment may be appropriate for these men.[27] More recent data across all ethnic groups shows PSA levels in midlife correlate future lethal PC suggesting that risk stratified screening may be valuable in men aged 45 to 59 years.[28] Considering these aspects of a patient's history are important when evaluating men for screening, diagnosis, and treatment.

ROLE OF IMAGING IN IDENTIFYING HIGH-RISK PATIENTS

The role of MRI in the diagnosis and management of localized PC is expanding rapidly,[29] because MRI can accurate identify men with potentially aggressive disease.[29,30] The use of ultrasound fusion biopsy, which uses MRI to identify regions

Table 1
Definitions of high-risk prostate cancer

Professional Organization	Definition(s)	Notes
American Urologic Association[16,17]	PSA $\geq$20 ng/mL or GS $\geq$8 or c $\geq$ T2c	Guidelines are based on the D'Amico Criteria.[14]
European Association of Urology[18]	PSA $\geq$20 ng/mL or GS $\geq$8 or c $\geq$ T3a	
National Comprehensive Cancer Network[19]	PSA >20 ng/mL or GS $\geq$8 or c $\geq$ T3a	Multiple adverse factors can be categorized in the next level. Very high risk includes: T3b-T4, primary GS = 5, or >4 cores with GS 8–10.
Radiation Therapy Oncology Group[20]	GS = 7 with cT3 or N1 GS $\geq$8 and cT1-2	Very high risk includes: T3b-T4.

Abbreviations: c, clinical stage; GS, Gleason score; PSA, prostate-specific antigen.

of suspicion that can later be targeted during traditional standard biopsy, has improved the accuracy of prostate biopsy.[31,32] A study of 1003 men undergoing both standard and targeted biopsy found that fusion biopsies using MRI were more likely to detect high-risk cancers (30% more high-risk cancers, P<.001) and less likely to detect low-risk cancers (17% fewer low-risk cancers, P<.001).[33] A retrospective analysis of 601 men found that MRI fusion biopsy resulted in a statistically significant increase in detection of clinically significant cancer (G7 and higher) in men with no biopsy, prior negative biopsy, and prior cancer diagnosis.[34] Additional studies have also supported the role of MRI in detecting clinically significant PC.[35–37] A metaanalysis of 21 studies demonstrated that MRI-ultrasound fusion biopsy detected more clinically significant cancers than standard biopsy (relative risk, 1.22; P = .01).[38]

Routine imaging for systemic disease has not evolved as rapidly, although there are new imaging modalities on the horizon. Bone scans are traditionally used to detect osseous metastases in men with PC. Judicious selection of patients is key to optimizing the identification of metastatic disease by bone scan. The likelihood of bone metastases in men with a PSA of less than 10 ng/mL is less than 1%.[39] However, for men with a PSA of greater than 20 ng/mL, the incidence of metastatic disease identified on bone scan may be as high as 16%.[40] Focused use of this test in men with high-risk disease can also help limit health care costs.[39] The role of computed tomography in detecting lymph node metastases is also of limited value in patients with low-risk disease.[41] Computed tomography has been found to be more useful in patients with Gleason 8 disease or a PSA of greater than 20 ng/mL.[40]

The use of imaging in PC is evolving and there are new imaging modalities on the horizon. Although beyond the scope of this article, for men with high-risk PC and concern for metastatic disease, additional imaging tools are being examined. Whole body MRI,[42] prostate-specific membrane antigen PET,[43,44] 18F-fluciclovine, and 18F-fluoride PET with or without computed tomography[45] are just a few examples of newer imaging modalities, but none have yet become a standard option in this patient population.

THERAPY

Men with high-risk PC are candidates for a number of treatments, including radical prostatectomy, androgen deprivation monotherapy, external-beam radiotherapy with hormone deprivation, and brachytherapy. Multimodal therapy is a cornerstone of management in men with high-risk disease. Robust randomized controlled trials attempting to determine the optimal therapy in men with high-risk disease with long-term follow-up are lacking. As a result, interpretation of subsets of clinical trials, case series, and retrospective analysis often inform decision making when considering management options.

Surgery

Historically, surgical therapy for high-risk disease was thought to be inappropriate owing to a poor likelihood of durable outcomes. However, the gradual accumulation of studies demonstrates beneficial clinical results for men undergoing radical prostatectomy. Briganti and colleagues[46] found that among 1366 patients with high-risk disease (PSA 20, cT3, G8) 10-year PC-specific survival was 91%. The high use of adjuvant androgen deprivation therapy (ADT) or radiation therapy (48%) demonstrates the need for multimodality therapy in these patients. Using the same high-risk definition, a multiinstitutional study by Stephenson and colleagues[47] reported a 10-year PC-specific survival of 92%. A third study of 1238 patients using identical high-risk criteria found a similar 10-year PC-specific survival of 92%. Again, high use of multimodality therapy with 40% receiving adjuvant therapy consisting of external beam radiation therapy with ADT or external beam radiation therapy alone.[48]

Other studies using different criteria for high-risk disease, such as cT3, corroborate a similar 10-year PC-specific survival of 90%.[49] Zwergel and colleagues[50] studied 275 patients with a PSA of greater than 20 ng/mL found a 10-year PC-specific survival of 83% with 47% receiving immediate ADT. Spahn and colleagues[51] studied 712 men with a PSA of greater than 20 ng/mL and found a 10-year estimated PC-specific survival of 90% with variability in administration of adjuvant external beam radiation therapy or ADT depending on clinical risk factors. In another study by Spahn and colleagues[52] of high-risk PC patients defined by a PSA of greater than 20 ng/mL, the investigators found a 10-year cancer-specific survival of 89%. Also, Lughezzani and colleagues[53] studied 580 consecutive patients with Gleason 8 to 10 disease at a single European institution and reported a 10-year PC-specific survival of 91.7% for patients with specimen confined disease at final pathology.

These are just a few of the retrospective studies of varying size that indicate improved PC-specific survival for high-risk patients who undergo radical prostatectomy. Although these studies are consistent with a 10-year PC-specific survival of approximately 90%, limitations to these data include retrospective analysis, variable definitions of high-risk disease, and heterogeneity of administration of adjuvant therapy. Nevertheless, these studies prove that men with high-risk disease can achieve durable cure with strategies that use surgical therapy.

Two prospective randomized trials provide evidence that surgery is effective for high-risk disease. In the SPCG-4 trial (Scandinavian Prostate Cancer Group 4 Trial), investigators randomly assigned 695 men with clinically localized disease to radical prostatectomy or watchful waiting.[54] Although the study did not focus on high-risk patients, the majority of the patients had high-risk features. At a median follow-up of 13 years, SPCG-4 found a significant reduction in mortality after radical prostatectomy was noted with a relative risk of 0.56 (95% CI, 0.41–0.77; $P = .001$) and an absolute risk difference of 11% (95% CI, 4.5–17.5).[55] Although PIVOT (Prostate Cancer Intervention versus Observation Trial) did not demonstrate a survival benefit to the entire cohort, subset analysis examining men with high-risk features demonstrated evidence of benefit. PC mortality was lower in the surgically treated men with a PSA of greater than 10 ng/mL (5.6% vs 12.8%; $P = .02$) and among men with D'Amico high-risk PC (9.1% vs 17.5%; $P = .04$).[56] Although the Prostate ProtecT trial (Testing for Cancer and Treatment) is being cited frequently, it is important to recognize that this study focused almost exclusively on low- and intermediate- risk disease; therefore, these results are not applicable to men with high-risk disease.[57]

In aggregate, many of these works provide valuable insights into the management of men with clinically localized PC. However, moving forward, as imaging technology evolves, biomarkers are developed, and biopsy accuracy improve, it may become progressively easier to identify these high-risk patients most likely to benefit from surgery. Also, studies conducted in other countries may not necessarily reflect clinical treatment norms for patients outside of those practice areas.

Neoadjuvant Therapy

There is also renewed interest in neoadjuvant therapy before surgery using new agents that can better achieve more complete androgen blockage. Older studies of neoadjuvant ADT failed to demonstrate an overall survival advantage, but these trials were limited by incomplete androgen ablation and overrepresentation of patients with low-risk cancer who were unlikely to die from their disease

(such as men with Gleason 6 disease).[58–70] New studies are focusing on complete androgen blockade (using agents such as abiraterone acetate and enzalutamide) in high-risk patients who are likely to fail local therapy.[71–74] Early results are promising in terms of achieving complete pathologic response and reduction in node-positive disease.[72,73]

Adjuvant Therapy After Surgery

Node-negative disease
Pathologic features of the prostatectomy specimen may allow identification of patients likely to benefit from adjuvant radiotherapy. In a study by Thompson and colleagues[75] (SWOG 8794) in men with pT3 cancer or positive margins, overall survival and metastasis free survival was improved with adjuvant therapy (60–65 Gy) at a median follow-up of 12 years. This study incorporated the standard treatment of the day, but unfortunately PSA was not available for many patients and, as a result, salvage radiation therapy was not routinely delivered in a timely manner. A second similar study, the EORTC trial 22,911 (European Organization for Research and Treatment of Cancer 22,911), also administered postoperative adjuvant therapy and demonstrated improved biochemical-free survival and decreased local failure at a median follow-up of 10.6 years.[76] Subset analysis suggested that adjuvant radiotherapy improved clinical progression free survival in patients with positive margins and patients younger than 70 years old. A third randomized trial by Wiegel and colleagues[77] demonstrated that adjuvant radiation therapy reduces biochemical recurrence but not PC-specific mortality or overall survival.

Although adjuvant radiotherapy clearly improves biochemical progression in men with high-risk disease after prostatectomy, use is variable.[78,79] In part this is because it is not clear that adjuvant therapy offers a survival advantage compared with observation followed by salvage radiation for an early increase in PSA (discussed elsewhere in this article). Discussion of salvage versus adjuvant radiation therapy should be undertaken with all men with high-risk features and referral to radiation oncologist if the patient is interested in the adjuvant approach.

Node-positive disease
The optimal timing of ADT is informed, in part, by a randomized trial by Messing and colleagues[80] examining the use of immediate versus delayed ADT in men with node-positive disease after prostatectomy. The benefits of immediate ADT were demonstrated with improvements in overall,

disease-specific, and progression-free survival being reported.[80] Other studies have examined the extent of node-positive disease to determine which men might benefit from ADT. Men with intermediate to high-risk disease (or positive margins) and 2 or fewer pelvic lymph nodes, and men with 3 to 4 pelvic lymph nodes involved had overall mortality with adjuvant radiotherapy based on a large retrospective analysis.[81] A second study examining Surveillance, Epidemiology, and End Results–Medicare data has suggested that adjuvant radiation therapy was not associated with a difference in overall survival.[82] However, this study did not include surgical margin status. Therefore, at the current time, use of ADT is recommended in this patient population, but use of radiation therapy is still in evolution.

Salvage Therapy After Surgery

Stringent monitoring of PSA in patients with high-risk features who opt for observation is essential because freedom from biochemical failure and metastasis-free survival is improved by earlier treatment.[83,84] Initial work by Stephenson and colleagues[84] demonstrated that earlier salvage radiation therapy improved biochemical-free survival. With longer follow-up, Tendulkar and colleagues[83] demonstrated an improvement in metastasis-free survival in addition to biochemical recurrence. The freedom from biochemical failure decreased from 71% for those with a presalvage PSA of 0.01 to 0.2 ng/mL to 37% for a presalvage PSA of greater than 2.0 ng/mL (P<.001). Metastasis-free survival also decreased from 9% for men with a presalvage PSA of 0.01 to 0.2 ng/mL to 37% for a presalvage PSA of greater than 2.0 ng/mL (P<.001). In addition to earlier use of radiation therapy, other factors associated with improved PC metastasis were lower score, absence of seminal vesicle invasion, positive surgical margins, and use of ADT. Others studies have supported the role of starting salvage radiotherapy for men with high-risk disease at even early PSA values, as low as 0.1 ng/mL, so it seems to be clear that earlier salvage radiation therapy is better.[85,86]

Shipley and colleagues[87] recently examined the impact of adding 24 months of daily bicalutamide versus salvage radiotherapy for men with positive margins or pT3 disease at prostatectomy. In this study, PSA levels varied from 0.2 to 4 ng/mL before the start of therapy and patients were reported to not have nodal involvement. Findings demonstrated that there was decreased death from PC (5.8% vs 13.4%; P<.001) and also improved overall survival. The fact that

bicalutamide monotherapy is considered inferior to standard ADT implies that standard ADT may provide an even greater survival advantage and therefore is becoming the preferred treatment.

Combination Radiation and Androgen Deprivation Therapy

Multiple large-scale studies have examined the impact of adding ADT to radiotherapy and have galvanized its role in this treatment approach. The EORTC 22,863 randomized 415 men with mostly cT3 and T4 disease to 70 Gy of radiotherapy with or without 3 years of concomitant goserelin. At the 5-year follow-up, men in the combination arm had improved outcomes including disease-specific survival of 74% versus 40% (P = .0001), and an overall survival of 78% versus 62% (P = .0002).[88] In 2005, in RTOG 8531 a total of 977 men were randomized to 60 to 70 Gy radiation alone or radiation with lifelong ADT. The patients who received combination therapy had improved clinical outcomes including a lower 10-year disease specific mortality of 16% versus 22% (P = .0052), and overall survival of 49% versus 39% (P = .002).[89]

The duration of ADT use has also been extensively studied and debated in men with advanced PC. In EORTC 22961 patients with locally advanced PC were randomized to 6 versus 36 months of ADT, and prolonged ADT resulted in improved PC-specific mortality (4.7% vs 3.2%; P = .002).[90] A second randomized study of cT2-4 disease also supported the role of extended ADT in radiotherapy including a comparison of 28 months versus 4 months favoring prolonged treatment.[91] A systematic review examining pooled data from 6 studies of varying duration in ADT use found that longer duration improves overall survival and disease-specific survival in intermediate- and high-risk disease patients.[92] For most men with high-risk disease treated with radiotherapy, the recommendation is to receive ADT for 2 or 3 years.[3]

Although many thought the improvements in survival was solely owing to the ADT, at least 2 randomized trials support the value of radiation in this clinical scenario. A randomized trial of 47 centers examining 875 patients with high-risk disease found that the addition of radiotherapy to ADT resulted in significant improvements in 10-year outcomes, including disease-specific survival (76% vs 88%; P<.001) and an overall survival (60% vs 70%; P = .004).[93] A second study of 1205 high-risk patients demonstrated that the addition of radiation (65–69 Gy to prostate, 45 Gy to pelvic nodes) to ADT resulted in improved overall survival

(74% vs 66%; $P = .03$) and disease-specific survival (90% vs 79%; $P = .0001$) compared with ADT alone.[94] It is clear that the synergy between ADT and radiation seems to be an important element of this treatment approach.

High-Dose Radiotherapy

Improvement in clinical outcomes with dose-escalated therapy for high-risk patients has been based on the value higher radiation doses in several studies. A randomized multicenter trial of 664 patients with stage T1b-4 disease found that use of 78 Gy versus 68 Gy was associated with a significant improvement in freedom from biochemical failure at 5 years.[95] Increased dosages, such as 78 versus 70 Gy, have been shown to result in decreased biochemical failure and PC deaths in patients with a pretreatment PSA of greater than 10 ng/mL or high-risk disease.[96] Zietman and colleagues[97] examined the use of 79.2 Gy versus 70.2 Gy without ADT in men with mostly low- and intermediate-risk disease and found improved biochemical-free rates at 10 years in the high-dose arm (32.4% vs 16.7%; $P<.0001$). Last, Dearnaley and colleagues[98] compared 843 men getting either 64 Gy versus 74 Gy external beam radiotherapy with ADT in each arm demonstrating improved 5-year biochemical recurrence with higher radiation doses.

Brachytherapy Boost to External Radiotherapy

Adding brachytherapy boost to external radiotherapy increases the total dose by approximately 50%. Although this may result in a local control benefit, it also comes at the cost of increased toxicity.[99–103] For example, Sathya and colleagues[104] demonstrated that the combination of external beam plus brachytherapy boost reduced biochemical failure (29% vs 66%; $P = .0024$) at a median follow-up of 8.2 years compared with radiation alone. Another study by Hoskin and colleagues[100] showed that at a median follow-up of 30 months the addition of high dose brachytherapy to external beam radiotherapy improved the duration of PSA-free relapse survival 5.1 years versus 4.3 years ($P = .03$). Studies examining the addition of ADT to high-dose brachytherapy with external beam radiotherapy have been mixed with some showing favorable results in terms of biochemical-free survival[105,106] and others showing no impact.[107,108] The National Comprehensive Cancer Network guidelines reports that, although the role of ADT remains to be determined, among men with high-risk disease receiving brachytherapy and external beam radiotherapy, the addition of 2 to 3 years of ADT is common.[109]

Local Therapy in Metastatic Disease

Aggressive treatment of advanced disease has even begun to play a role in metastatic disease. Two retrospective queries suggest there may be a survival benefit to definitive treatment of the prostate. Culp and colleagues[110] studied 8185 patients in the Surveillance, Epidemiology, and End Results database and demonstrated an improved 5-year overall survival in patients undergoing radical prostatectomy or brachytherapy versus no therapy. Although unable to determine the impact of systemic therapy, this work demonstrates the potential impact of local therapy in the setting of metastatic disease. A second study using the National Cancer Database identified 6382 men with metastatic PC, finding that those treated with radiation therapy and ADT versus ADT alone had an improved 5-year overall survival.[111] In the future, trials examining the potential of local therapy in metastatic disease settings may improve our understanding and local treatment with radiation therapy or surgery could become a standard of care. At the current time, it remains investigational.

SUMMARY

The diagnosis and management of high-risk PC is central to improving survival in men with this disease. Curative therapy achieves durable cure rates in this patient population. Judicious use of imaging and considerations of risk factors are essential when caring for these men. An integrated approach including surgery, radiation therapy, and systemic therapy is pivotal and men may need multiple modalities to achieve cure. The optimal combinations of therapeutic regimens are an evolving area of study and future work examining novel therapies this patient population is a critical need.

REFERENCES

1. Siegel RL, Miller KD, Jemal A. Cancer statistics, 2016. CA Cancer J Clin 2016;66(7):7–30.
2. Cooperberg MR, Cowan J, Broering JM, et al. High-risk prostate cancer in the United States, 1990-2007. World J Urol 2008;26:211.
3. Chang AJ, Autio KA, Roach M 3rd, et al. High-risk prostate cancer-classification and therapy. Nat Rev Clin Oncol 2014;11:308.
4. Punnen S, Cooperberg MR. The epidemiology of high-risk prostate cancer. Curr Opin Urol 2013; 23:331.

5. Weiner AB, Matulewicz RS, Eggener SE, et al. Increasing incidence of metastatic prostate cancer in the United States (2004-2013). Prostate Cancer Prostatic Dis 2016;19:395–7.

6. Jemal A, Fedewa SA, Ma J, et al. Prostate cancer incidence and PSA testing patterns in relation to USPSTF screening recommendations. JAMA 2015;314:2054–61.

7. Cooperberg MR, Broering JM, Carroll PR. Time trends and local variation in primary treatment of localized prostate cancer. J Clin Oncol 2010; 28:1117.

8. D'Amico AV, Moul J, Carroll PR, et al. Cancer-specific mortality after surgery or radiation for patients with clinically localized prostate cancer managed during the prostate-specific antigen era. J Clin Oncol 2003;21:2163.

9. Hamilton AS, Fleming ST, Wang D, et al. Clinical and demographic factors associated with receipt of non guideline-concordant initial therapy for nonmetastatic prostate cancer. Am J Clin Oncol 2016; 39:55.

10. Goldberg H, Baniel J, Yossepowitch O. Defining high-risk prostate cancer. Curr Opin Urol 2013; 23:337.

11. Cooperberg MR, Pasta DJ, Elkin EP, et al. The University of California, San Francisco Cancer of the Prostate Risk Assessment score: a straightforward and reliable preoperative predictor of disease recurrence after radical prostatectomy. J Urol 2005;173:1938.

12. Kattan MW, Eastham JA, Stapleton AM, et al. A preoperative nomogram for disease recurrence following radical prostatectomy for prostate cancer. J Natl Cancer Inst 1998;90:766.

13. Yossepowitch O, Eggener SE, Bianco FJ Jr, et al. Radical prostatectomy for clinically localized, high risk prostate cancer: critical analysis of risk assessment methods. J Urol 2007;178:493.

14. Rodrigues G, Warde P, Pickles T, et al. Pre-treatment risk stratification of prostate cancer patients: A critical review. Can Urol Assoc J 2012;6:121.

15. Mano R, Eastham J, Yossepowitch O. The very-high-risk prostate cancer: a contemporary update. Prostate Cancer Prostatic Dis 2016;19:340–8.

16. D'Amico AV, Whittington R, Malkowicz SB, et al. Biochemical outcome after radical prostatectomy, external beam radiation therapy, or interstitial radiation therapy for clinically localized prostate cancer. JAMA 1998;280:969.

17. Thompson I, Thrasher JB, Aus G, et al. Guideline for the management of clinically localized prostate cancer: 2007 update. J Urol 2007;177:2106.

18. Heidenreich A, Bellmunt J, Bolla M, et al. EAU guidelines on prostate cancer. Part 1: screening, diagnosis, and treatment of clinically localised disease. Eur Urol 2011;59:61.

19. Bahnson RR, Hanks GE, Huben RP, et al. NCCN practice guidelines for prostate cancer. Oncology (Williston Park) 2000;14:111.

20. Roach M, Lu J, Pilepich MV, et al. Four prognostic groups predict long-term survival from prostate cancer following radiotherapy alone on Radiation Therapy Oncology Group clinical trials. Int J Radiat Oncol Biol Phys 2000;47:609.

21. Zavaski ME, Meyer CP, Sammon JD, et al. Differences in prostate-specific antigen testing among urologists and primary care physicians following the 2012 USPSTF recommendations. JAMA Intern Med 2016;176:546.

22. Lindstrom LS, Hall P, Hartman M, et al. Familial concordance in cancer survival: a Swedish population-based study. Lancet Oncol 2007;8:1001.

23. Hemminki K, Ji J, Forsti A, et al. Concordance of survival in family members with prostate cancer. J Clin Oncol 2008;26:1705.

24. Kheirandish P, Chinegwundoh F. Ethnic differences in prostate cancer. Br J Cancer 2011;105:481.

25. Brawley OW. Trends in prostate cancer in the United States. J Natl Cancer Inst Monogr 2012; 152:2012.

26. Jindal T, Kachroo N, Sammon J, et al. Racial differences in prostate-specific antigen-based prostate cancer screening: State-by-state and region-by-region analyses. Urol Oncol 2017;35:460.e9-20.

27. Taksler GB, Keating NL, Cutler DM. Explaining racial differences in prostate cancer mortality. Cancer 2012;118:4280.

28. Preston MA, Batista JL, Wilson KM, et al. Baseline prostate-specific antigen levels in midlife predict lethal prostate cancer. J Clin Oncol 2016;34:2705.

29. Mendhiratta N, Taneja SS, Rosenkrantz AB. The role of MRI in prostate cancer diagnosis and management. Future Oncol 2016;12:2431.

30. Hoeks CM, Barentsz JO, Hambrock T, et al. Prostate cancer: multiparametric MR imaging for detection, localization, and staging. Radiology 2011; 261:46.

31. Jones TA, Radtke JP, Hadaschik B, et al. Optimizing safety and accuracy of prostate biopsy. Curr Opin Urol 2016;26:472.

32. Bjurlin MA, Mendhiratta N, Wysock JS, et al. Multiparametric MRI and targeted prostate biopsy: Improvements in cancer detection, localization, and risk assessment. Cent European J Urol 2016;69:9.

33. Siddiqui MM, Rais-Bahrami S, Turkbey B, et al. Comparison of MR/ultrasound fusion-guided biopsy with ultrasound-guided biopsy for the diagnosis of prostate cancer. JAMA 2015;313:390.

34. Meng X, Rosenkrantz AB, Mendhiratta N, et al. Relationship between prebiopsy multiparametric magnetic resonance imaging (MRI), biopsy indication, and MRI-ultrasound fusion-targeted prostate biopsy outcomes. Eur Urol 2016;69:512.

35. Filson CP, Natarajan S, Margolis DJ, et al. Prostate cancer detection with magnetic resonance-ultrasound fusion biopsy: the role of systematic and targeted biopsies. Cancer 2016;122:884.

36. Kuru TH, Roethke MC, Seidenader J, et al. Critical evaluation of magnetic resonance imaging targeted, transrectal ultrasound guided transperineal fusion biopsy for detection of prostate cancer. J Urol 2013;190:1380.

37. Mendhiratta N, Rosenkrantz AB, Meng X, et al. Magnetic resonance imaging-ultrasound fusion targeted prostate biopsy in a consecutive cohort of men with no previous biopsy: reduction of over detection through improved risk stratification. J Urol 2015;194:1601.

38. Jiang X, Zhang J, Tang J, et al. Magnetic resonance imaging - ultrasound fusion targeted biopsy outperforms standard approaches in detecting prostate cancer: a meta-analysis. Mol Clin Oncol 2016;5:301.

39. Oesterling JE. Using PSA to eliminate the staging radionuclide bone scan. Significant economic implications. Urol Clin North Am 1993;20:705.

40. Abuzallouf S, Dayes I, Lukka H. Baseline staging of newly diagnosed prostate cancer: a summary of the literature. J Urol 2004;171:2122.

41. Taneja SS. Imaging in the diagnosis and management of prostate cancer. Rev Urol 2004;6:101.

42. Lecouvet FE, El Mouedden J, Collette L, et al. Can whole-body magnetic resonance imaging with diffusion-weighted imaging replace Tc 99m bone scanning and computed tomography for single-step detection of metastases in patients with high-risk prostate cancer? Eur Urol 2012;62:68.

43. Rowe SP, Macura KJ, Ciarallo A, et al. Comparison of prostate-specific membrane antigen-based 18F-DCFBC PET/CT to conventional imaging modalities for detection of hormone-naive and castration-resistant metastatic prostate cancer. J Nucl Med 2016;57:46.

44. Rowe SP, Macura KJ, Mena E, et al. PSMA-based [(18)F]DCFPyL PET/CT is superior to conventional imaging for lesion detection in patients with metastatic prostate cancer. Mol Imaging Biol 2016;18:411.

45. Even-Sapir E, Metser U, Mishani E, et al. The detection of bone metastases in patients with high-risk prostate cancer: 99mTc-MDP Planar bone scintigraphy, single- and multi-field-of-view SPECT, 18F-fluoride PET, and 18F-fluoride PET/CT. J Nucl Med 2006;47:287.

46. Briganti A, Joniau S, Gontero P, et al. Identifying the best candidate for radical prostatectomy among patients with high-risk prostate cancer. Eur Urol 2012;61:584.

47. Stephenson AJ, Kattan MW, Eastham JA, et al. Prostate cancer-specific mortality after radical prostatectomy for patients treated in the prostate-specific antigen era. J Clin Oncol 2009;27:4300.

48. Boorjian SA, Karnes RJ, Viterbo R, et al. Long-term survival after radical prostatectomy versus external-beam radiotherapy for patients with high-risk prostate cancer. Cancer 2011;117:2883.

49. Ward JF, Slezak JM, Blute ML, et al. Radical prostatectomy for clinically advanced (cT3) prostate cancer since the advent of prostate-specific antigen testing: 15-year outcome. BJU Int 2005;95:751.

50. Zwergel U, Suttmann H, Schroeder T, et al. Outcome of prostate cancer patients with initial PSA> or =20 ng/ml undergoing radical prostatectomy. Eur Urol 2007;52:1058.

51. Spahn M, Joniau S, Gontero P, et al. Outcome predictors of radical prostatectomy in patients with prostate-specific antigen greater than 20 ng/ml: a European multi-institutional study of 712 patients. Eur Urol 2010;58:1.

52. Spahn M, Weiss C, Bader P, et al. Long-term outcome of patients with high-risk prostate cancer following radical prostatectomy and stage-dependent adjuvant androgen deprivation. Urol Int 2010;84:164.

53. Lughezzani G, Gallina A, Larcher A, et al. Radical prostatectomy represents an effective treatment in patients with specimen-confined high pathological Gleason score prostate cancer. BJU Int 2013;111:723.

54. Bill-Axelson A, Holmberg L, Ruutu M, et al. Radical prostatectomy versus watchful waiting in early prostate cancer. N Engl J Med 2011;364:1708.

55. Bill-Axelson A, Holmberg L, Garmo H, et al. Radical prostatectomy or watchful waiting in early prostate cancer. N Engl J Med 2014;370:932.

56. Wilt TJ, Brawer MK, Jones KM, et al. Radical prostatectomy versus observation for localized prostate cancer. N Engl J Med 2012;367:203.

57. Hamdy FC, Donovan JL, Lane JA, et al. 10-year outcomes after monitoring, surgery, or radiotherapy for localized prostate cancer. N Engl J Med 2016;375:1415.

58. Dalkin BL, Ahmann FR, Nagle R, et al. Randomized study of neoadjuvant testicular androgen ablation therapy before radical prostatectomy in men with clinically localized prostate cancer. J Urol 1996;155:1357.

59. Labrie F, Cusan L, Gomez JL, et al. Neoadjuvant hormonal therapy: the Canadian experience. Urology 1997;49:56.

60. Fair WR, Rabbani F, Bastar A, et al. Neoadjuvant hormone therapy before radical prostatectomy: update on the Memorial Sloan-Kettering Cancer Center trials. Mol Urol 1999;3:253.

61. van der Kwast TH, Tetu B, Candas B, et al. Prolonged neoadjuvant combined androgen blockade

leads to a further reduction of prostatic tumor volume: three versus six months of endocrine therapy. Urology 1999;53:523.

62. Schulman CC, Debruyne FM, Forster G, et al. 4-Year follow-up results of a European prospective randomized study on neoadjuvant hormonal therapy prior to radical prostatectomy in T2-3N0M0 prostate cancer. European Study Group on Neoadjuvant Treatment of Prostate Cancer. Eur Urol 2000; 38:706.

63. Gleave ME, Goldenberg SL, Chin JL, et al. Randomized comparative study of 3 versus 8-month neoadjuvant hormonal therapy before radical prostatectomy: biochemical and pathological effects. J Urol 2001;166:500.

64. Soloway MS, Pareek K, Sharifi R, et al. Neoadjuvant androgen ablation before radical prostatectomy in cT2bNxMo prostate cancer: 5-year results. J Urol 2002;167:112.

65. Selli C, Montironi R, Bono A, et al. Effects of complete androgen blockade for 12 and 24 weeks on the pathological stage and resection margin status of prostate cancer. J Clin Pathol 2002;55:508.

66. Aus G, Abrahamsson PA, Ahlgren G, et al. Three-month neoadjuvant hormonal therapy before radical prostatectomy: a 7-year follow-up of a randomized controlled trial. BJU Int 2002;90:561.

67. Klotz LH, Goldenberg SL, Jewett MA, et al. Long-term followup of a randomized trial of 0 versus 3 months of neoadjuvant androgen ablation before radical prostatectomy. J Urol 2003;170:791.

68. Prezioso D, Lotti T, Polito M, et al. Neoadjuvant hormone treatment with leuprolide acetate depot 3.75 mg and cyproterone acetate, before radical prostatectomy: a randomized study. Urol Int 2004;72:189.

69. Gravina GL, Festuccia C, Galatioto GP, et al. Surgical and biologic outcomes after neoadjuvant bicalutamide treatment in prostate cancer. Urology 2007;70:728.

70. Yee DS, Lowrance WT, Eastham JA, et al. Long-term follow-up of 3-month neoadjuvant hormone therapy before radical prostatectomy in a randomized trial. BJU Int 2010;105:185.

71. Mostaghel EA, Nelson PS, Lange P, et al. Targeted androgen pathway suppression in localized prostate cancer: a pilot study. J Clin Oncol 2014;32:229.

72. Taplin ME, Montgomery B, Logothetis CJ, et al. Intense androgen-deprivation therapy with abiraterone acetate plus leuprolide acetate in patients with localized high-risk prostate cancer: results of a randomized phase II neoadjuvant study. J Clin Oncol 2014;32:3705.

73. Montgomery B, Tretiakova MS, Joshua AM, et al. Neoadjuvant enzalutamide prior to prostatectomy. Clin Cancer Res 2016;23:2169.

74. Dana-Farber Cancer Institute, Medivation Inc.: Enzalutamide/leuprolide +/- abiraterone/Pred in prostate. 2014. Available at: https://clinicaltrials.gov/show/NCT02268175. Accessed January 11, 2016.

75. Thompson IM, Tangen CM, Paradelo J, et al. Adjuvant radiotherapy for pathological T3N0M0 prostate cancer significantly reduces risk of metastases and improves survival: long-term followup of a randomized clinical trial. J Urol 2009; 181:956.

76. Bolla M, van Poppel H, Tombal B, et al. Postoperative radiotherapy after radical prostatectomy for high-risk prostate cancer: long-term results of a randomised controlled trial (EORTC trial 22911). Lancet 2012;380:2018.

77. Wiegel T, Bartkowiak D, Bottke D, et al. Adjuvant radiotherapy versus wait-and-see after radical prostatectomy: 10-year follow-up of the ARO 96-02/AUO AP 09/95 trial. Eur Urol 2014;66:243.

78. Showalter TN, Ohri N, Teti KG, et al. Physician beliefs and practices for adjuvant and salvage radiation therapy after prostatectomy. Int J Radiat Oncol Biol Phys 2012;82:e233.

79. Taggar A, Alghamdi M, Tilly D, et al. Assessing guideline impact on referral patterns of post-prostatectomy patients to radiation oncologists. Can Urol Assoc J 2016;10:314.

80. Messing EM, Manola J, Yao J, et al. Immediate versus deferred androgen deprivation treatment in patients with node-positive prostate cancer after radical prostatectomy and pelvic lymphadenectomy. Lancet Oncol 2006;7:472.

81. Abdollah F, Karnes RJ, Suardi N, et al. Impact of adjuvant radiotherapy on survival of patients with node-positive prostate cancer. J Clin Oncol 2014; 32:3939.

82. Kaplan JR, Kowalczyk KJ, Borza T, et al. Patterns of care and outcomes of radiotherapy for lymph node positivity after radical prostatectomy. BJU Int 2013;111:1208.

83. Tendulkar RD, Agrawal S, Gao T, et al. Contemporary update of a multi-institutional predictive nomogram for salvage radiotherapy after radical prostatectomy. J Clin Oncol 2016;34:3648.

84. Stephenson AJ, Scardino PT, Kattan MW, et al. Predicting the outcome of salvage radiation therapy for recurrent prostate cancer after radical prostatectomy. J Clin Oncol 2007;25: 2035–41.

85. Karlin JD, Koontz BF, Freedland SJ, et al. Identifying appropriate patients for early salvage radiotherapy after prostatectomy. J Urol 2013; 190:1410.

86. Nguyen PL. Value of extra-early initiation of salvage radiation for increasing prostate-specific antigen after prostatectomy. J Clin Oncol 2016;34:3598.

87. Shipley WU, Seiferheld W, Lukka HR, et al. Radiation with or without Antiandrogen Therapy in Recurrent Prostate Cancer. N Engl J Med 2017;376:417.

88. Bolla M, Collette L, Blank L, et al. Long-term results with immediate androgen suppression and external irradiation in patients with locally advanced prostate cancer (an EORTC study): a phase III randomised trial. Lancet 2002;360:103.

89. Pilepich MV, Winter K, Lawton CA, et al. Androgen suppression adjuvant to definitive radiotherapy in prostate carcinoma–long-term results of phase III RTOG 85-31. Int J Radiat Oncol Biol Phys 2005; 61:1285.

90. Bolla M, de Reijke TM, Van Tienhoven G, et al. Duration of androgen suppression in the treatment of prostate cancer. N Engl J Med 2009; 360:2516.

91. Horwitz EM, Bae K, Hanks GE, et al. Ten-year follow-up of radiation therapy oncology group protocol 92-02: a phase III trial of the duration of elective androgen deprivation in locally advanced prostate cancer. J Clin Oncol 2008;26:2497.

92. Leal F, Figueiredo MA, Sasse AD. Optimal duration of androgen deprivation therapy following radiation therapy in intermediate- or high-risk nonmetastatic prostate cancer: A systematic review and metaanalysis. Int Braz J Urol 2015;41:425.

93. Widmark A, Klepp O, Solberg A, et al. Endocrine treatment, with or without radiotherapy, in locally advanced prostate cancer (SPCG-7/SFUO-3): an open randomised phase III trial. Lancet 2009; 373:301.

94. Warde P, Mason M, Ding K, et al. Combined androgen deprivation therapy and radiation therapy for locally advanced prostate cancer: a randomised, phase 3 trial. Lancet 2011;378:2104.

95. Peeters ST, Heemsbergen WD, Koper PC, et al. Dose-response in radiotherapy for localized prostate cancer: results of the Dutch multicenter randomized phase III trial comparing 68 Gy of radiotherapy with 78 Gy. J Clin Oncol 1990;24: 2006.

96. Kuban DA, Levy LB, Cheung MR, et al. Long-term failure patterns and survival in a randomized dose-escalation trial for prostate cancer. Who dies of disease? Int J Radiat Oncol Biol Phys 2011;79:1310.

97. Zietman AL, Bae K, Slater JD, et al. Randomized trial comparing conventional-dose with high-dose conformal radiation therapy in early-stage adenocarcinoma of the prostate: long-term results from Proton Radiation Oncology Group/American College of Radiology 95-09. J Clin Oncol 2010;28:1106.

98. Dearnaley DP, Sydes MR, Graham JD, et al. Escalated-dose versus standard-dose conformal radiotherapy in prostate cancer: first results from the MRC RT01 randomised controlled trial. Lancet Oncol 2007;8:475.

99. Fang FM, Wang YM, Wang CJ, et al. Comparison of the outcome and morbidity for localized or locally advanced prostate cancer treated by high-dose-rate brachytherapy plus external beam radiotherapy (EBRT) versus EBRT alone. Jpn J Clin Oncol 2008;38:474.

100. Hoskin PJ, Motohashi K, Bownes P, et al. High dose rate brachytherapy in combination with external beam radiotherapy in the radical treatment of prostate cancer: initial results of a randomised phase three trial. Radiother Oncol 2007;84:114.

101. Hoskin PJ, Rojas AM, Bownes PJ, et al. Randomised trial of external beam radiotherapy alone or combined with high-dose-rate brachytherapy boost for localised prostate cancer. Radiother Oncol 2012;103:217.

102. Soumarova R, Homola L, Perkova H, et al. Three-dimensional conformal external beam radiotherapy versus the combination of external radiotherapy with high-dose rate brachytherapy in localized carcinoma of the prostate: comparison of acute toxicity. Tumori 2007;93:37.

103. Morris WJ, Tyldesley S, Rodda S, et al. Androgen Suppression Combined with Elective Nodal and Dose Escalated Radiation Therapy (the ASCENDE-RT Trial): an analysis of survival endpoints for a randomized trial comparing a low-dose-rate brachytherapy boost to a dose-escalated external beam boost for high- and intermediate-risk prostate cancer. Int J Radiat Oncol Biol Phys 2016;98(2):275–85.

104. Sathya JR, Davis IR, Julian JA, et al. Randomized trial comparing iridium implant plus external-beam radiation therapy with external-beam radiation therapy alone in node-negative locally advanced cancer of the prostate. J Clin Oncol 2005;23:1192.

105. Martinez-Monge R, Moreno M, Ciervide R, et al. External-beam radiation therapy and high-dose rate brachytherapy combined with long-term androgen deprivation therapy in high and very high prostate cancer: preliminary data on clinical outcome. Int J Radiat Oncol Biol Phys 2012;82:e469.

106. Bittner N, Merrick GS, Butler WM, et al. Long-term outcome for very high-risk prostate cancer treated primarily with a triple modality approach to include permanent interstitial brachytherapy. Brachytherapy 2012;11:250.

107. Demanes DJ, Brandt D, Schour L, et al. Excellent results from high dose rate brachytherapy and external beam for prostate cancer are not improved by androgen deprivation. Am J Clin Oncol 2009;32:342.

108. D'Amico AV, Moran BJ, Braccioforte MH, et al. Risk of death from prostate cancer after brachytherapy alone or with radiation, androgen

suppression therapy, or both in men with high-risk disease. J Clin Oncol 2009;27:3923.

109. O'Keefe D, Dao D, Zhao L, et al. Coding mutations in p57KIP2 are present in some cases of Beckwith-Wiedemann syndrome but are rare or absent in Wilms tumors. Am J Hum Genet 1997;61:295.

110. Culp SH, Schellhammer PF, Williams MB. Might men diagnosed with metastatic prostate cancer benefit from definitive treatment of the primary tumor? A SEER-based study. Eur Urol 2014;65:1058.

111. Rusthoven CG, Jones BL, Flaig TW, et al. Improved survival with prostate radiation in addition to androgen deprivation therapy for men with newly diagnosed metastatic prostate cancer. J Clin Oncol 2016;34:2835.

Castration-Resistant Prostate Cancer
An Algorithmic Approach

Kelly Stratton, MD*, Michael Cookson, MD, MMHC

KEYWORDS

- Prostate cancer • Castration resistance • Guidelines • Metastases • Androgen antagonist

KEY POINTS

- Metastatic castrate-resistant prostate cancer (CRPC) is the final step in cancer progression that represents a lethal and treatment-resistant clinical state.
- Multiple therapeutics have been approved for treatment, but some have narrow windows of clinical indication.
- Urologists play an integral part in a multidisciplinary team that manages CRPC.
- The American Urologic Association Guidelines for CRPC provide recommended treatments based on 6 Index cases delineated by clinical factors.
- Understanding both indications and mechanism of action can provide further guidance for treatment sequencing in men with CRPC.

INTRODUCTION

In 2016, nearly 200,000 new cases of prostate cancer were predicted with more than 25,000 deaths.[1] Although only a small percentage of men are initially diagnosed with advanced or metastatic prostate cancer, nearly one-third eventually progress to metastatic disease.[2] Before 2004, treatment options for patients with metastatic castration-resistant prostate cancer (mCRPC) were limited to symptom relief and palliation. The approval of docetaxel, which demonstrated survival advantage in men with mCRPC, was a major advancement in treatment.[3] However, since 2010, 5 new agents with varied mechanisms of action have been approved for treatment of mCRPC.[4] As new treatments became available, patient selection and drug sequencing became increasingly complex. In 2013, the American Urologic Association (AUA) published guidelines for the management of patients with CRPC.[5] Since that time, new trial results and broadening indications have resulted in 2 amendment updates for these AUA CRPC guidelines.[6,7] The guidelines identify 6 index patients that were created based on the criteria used for clinical trial enrollment in the studies that led to each drug's approval. The mechanisms of action, clinical indications, and side-effect profiles of each agent allow for sequencing and combination therapy. However, the lack of comparative effectiveness coupled with the heterogeneous population that encompasses mCRPC makes treatment selection challenging. Clinicians have noted that as the newly approved agents are increasingly used, some patients do remarkably better than others. Predicting response to therapy and understanding resistance that some cancers have for treatment has become both a growing concern and an area of active research.

Department of Urology, Stephenson Cancer Center, University of Oklahoma Health Sciences Center, 920 Stanton L. Young BLVD, WP 3150, Oklahoma City, OK 73104, USA
* Corresponding author.
E-mail address: kelly-stratton@ouhsc.edu

Urol Clin N Am 44 (2017) 647–655
http://dx.doi.org/10.1016/j.ucl.2017.07.010

DEFINING THE PATIENT WITH METASTATIC CASTRATION-RESISTANT PROSTATE CANCER

Understanding the therapeutic approach to patients with advanced prostate cancer remains difficult because of the long and nuanced path that has resulted in our currently approved agents. Since the time of the work by Huggins[8] and Hodges on the endocrine manipulation of prostate cancer, castration therapy has been the principal first-line treatment of metastatic prostate cancer. This foundation of therapy creates a division between patients who are responding to castration and those who have disease progression despite low testosterone levels. To ensure a measure of consistency, castration from androgen deprivation therapy (ADT) has been defined as a serum testosterone less than 50 ng/dL. For patients treated with ADT, at some point during therapy the cancer cells may become resistant to the low levels of testosterone and begin to proliferate with the resultant progression of disease and possibility of symptoms. This state is referred to as castrate-resistance and is felt to arise from changes in the androgen receptor that allow continued receptor activity despite the low levels of androgens. Some proposed mechanisms for this resistance include induced hypersensitivity of the androgen receptor to residual low levels of testosterone or alterations that result in ligand-independent androgen receptor activity.[9] Many patients undergoing transition to castrate-resistance will have an initial increase in prostate-specific antigen (PSA). Biochemical progression in the castrate patient is defined by the Prostate Cancer Clinical Trials Working Group 3 as a PSA increase at least 25% and at least 2 ng/dL above the nadir with a confirmed second value at least 3 weeks later.[10]

Decades after the discovery of ADT for metastatic prostate cancer, the chemotherapy drug docetaxel was found to provide a significant survival benefit to patients with mCRPC. The approval of docetaxel was based on the results of TAX-327 and SWOG 9916.[3,11] The approval of chemotherapy provided hope for additional treatments that could improve patient survival. However, drug approval was complicated by limitations in outcomes measurements that would ensure new agents provided survival benefit. Development of the Prostate Cancer Clinical Trials Working Group was aimed at improving the standardization of clinical trials for mCRPC. Following the approval of docetaxel, clinical trials shifted to agents that could be used following chemotherapy failure. Although some more traditional agents focused on moving the drug indications from the

postchemotherapy to prechemotherapy settings, more novel agents considered substratification by symptomatology and disease location. The result is a complex landscape of drugs with unique indications, variable routes of administration, narrow windows of opportunity, and a wide range of side effects. However, in creating an approach to patient care, treatment guidelines and algorithms can be useful for creating a treatment plan. Although not without limitation, these guidelines can be further enhanced by considering the drug class mechanism of action and aligning these with the patient's clinical situation and treatment goals.

LIMITATIONS TO THE SYSTEMATIC APPROACH TO PATIENTS WITH METASTATIC CASTRATION-RESISTANT PROSTATE CANCER

Many attempts have been made to guide clinical treatment decision making for patients who present with mCRPC. The increase in new drug approvals was spurred by a transition in the approach to clinical trials brought about by the Prostate Cancer Urology Group and a clinical states model of evaluating men with mCRPC.[10,12] Although important to guide clinical trial design, the clinical states lack applicability to patients seen in practice. In 2013, the AUA developed the Castration-resistant Prostate Cancer Guidelines.[5] The guidelines were written to include index patients and to consider groups enrolled in the clinical trials. These guidelines relied on 6 index patients who could be used to guide clinical practice. Amendment updates to the guidelines have since been published to reflect new indications and results from ongoing trials.[6,7] The guidelines are based on a rigorous evidence-based approach to clinical trials published in the literature followed by peer-review. The index patients were created based on the presence of metastatic disease, symptoms, performance status, and prior docetaxel chemotherapy. Index Patient 1 is castrate resistant but does not have metastatic disease. The remaining patients have confirmed metastatic disease, but differ by prior treatments, symptomatology, and performance status. Index Patients 2, 3, and 4 are chemotherapy naïve. Patients 5 and 6 have previously received docetaxel, but differ by performance status. In practice, it may be difficult to classify patients as 1 distinct index patient. Symptoms may come and go, usage of narcotic pain medication may be variable, and patients may have reduced performance status but appear fit for additional treatment. Further, even for patients who are clearly identified as a particular index patient, the number of available agents for treatment makes drug selection challenging.

The National Comprehensive Cancer Network (NCCN) and the European Association of Urology (EAU) each publish guidelines for the treatment of patients with mCRPC as part of larger guidelines for the management of prostate cancer. The NCCN guidelines (http://www.nccn.org) divide treatment options by the presence of visceral metastases and subsequent treatments are stratified by initial exposure to chemotherapy or to a secondary hormonal agent such as abiraterone or enzalutamide. The EAU describes the available first-line options for patients with mCRPC but lists the drugs alphabetically and recommends treatment choice based on clinical factors.[13] Although all 3 guidelines have similarities, there are also distinct differences, including mention of older drugs, such as diethylstilbestrol in the NCCN guidelines and alternative dosing regimens for docetaxel in the EAU guidelines. Even within the guidelines, the lack of mature data to strongly support a treatment strategy results in a lack of consensus. For instance, in the NCCN guidelines, the decision to recommend docetaxel chemotherapy to all patients presenting with hormone-naïve metastatic disease was not clearly decided.[14]

MECHANISM OF ACTION–BASED ALGORITHMIC APPROACH

Although clinical guidelines have provided a best practice overview of managing patients with mCRPC, the clinician must consider additional factors when making the final decision. For some, the complexity of managing these patients may result in referral to another provider. Others may consider creating a multidisciplinary team to manage patients. Several clinic structures have been proposed to help clinicians provide the required services.[15] Regardless of the clinical structure, creating an algorithmic approach to disease management provides options and sequencing combinations for optimal patient management. In the absence of level 1 evidence for sequencing and coupled with overlapping indications for some, many clinicians have considered combining therapies with unique mechanisms of action and differing adverse event profiles. **Fig. 1** shows the drug classes available for the management of CRPC along with appropriate indications for use based on burden of disease, presence of symptoms, and performance status.

ANDROGEN AXIS TREATMENTS

Continued manipulation of the androgen axis has been a proposed to overcome disease progression. After variable periods of castrate levels of testosterone using Luteinizing Hormone - Releasing Hormone agonist ADT such as leuprolide or goserelin, a noticeable rise in the PSA will signify the start of the castrate-resistant state. Consensus among the clinical guidelines recommends monitoring for development of mCRPC before additional lines of therapy due to a lack of benefit from additional agents. However, starting a first-line androgen axis agent is an option and may be suitable for patients who are reluctant to continue with observation alone. Specifically, the AUA guidelines mention the first-generation androgen synthesis inhibitor (ketoconazole) and first-generation antiandrogens (bicalutamide, flutamide, nilutamide). Ketoconazole is an antifungal medication that disrupts the androgen synthesis pathway by inhibiting the function of the CYP-11A and CYP-17A enzymes. In studies, ketoconazole at doses up to 400 mg every 8 hours along

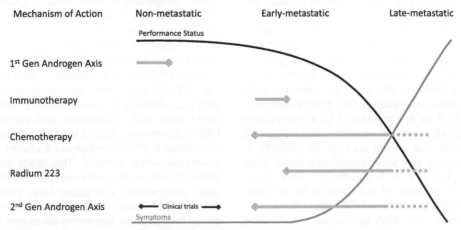

Fig. 1. Opportunities for treatment of mCRPC across indications.

with steroid support have been shown to reduce PSA levels in more than 50% of patients.[16] Bicalutamide is a highly selective antagonist of the androgen receptor that can be added to ADT to generate a PSA response.[17] Most patients are treated at the approved 50 mg per day dose with a potential PSA response in up to 40% of patients.[18] Each of these medications represents options in the first generation of androgen axis drugs. From **Fig. 1**, use of these medications are limited to patients without metastatic disease who generally have good performance status and no symptoms.

The second-generation androgen axis treatments include the androgen synthesis inhibitor abiraterone and the androgen receptor antagonist enzalutamide. Abiraterone works to further reduce androgen production by blocking the enzymes 17-alpha hydroxylase and C17, 20-lyase. The widespread effect is reduced androgen production by the testicles, adrenals, and tumor. Increased mineralocorticoid production can result from the enzymatic blockade with resultant hypokalemia, fluid retention, and hypertension. The addition of twice-daily prednisone is used to reduce these side effects. The initial approval of abiraterone was based on the COU-AA-301 trial of abiraterone plus prednisone compared with placebo plus prednisone in patients who had previously received docetaxel.[19] The primary endpoint was overall survival. At a median follow-up of 12.8 months, survival was longer in the patients who received abiraterone than placebo (14.8 months vs 10.9 months). Progression-free survival was also longer in the treatment group (5.6 months vs 3.6 months). In an exploratory analysis of patients enrolled in the COU-AA-301 trial, abiraterone provided significantly better pain relief and reductions in pain progression and skeletal-related events.[20] Based on these studies, abiraterone was approved for mCRPC following docetaxel in 2011. A follow-up study, COU-AA-302 was undertaken in patients with asymptomatic or minimally symptomatic mCRPC before chemotherapy. This study evaluated both radiographic progression-free survival and overall survival. At an interim analysis, the trial was stopped early due to improved radiographic progression-free survival (16.5 vs 8.3 months).[21] In a subsequent final analysis with a median follow-up of 49.2 months, the overall survival for patients in the abiraterone arm was significantly longer than placebo (34.7 vs 30.3 months).[22] This study resulted in approval of abiraterone for patients with mCRPC before chemotherapy. Based on these studies, the AUA guidelines recommend abiraterone for all patients with mCRPC who

have good performance status. Further, based on improvements in pain and reduced skeletal-related events in patients on COU-AA-301, the guidelines suggest that abiraterone is an option for patients with poor performance status.

Enzalutamide is a second-generation androgen axis treatment that works as an androgen receptor inhibitor, but unlike the first-generation antagonists, also prevents androgen receptor translocation, DNA binding, and interaction with coactivators.[23] These additional activities allow enzalutamide to remain effective even in the conditions of androgen receptor overexpression.[24] Similar to abiraterone, enzalutamide was initially evaluated in patients who had previously been treated with chemotherapy. In the AFFIRM trial, enzalutamide was compared with placebo in a group of patients with mCRPC with disease progression after docetaxel. During an interim analysis, the AFFIRM trial was stopped due to an overall survival benefit in the enzalutamide arm compared with placebo (18.4 vs 13.6 months).[25] Enzalutamide also produced improvement in each of the secondary endpoints including PSA reduction, soft tissue response, radiographic and PSA progression, and skeletal-related events. In the PREVAIL trial, enzalutamide was compared with placebo in patients without previous chemotherapy.[26] This trial enrolled 1717 patients and evaluated co-primary endpoints radiographic progression-free and overall survival. The trial was also stopped after an interim analysis found an improvement in 12-month freedom from radiographic progression with 14% in the placebo compared with 65% undergoing treatment. There was also a 29% decrease in the risk of death for patients on enzalutamide. In the more recent TERRAIN study, enzalutamide was compared with bicalutamide in patients with mCRPC. The study included 375 asymptomatic or minimally symptomatic men who received either 160 mg/d enzalutamide or 50 mg/d bicalutamide. The primary endpoint was progression-free survival. Patients who received enzalutamide had a significantly improved median progression-free survival (15.7 vs 5.8 months).[27] Another study, the STRIVE trial, also compared enzalutamide with bicalutamide. However, STRIVE included patients with both metastatic and nonmetastatic CRPC. In this trial, 139 of the 396 men were nonmetastatic CRPC. The primary endpoint was also progression-free survival. The study found that enzalutamide significantly reduced the risk of disease progression compared with bicalutamide (19.4 vs 5.7 months). Enzalutamide also significantly improved all secondary endpoints including PSA response, PSA progression, and radiographic progression.[28] Similar to abiraterone, the AUA guidelines recommend enzalutamide for all patients with mCRPC who have good performance status and select patients with poor performance status.

Both second-generation androgen axis treatments have unique side effects that should be considered before starting treatment. Abiraterone inhibition of CYP17 causes increased mineralocorticoid production that can result in side effects, including hypokalemia, fluid retention, and hypertension. These effects are reduced by coadministration of prednisone with abiraterone. Elevations in serum aminotransferase levels were also observed, necessitating monitoring of liver function tests during abiraterone therapy.[19] In the enzalutamide trials, side effects included fatigue, diarrhea, and hot flashes. Five patients (0.6%) receiving enzalutamide in the AFFIRM trial experienced a seizure compared with none in the placebo arm.[25] Although an increase in seizures was not identified in the PREVAIL trial, enzalutamide should not be used for patients with a prior history of seizures, stroke, or transient ischemic attack.

IMMUNOTHERAPY

Sipuleucel-T became the first immunotherapy for prostate cancer following its approval by the Food and Drug Administration (FDA) in 2010. This treatment uses filtered antigen-presenting cells that have been activated against a recombinant fusion protein consisting of prostate acid phosphatase and granulocyte-macrophage colony-stimulating factor.[29] In the IMPACT trial, men with asymptomatic or minimally symptomatic mCRPC were randomized to sipuleucel-T or placebo. The treatment group experienced a 22% reduction in the relative risk of death and a 4.1-month improvement in median overall survival. However, few patients experienced significant reductions in PSA and disease progression rates were similar between groups.[29] In an exploratory analysis of the IMPACT trial to identify prognostic factors associated with response to sipuleucel-T treatment, lower PSA at baseline was found to predict the best response to therapy.[30] The most common adverse events associated with sipuleucel-T therapy include fever, chills, and headache. Up to 23% of patients will require central venous catheter for leukapheresis due to inadequate venous access. Based on the IMPACT study inclusion criteria, the AUA guidelines recommend sipuleucel-T for men with mCRPC who have asymptomatic or minimally symptomatic disease not requiring narcotic pain medication and good performance status.

CHEMOTHERAPY

The first-line chemotherapy for mCRPC is docetaxel. First approved in 2004, the survival benefits of docetaxel have made it a central focus in the treatment of mCRPC. In the TAX-327 trial, patients experienced a median overall survival benefit of 2.4 months compared with mitoxantrone.[3] There was also improvement in the secondary endpoints of pain, PSA reduction, and quality of life. Based on these results, clinical trials and drug approvals were dependent on either benefit after chemotherapy failure or for patients in the chemotherapy-naïve state. The AUA guidelines recommend docetaxel for patients with asymptomatic or minimally symptomatic mCRPC and for those with symptomatic disease and good performance status. For patients with poor performance status, docetaxel can be considered in select cases, with potentially the most benefit for patients with limitations due to pain caused directly from bone metastases.

Cabazitaxel is a second-line chemotherapy for mCRPC that was approved in 2010. In the TROPIC trial, men with mCRPC who had progressed after docetaxel were randomized to cabazitaxel plus prednisone or mitoxantrone plus prednisone. Cabazitaxel provided a median overall survival benefit of 2.4 months.[31] The most common significant adverse events were neutropenia and diarrhea. Febrile neutropenia occurred in 8% of patients. The AUA guidelines recommend cabazitaxel for patients who have previously received docetaxel who have good performance status. The FDA indication recommends addition of prophylactic neutrophil growth factor support, particularly in patients who may be at risk for neutropenia.[5]

BONE-TARGETING AGENTS

Radium-223 is an alpha-particle emitter that functions as a calcium memetic and selectively targets areas of high bone turnover, such as metastatic deposits. In the ALSYMPCA trial, Radium-223 was compared with placebo in patients with CRPC and bony metastases who had either previously received, declined, or were not eligible for docetaxel. Patients in both arms remained on best standard of care during the trial. The study found a median overall survival benefit of 3.6 months. Radium-223 also provided significant improvement in time to first symptomatic skeletal event and time to PSA elevation.[32] Radium-223 was well tolerated with no significant difference in grade 3 or 4 adverse events. Side effects for patients on radium-223 included nausea, diarrhea, and hematologic changes. The AUA guidelines recommend radium-223 as a standard for men with mCRPC with symptomatic bone lesions, no visceral metastases, and good performance status. Select patients with poor performance status may also benefit from radium-223, particularly when limitations are due to painful bone metastases. Although radium-223 was approved as additional treatment with best standard of care, concurrent administration with chemotherapy is not recommended due to concern for hematologic complications.

SEQUENCING OF THERAPY

As new agents have become available, the optimal sequencing of treatments has become increasingly important. There are currently no recommendations for the sequencing of therapies. Clinicians consider several factors when discussing treatment options with patients, including symptomatology, location of metastases, and performance status. One of the most important factors is patient preference. Many patients desire to start a therapy that is not disruptive to their normal routine and that will be well tolerated with a low risk of side effects. **Fig. 2** represents a treatment algorithm that can be considered when initiating therapy and moving to a next line of treatment. The figure is meant to supplement the index patients discussed in the AUA guidelines. By categorizing a patient within these groups, treatment choices become clearer. For patients who desire to avoid initial treatment with chemotherapy, the advanced androgen axis therapies or immunotherapy are recommended first-line treatments. The presence of symptoms requiring narcotic pain medication would preclude the use of immunotherapy. Otherwise, the brief duration of therapy (6 weeks) and the limited therapeutic window

(before symptoms) makes sipuleucel-T a good initial therapy. There is also evidence to support use of immunotherapy earlier in the course of the disease when PSA levels are low.[30] At the time of treatment completion, the patient can be transitioned to one of the androgen axis treatments. Simultaneous administration of sipuleucel-T with androgen axis agents has been evaluated and may be well tolerated, but it remains unclear if this improves response.[33] For patients who have experienced treatment failure while on abiraterone or enzalutamide, transition to chemotherapy would be a reasonable next step. However, for patients who develop symptomatic bone metastases, a reasonable alternative therapy would be radium-223. The presence or absence of visceral metastases may be considered in determining the best sequencing of therapy.

Patients who have completed docetaxel, either as initial treatment of mCRPC or as second-line therapy are often transitioned to one of the androgen axis therapies. These agents are generally well tolerated and have side-effect profiles that allow for continued treatment even if chemotherapy was complicated by intolerance or adverse events. For patients taking prednisone along with docetaxel therapy, transition to abiraterone is often considered because it is a co-administered agent. Although the AUA guidelines do not list sipuleucel-T as a recommended agent after docetaxel, 19% of patients had prior chemotherapy in the IMPACT study.[29] Movement into third-line and fourth-line therapy is typically influenced by symptomatology and performance status. The second-line chemotherapy, cabazitaxel, is frequently used to improve symptoms and obtain maximal survival benefit before limiting reductions in performance status. Importantly, some patients who have previously been treated

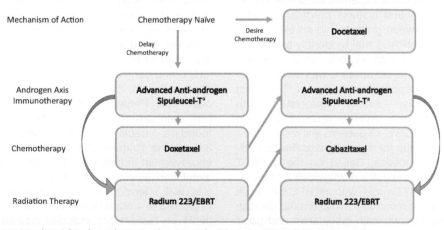

Fig. 2. Treatment algorithm based on mechanism of action. [a] Minimally symptomatic.

with docetaxel may continue to benefit from retreatment after additional drug failures and progression.[34]

Drug resistance has also been considered when determining treatment sequencing. In a study of patients undergoing treatment with abiraterone and enzalutamide, the resistant androgen receptor variant, AR-V7, was evaluated in circulating tumor cells. AR-V7 was identified in 19% of abiraterone-treated and 39% of enzalutamide-treated patients. The presence of AR-V7 was associated with worse biochemical progression-free, radiographic progression-free, and overall survival in both groups.[35] For patients who have failed initial androgen axis agents and may be at risk for androgen receptor variants, next-line therapy with a new drug class, such as chemotherapy, may be advantageous. A follow-up study of the patients with AR-V7 found that chemotherapy remained effective in these patients.[36]

NEW ROLE FOR CHEMOTHERAPY

Early use of chemotherapy has been proposed to improve survival for patients who present with metastatic disease in the castration-sensitive state. Recent clinical trials have shown that some patients may benefit from early chemotherapy. In the CHAARTED trail, 790 men were randomized to 6 cycles of docetaxel plus ADT or ADT alone. Patients were stratified by the "volume" of disease. Patients who received docetaxel, particularly those with high-volume disease, had significantly improved median overall survival.[37] Two additional studies, the STAMPEDE and GETUG-AFU15, have been published. The STAMPEDE trial confirmed a significant survival advantage in patients who undergo early treatment with docetaxel.[38] However, GETUG-15 showed a nonsignificant survival benefit for high-volume disease, but no clear benefit for low-volume disease.[39]

Enthusiasm for chemotherapy in the castrate-sensitive state will result in a growing population of patients with mCRPC who have had prior chemotherapy. For these patients, second-line therapy with an androgen axis agent or immunotherapy would be a strong consideration. Similarly, these patients will likely be candidates for retreatment with docetaxel.

IMPACT FROM ONGOING AND FUTURE STUDIES

The current recommendation to continue observation in patients with a rising PSA and castration resistance remains an area of research and development. For most men, it is a matter of time until metastatic disease is identified. Improved imaging has reduced the lag between castration resistance and treatment. However, new drug approvals are being evaluated to reduce radiographic progression rates and improve survival. At least 3 trials are ongoing for men with nonmetastatic CRPC. The SPARTAN trial is evaluating a novel androgen receptor inhibitor ARN-509 with a primary outcome of metastasis-free survival.[40] Similarly, the PROSPER trial is enrolling men with nonmetastatic CRPC to undergo treatment with enzalutamide. Last, the ARAMIS trial is evaluating another androgen receptor inhibitor, ODM-201 in a similar group of men.[4] New combination strategies are also being considered, including the addition of second-generation androgen axis agents with radium-223. The ERA-223 trial is evaluating the combination of abiraterone and radium-223 for the prevention of symptomatic skeletal events. Similarly, the PEACE-III trial is combining enzalutamide with radium-223 to evaluate radiographic progression-free survival.[4] The addition of new agents, broadening indications for currently available drugs, and new drug combinations could further increase the survival benefit anticipated for patients with mCRPC.

SUMMARY

Patients with mCRPC have benefited from the development of several new agents with differing mechanisms of action and toxicity profiles. Appropriate and thoughtful use of these treatments could lead to stable disease responses. In addition to consideration of guideline recommendations for treatment, each drug mechanism of action can be used to provide a rational approach to drug sequencing. By sharing in decision making, patients can prioritize treatment based on symptom relief, survival benefit, and expected side effects. As newer agents are developed and drugs get updated indications, patients will potentially benefit from increasing choices in treatment, as well as introduction of therapies earlier in the disease spectrum. With a continued desire to provide patients with advanced prostate cancer with the most up-to-date therapy and optimal sequencing, urologists will continue to play a vital role in the management of patients with CRPC.

REFERENCES

1. Siegel RL, Miller KD, Jemal A. Cancer statistics, 2016. CA Cancer J Clin 2016;66(1):7–30.

2. Pound CR, Partin AW, Eisenberger MA, et al. Natural history of progression after PSA elevation following radical prostatectomy. JAMA 1999; 281(17):1591–7.

3. Tannock IF, de Wit R, Berry WR, et al. Docetaxel plus prednisone or mitoxantrone plus prednisone for advanced prostate cancer. N Engl J Med 2004; 351(15):1502–12.

4. Ritch CR, Cookson MS. Advances in the management of castration resistant prostate cancer. BMJ 2016;355:i4405.

5. Cookson MS, Roth BJ, Dahm P, et al. Castration-resistant prostate cancer: AUA guideline. J Urol 2013;190(2):429–38.

6. Cookson MS, Lowrance WT, Murad MH, et al. Castration-resistant prostate cancer: AUA guideline amendment. J Urol 2015;193(2):491–9.

7. Lowrance WT, Roth BJ, Kirkby E, et al. Castration-resistant prostate cancer: AUA guideline amendment 2015. J Urol 2016;195(5):1444–52.

8. Huggins C. Endocrine control of prostatic cancer. Science 1943;97(2529):541–4.

9. Pienta KJ, Bradley D. Mechanisms underlying the development of androgen-independent prostate cancer. Clin Cancer Res 2006;12(6):1665–71.

10. Scher HI, Morris MJ, Stadler WM, et al. Trial design and objectives for castration-resistant prostate cancer: updated recommendations from the prostate cancer clinical trials working group 3. J Clin Oncol 2016;34:1402–18.

11. Petrylak DP, Tangen CM, Hussain MHA, et al. Docetaxel and estramustine compared with mitoxantrone and prednisone for advanced refractory prostate cancer. N Engl J Med 2004;351(15):1513–20.

12. Scher HI, Halabi S, Tannock I, et al. Design and end points of clinical trials for patients with progressive prostate cancer and castrate levels of testosterone: recommendations of the Prostate Cancer Clinical Trials Working Group. J Clin Oncol 2008;26(7): 1148–59.

13. Cornford P, Bellmunt J, Bolla M, et al. EAU-ESTRO-SIOG guidelines on prostate cancer. Part II: treatment of relapsing, metastatic, and castration-resistant prostate cancer. Eur Urol 2017;71(4): 630–42.

14. Mohler JL, Armstrong AJ, Bahnson RR, et al. Prostate cancer, Version 1.2016. J Natl Compr Canc Netw 2016;14(1):19–30.

15. Stratton K, Moeller AM, Cookson MS. Implementation of the AUA castration resistant prostate cancer guidelines into practice: establishing a multidisciplinary clinic. Urol Pract 2016;3(3):203–9.

16. Keizman D, Huang P, Carducci MA, et al. Contemporary experience with ketoconazole in patients with metastatic castration-resistant prostate cancer: clinical factors associated with PSA response and disease progression. Prostate 2012;72(4):461–7.

17. Joyce R, Fenton MA, Rode P, et al. High dose bicalutamide for androgen independent prostate cancer: effect of prior hormonal therapy. J Urol 1998;159(1): 149–53.

18. Scher HI, Liebertz C, Kelly WK, et al. Bicalutamide for advanced prostate cancer: the natural versus treated history of disease. J Clin Oncol 1997;15(8): 2928–38.

19. de Bono JS, Logothetis CJ, Molina A, et al. Abiraterone and increased survival in metastatic prostate cancer. N Engl J Med 2011;364(21):1995–2005.

20. Logothetis CJ, Basch E, Molina A, et al. Effect of abiraterone acetate and prednisone compared with placebo and prednisone on pain control and skeletal-related events in patients with metastatic castration-resistant prostate cancer: exploratory analysis of data from the COU-AA-301 randomised trial. Lancet Oncol 2012;13(12):1210–7.

21. Ryan CJ, Smith MR, de Bono JS, et al. Abiraterone in metastatic prostate cancer without previous chemotherapy. N Engl J Med 2012;368(2):138–48.

22. Ryan CJ, Smith MR, Fizazi K, et al. Abiraterone acetate plus prednisone versus placebo plus prednisone in chemotherapy-naive men with metastatic castration-resistant prostate cancer (COU-AA-302): final overall survival analysis of a randomised, double-blind, placebo-controlled phase 3 study. Lancet Oncol 2015;16(2):152–60.

23. Rodriguez-Vida A, Galazi M, Rudman S, et al. Enzalutamide for the treatment of metastatic castration-resistant prostate cancer. Drug Des Devel Ther 2015;9:3325–39.

24. Tran C, Ouk S, Clegg NJ, et al. Development of a second-generation antiandrogen for treatment of advanced prostate cancer. Science 2009; 324(5928):787–90.

25. Scher HI, Fizazi K, Saad F, et al. Increased survival with enzalutamide in prostate cancer after chemotherapy. N Engl J Med 2012;367(13):1187–97.

26. Beer TM, Armstrong AJ, Rathkopf DE, et al. Enzalutamide in metastatic prostate cancer before chemotherapy. N Engl J Med 2014;371(5):424–33.

27. Shore ND, Chowdhury S, Villers A, et al. Efficacy and safety of enzalutamide versus bicalutamide for patients with metastatic prostate cancer (TERRAIN): a randomised, double-blind, phase 2 study. Lancet Oncol 2016;17(2):153–63.

28. Penson DF, Armstrong AJ, Concepcion R, et al. Enzalutamide versus bicalutamide in castration-resistant prostate cancer: the STRIVE trial. J Clin Oncol 2016;34(18):2098–106.

29. Kantoff PW, Higano CS, Shore ND, et al. Sipuleucel-T immunotherapy for castration-resistant prostate cancer. N Engl J Med 2010;363(5):411–22.

30. Schellhammer PF, Chodak G, Whitmore JB, et al. Lower baseline prostate-specific antigen is associated with a greater overall survival benefit from

sipuleucel-T in the Immunotherapy for Prostate Adenocarcinoma Treatment (IMPACT) trial. Urology 2013;81(6):1297–302.

31. de Bono JS, Oudard S, Ozguroglu M, et al. Prednisone plus cabazitaxel or mitoxantrone for metastatic castration-resistant prostate cancer progressing after docetaxel treatment: a randomised open-label trial. Lancet 2010;376(9747):1147–54.

32. Parker C, Nilsson S, Heinrich D, et al. Alpha emitter radium-223 and survival in metastatic prostate cancer. N Engl J Med 2013;369(3):213–23.

33. Small EJ, Lance RS, Gardner TA, et al. A randomized phase II trial of Sipuleucel-T with concurrent versus sequential abiraterone acetate plus prednisone in metastatic castration-resistant prostate cancer. Clin Cancer Res 2015;21(17):3862–9.

34. Di Lorenzo G, Buonerba C, Faiella A, et al. Phase II study of docetaxel re-treatment in docetaxel-pretreated castration-resistant prostate cancer. BJU Int 2011;107(2):234–9.

35. Antonarakis ES, Lu C, Wang H, et al. AR-V7 and resistance to enzalutamide and abiraterone in prostate cancer. N Engl J Med 2014;371(11):1028–38.

36. Antonarakis ES, Lu C, Luber B, et al. Androgen Receptor Splice Variant 7 and efficacy of taxane chemotherapy in patients with metastatic castration-resistant prostate cancer. JAMA Oncol 2015;1(5): 582–91.

37. Sweeney CJ, Chen Y-H, Carducci M, et al. Chemohormonal therapy in metastatic hormone-sensitive prostate cancer. N Engl J Med 2015; 373(8):737–46.

38. James ND, Sydes MR, Clarke NW, et al. Addition of docetaxel, zoledronic acid, or both to first-line long-term hormone therapy in prostate cancer (STAMPEDE): survival results from an adaptive, multiarm, multistage, platform randomised controlled trial. Lancet 2016;387(10024):1163–77.

39. Gravis G, Boher J-M, Joly F, et al. Androgen deprivation therapy (ADT) plus docetaxel versus ADT alone in metastatic non castrate prostate cancer: impact of metastatic burden and long-term survival analysis of the randomized phase 3 GETUG-AFU15 Trial. Eur Urol 2016;70(2):256–62.

40. Smith MR, Antonarakis ES, Ryan CJ, et al. Phase 2 Study of the Safety and Antitumor Activity of Apalutamide (ARN-509), a potent androgen receptor antagonist, in the high-risk nonmetastatic castration-resistant prostate cancer cohort. Eur Urol 2016;70(6):963–70.

UNITED STATES POSTAL SERVICE®
Statement of Ownership, Management, and Circulation
(All Periodicals Publications Except Requester Publications)

1. Publication Title	2. Publication Number	3. Filing Date
UROLOGIC CLINICS OF NORTH AMERICA	000 – 711	9/18/2017

4. Issue Frequency	5. Number of Issues Published Annually	6. Annual Subscription Price
FEB, MAY, AUG, NOV	4	$360.00

7. Complete Mailing Address of Known Office of Publication (Not printer) (Street, city, county, state, and ZIP+4®)

ELSEVIER INC.
230 Park Avenue, Suite 800
New York, NY 10169

Contact Person
STEPHEN R. BUSHING

Telephone (Include area code)
215-239-3688

8. Complete Mailing Address of Headquarters or General Business Office of Publisher (Not printer)

ELSEVIER INC.
230 Park Avenue, Suite 800
New York, NY 10169

9. Full Names and Complete Mailing Addresses of Publisher, Editor, and Managing Editor (Do not leave blank)

Publisher (Name and complete mailing address)

ADRIANNE BRIGIDO, ELSEVIER INC.
1600 JOHN F KENNEDY BLVD. SUITE 1800
PHILADELPHIA, PA 19103-2899

Editor (Name and complete mailing address)

KERRY HOLLAND, ELSEVIER INC.
1600 JOHN F KENNEDY BLVD. SUITE 1800
PHILADELPHIA, PA 19103-2899

Managing Editor (Name and complete mailing address)

PATRICK MANLEY, ELSEVIER INC.
1600 JOHN F KENNEDY BLVD. SUITE 1800
PHILADELPHIA, PA 19103-2899

10. Owner (Do not leave blank. If the publication is owned by a corporation, give the name and address of the corporation immediately followed by the names and addresses of all stockholders owning or holding 1 percent or more of the total amount of stock. If not owned by a corporation, give the names and addresses of the individual owners. If owned by a partnership or other unincorporated firm, give its name and address as well as those of each individual owner. If the publication is published by a nonprofit organization, give its name and address.)

Full Name	Complete Mailing Address
WHOLLY OWNED SUBSIDIARY OF REED/ELSEVIER, US HOLDINGS	1600 JOHN F KENNEDY BLVD. SUITE 1800 PHILADELPHIA, PA 19103-2899

11. Known Bondholders, Mortgagees, and Other Security Holders Owning or Holding 1 Percent or More of Total Amount of Bonds, Mortgages, or Other Securities. If none, check box.   ▶ ☐ None

Full Name	Complete Mailing Address
N/A	

12. Tax Status (For completion by nonprofit organizations authorized to mail at nonprofit rates) (Check one)
The purpose, function, and nonprofit status of this organization and the exempt status for federal income tax purposes:
☒ Has Not Changed During Preceding 12 Months
☐ Has Changed During Preceding 12 Months (Publisher must submit explanation of change with this statement)

PS Form **3526**, July 2014 [Page 1 of 4 (see instructions page 4)]   PSN: 7530-01-000-9931   PRIVACY NOTICE: See our privacy policy on www.usps.com.

---

13. Publication Title	14. Issue Date for Circulation Data Below
UROLOGIC CLINICS OF NORTH AMERICA	FEBRUARY 2017

15. Extent and Nature of Circulation		Average No. Copies Each Issue During Preceding 12 Months	No. Copies of Single Issue Published Nearest to Filing Date
a. Total Number of Copies (Net press run)		744	664
b. Paid Circulation (By Mail and Outside the Mail)	(1) Mailed Outside-County Paid Subscriptions Stated on PS Form 3541 (Include paid distribution above nominal rate, advertiser's proof copies, and exchange copies)	275	265
	(2) Mailed In-County Paid Subscriptions Stated on PS Form 3541 (Include paid distribution above nominal rate, advertiser's proof copies, and exchange copies)	0	0
	(3) Paid Distribution Outside the Mails Including Sales Through Dealers and Carriers, Street Vendors, Counter Sales, and Other Paid Distribution Outside USPS®	201	121
	(4) Paid Distribution by Other Classes of Mail Through the USPS (e.g., First-Class Mail®)	0	0
c. Total Paid Distribution (Sum of 15b (1), (2), (3), and (4))	▶	476	386
d. Free or Nominal Rate Distribution (By Mail and Outside the Mail)	(1) Free or Nominal Rate Outside-County Copies included on PS Form 3541	80	78
	(2) Free or Nominal Rate In-County Copies Included on PS Form 3541	0	0
	(3) Free or Nominal Rate Copies Mailed at Other Classes Through the USPS (e.g., First-Class Mail)	0	0
	(4) Free or Nominal Rate Distribution Outside the Mail (Carriers or other means)	0	0
e. Total Free or Nominal Rate Distribution (Sum of 15d (1), (2), (3) and (4))	▶	80	78
f. Total Distribution (Sum of 15c and 15e)	▶	556	464
g. Copies not Distributed (See Instructions to Publishers #4 (page #3))	▶	188	200
h. Total (Sum of 15f and g)	▶	744	664
i. Percent Paid (15c divided by 15f times 100)	▶	85.61%	83.19%

* If you are claiming electronic copies, go to line 16 on page 3. If you are not claiming electronic copies, skip to line 17 on page 3.

16. Electronic Copy Circulation		Average No. Copies Each Issue During Preceding 12 Months	No. Copies of Single Issue Published Nearest to Filing Date
a. Paid Electronic Copies	▲	0	0
b. Total Paid Print Copies (Line 15c) + Paid Electronic Copies (Line 16a)	▲	476	386
c. Total Print Distribution (Line 15f) + Paid Electronic Copies (Line 16a)	▲	556	464
d. Percent Paid (Both Print & Electronic Copies) (16b divided by 16c × 100)	▲	85.61%	83.19%

☒ I certify that 50% of all my distributed copies (electronic and print) are paid above a nominal price.

17. Publication of Statement of Ownership
☒ If the publication is a general publication, publication of this statement is required. Will be printed in the NOVEMBER 2017 issue of this publication.   ☐ Publication not required.

18. Signature and Title of Editor, Publisher, Business Manager, or Owner

STEPHEN R. BUSHING - INVENTORY DISTRIBUTION CONTROL MANAGER

Date 9/18/2017

I certify that all information furnished on this form is true and complete. I understand that anyone who furnishes false or misleading information on this form or who omits material or information requested on the form may be subject to criminal sanctions (including fines and imprisonment) and/or civil sanctions (including civil penalties).

PS Form **3526**, July 2014 (Page 3 of 4)   PRIVACY NOTICE: See our privacy policy on www.usps.com.

Moving?

Make sure your subscription moves with you!

To notify us of your new address, find your **Clinics Account Number** (located on your mailing label above your name), and contact customer service at:

Email: journalscustomerservice-usa@elsevier.com

800-654-2452 (subscribers in the U.S. & Canada)
314-447-8871 (subscribers outside of the U.S. & Canada)

Fax number: 314-447-8029

Elsevier Health Sciences Division
Subscription Customer Service
3251 Riverport Lane
Maryland Heights, MO 63043

*To ensure uninterrupted delivery of your subscription, please notify us at least 4 weeks in advance of move.

Printed and bound by CPI Group (UK) Ltd, Croydon, CR0 4YY

03/10/2024

01040384-0007